The Royal Protomedicato

The Royal Protomedicato

The Regulation of the Medical Professions

in the Spanish Empire ❧

❧ *by John Tate Lanning*

---

edited by John Jay TePaske

For Georgette Dorn,
With the greatest respect and
affection,

John Jay TePaske

Duke University Press   *Durham 1985*

Printed in the United States of America
Library of Congress Cataloging in Publication Data
Lanning, John Tate, 1902–
The royal protomedicato.
Bibliography: p.
Includes index.
1. Medical care—Latin America—Quality control.
2. Physicians—Latin America—Discipline.   3. Medicine—
Latin America—History.   I. TePaske, John Jay.
II. Title.   III. Title: Protomedicato.
RA399.L29L36   1985   362.1′098   85-4611
ISBN 0-8223-0651-4

Publication of this book was supported by grants from the
Josiah Charles Trent Foundation and the Duke University
Center for International Studies Publications.

Contents

T HE LATE John Tate Lanning spent virtually a lifetime studying the cultural and intellectual life of colonial Spanish America; this work is the capstone to his distinguished scholarly career. Although he made his mark in the mid-1930s with books on the Spanish missions of Georgia and the diplomatic history of the War of Jenkins' Ear in the Southeast,[1] the publication of a series of essays, *Academic Culture in the Spanish Colonies* (New York, 1940), established him as the major authority on Spanish colonial universities. His pioneering research on teaching, learning, and intellectual life in these universities led him also to investigation of medical schools and medical practice in the Spanish Indies. In 1953 his sprightly biography of the Venezuelan doctor and medical innovator, Narciso Esparragosa, demonstrated the rich rewards of using changes in medical practices and medical curricula to show the flow of new ideas into the Spanish colonies.[2] Three years later his prizewinning *The Eighteenth-Century Enlightenment in the University of San Carlos de Guatemala* (Ithaca, 1956) reinforced the validity of this approach for analysis of the changes in Spanish American intellectual currents.

By the time his book on the Enlightenment in San Carlos appeared, Lanning was well into his new, massive research project on the royal *protomedicato*[3] and regulation of medical practice in the Spanish empire. Carrying on his investigations in archives in Spain, Mexico, Guatemala, Venezuela, Colombia, Ecuador, Peru, and Chile, he assembled a massive amount of documentation that forms the basis of this book. In the 1960s he drew on some of these materials for articles on the illicit practice of medicine and on the purity of blood of medical practitioners in the Indies[4] and in 1974 published his charming little book on *Pedro de la Torre: Doctor to Conquerors* (Baton Rouge), which he considered an important footnote to his ongoing work on the protomedicato.

In March 1973, a little less than a year after his retirement from Duke University, perhaps with an inkling of the illness that would soon beset him, Lanning wrote to his lawyer, Alston Stubbs, reviewing the status of his scholarly work. He stated, among other things, that his manuscript on the protomedicato and the regulation of medical practice was his last major piece of scholarship, but as yet it was not ready for publication: "I should not be willing to see the work published as is . . . ," he wrote. Still, since retirement had relieved him of teaching and institutional responsibilities, he was able to give full attention to the manuscript and continued to work steadily on it until he was diagnosed with bone cancer in December 1973. By this time, however, he felt he had done enough on the proposed book to prepare it for publication, and he called me in to ask if I would assume that task if he should die. In the meantime, though, late in 1974 and into the following year, he got a temporary reprieve from the onslaught of the disease and was able to devote time to his writing once again, albeit with less vigor and energy than before.

In August 1976 Lanning finally succumbed to the bone cancer, leaving me with his manuscript in a large box containing seventeen or eighteen massive envelopes. Some of these contained fairly finished chapters or sections of chapters that Lanning himself had revised and polished and prepared for publication. This was true of the chapters on the illicit practice of medicine and on legitimacy and the purity of blood of medical practitioners in the Indies, which had already appeared in part as articles elsewhere. Others such as those on the pre-protomedicato municipal phase of medical regulation, the formation and functioning of the protomedicato, and the jurisdictional problems which beset that institution, albeit long, had also received a good deal of his critical attention and needed little revision. Others, however, were in terrible disarray. These envelopes contained notes, sparse outlines, suggestions for organization, bits and pieces of manuscript on topics pertaining to that particular chapter, and pertinent information that he hoped could be welded together into a coherent whole. This was especially true of the chapters on the regulation of the apothecary, surgeon, phlebotomist, and midwife and those on public health and medical learning and research.

With approximately two thousand manuscript pages to edit and prepare for publication, I decided at the outset to establish certain guidelines. The first of these was to adhere strictly to the written instructions Lanning included in each envelope. The second was to preserve the integrity of the manuscript as Lanning wrote and conceived it without intruding any of my own views. This was difficult at times. In the chapter on the regulation of obstetrics, for example, my own opinion of the role of the midwife in Spanish colonial towns and villages differs markedly from his, but his views, for which he has marshaled a good deal of evidence, stand. A third guideline was to preserve as much of his research as possible as a base for further investigation by other scholars. In addition to the protomedicato and the regulation of medical practice, Lanning's work focuses on society, law, institutions, and values in colonial Hispanic America, and he provides many new avenues for understanding the reality of Spanish colonial society. Also, because his research breaks so much new ground, he provides vital new points of departure for other scholars involved in medical, social, institutional, or cultural history.

A number of other issues arose also that should be pointed out here. One was my decision not to do any further research or incorporate into this study any new works that appeared after Lanning's death, except to cite as books those dissertations that ultimately became books. This meant adherence to the guideline of preserving the work as Lanning conceived and wrote it. References have also constituted a problem. Since Lanning had worked in the archives of eight countries, it was impossible to retrace his steps to these repositories to check his sources, forcing me to rely solely on his citations, which in some cases may not be accurate. Lanning, though, was a scrupulous scholar, who could be trusted implicitly, and I feel that most of the references will be correct. Last, in most of his later works, because he wrote primarily from manuscript sources, Lanning did not include a bibliography. I have included a bibliography of works cited, however, to make it easier for those who might wish to use these citations for further research.

In his own preface to this work, John Tate Lanning is emphatic about what this book is *not*. He stresses that it is *not* a "history of medicine or of the medical sciences in the Spanish empire." The title makes that clear. Lanning knew he was not an historian of medicine, nor did he have any such pretensions. Thus it must be reiterated as emphatically as possible that he did not focus primarily on what physicians, apothecaries, surgeons, algebraists, phlebotomists, or midwives did; rather his preoccupation was on how these practitioners were or were not regulated. Still because of his interest in regulation, there is much in this work to throw new light on medical practice and suggest new avenues for further research on this subject. Also, this book does not deal with folk medicine. Lanning provides only a few references to indigenous contributions to the pharmacopoeia and to what he considered the barbaric practices of indigenous midwives, but otherwise he has willingly left this important subject to anthropologists or historians of medicine.

What then are his central themes? First and foremost this book is an institutional study of the protomedicato—its formation, structure, and functions, particularly in the major centers of Lima and Mexico City. Second, this is a social history of medical practitioners, explaining the duties and obligations of legally licensed physicians and their role in colonial society. Also included in this social history are analyses of the roles of foreign and illicit practitioners in colonial Hispanic America. Third, this is a history of the *regulation* of medical practice and methods used to control the surgeon, apothecary, phlebotomist, and midwife. Wherever possible Lanning also provides Peninsular precedents and models for such regulation, although he readily admits this is not a study of the Spanish protomedicato or of Spanish regulatory practices. Fourth, Lanning discusses medical training and medical research, a realm in which he is very much at home—the education of doctors, medical curricula, and medical research. Last, and far more tentatively, he discusses public health and sanitation, the handling of epidemics, and the control of medical publicity on new drugs, all for the late eighteenth and early nineteenth centuries. On balance, however, this is a monumental, magisterial work that opens up a totally new dimension in Spanish colonial history. The great tragedy is that John Tate Lanning did not live to see it through to publication himself.

For this massive project Lanning received help from a vast number of individuals and institutions. To his German friend and colleague in Cologne, Richard Konetzke, he felt deeply indebted for the insights he provided into the social history of the Spanish Indies and for bibliographic and archival references. The historian of Guatemalan medicine, Carlos Martínez Durán, was most helpful to Lanning when he worked in Guatemala City in the Archivo de Gobierno. In tracking down information on Italian doctors practicing medicine in Spanish America and supposedly holding medical degrees from Italian universities, he received the assistance of Professors Giorgio Abetti, Cesira Gasparotto, Elda Martellozzo Forin, and Lucia Rosetti, also Mr. B. Attolico. In Mexico City, a major focus of his research, he was aided by Beatriz Arteaga; the historians of Mexican medicine, Francisco Fernández del Castillo and Alicia Hernández Torres; Francisco A. Icaza; Jorge Ignacio Rubio Mañé, former Director of the Archivo General de la Nación Mexicana; and Antonio Pompa y Pompa, Director of the Archivo Histórico del Instituto Nacional de Antropología e Historia. In Peru the Director of the Archivo General de la Nación in Lima, Guillermo Durán Flórez, rendered invaluable assistance, while Eduardo A. Camps Vega, Dr. Ildefonso Leal, Marina Vega G., and librarians at the Universidad Central did the same in Caracas. In Spanish archives Lanning had the assistance of Teresa Pacheco of the Archivo Histórico Nacional in Madrid; Alfredo Paris Aceña, administrator of the Real Academia de Farmacia, also in Madrid; and Gloria Tejada in the Archivo General de Simancas. In Sevilla at the Archivo General de Indias, a number of individuals gave of their time and expertise to his project, including the present Director of the Archive of the Indies, Rosario Parra Cala; the former Director, José de la Peña y Cámara; Julia Herráez; and Rafael Sánchez Montero.

The list of Lanning's American colleagues, students, and associates who assisted in the research for this project is a long one. Colleagues who helped because of their archival knowledge, contacts, and notes included Ernest Burrus, S.J., Donald Cooper, Earl J. Hamilton, Ernest W. Nelson, and Robert Sydney Smith. Students of Lanning—"my boys," he called them—Stephen K. Ainsworth, Michael Burke, Arthur Steele, and John Woodham, contributed either their expertise or archival references needed by their mentor. At Duke University Jesús Leyte-Vidal often provided hard-to-find references, while Joan Furlow and Vivian Jackson helped prepare the early drafts of the manuscript. Last, the American Philosophical Society, Duke University Research Council, and National Library of Medicine provided the monetary support essential for carrying on a project of this magnitude. Many others also contributed to this work, but because of Lanning's death they will unfortunately remain nameless.

As editor of the manuscript, I have also received a great deal of help. First, my friend and colleague, Dr. Peter English, historian of medicine and pediatrician at Duke University, read and criticized the entire manuscript. Professor Michael McVaugh of the University of North Carolina at Chapel Hill did the same. I benefited greatly from their comments and criticisms but deeply regret that I was unable to take many of their timely and well-warranted suggestions, simply because I could not put myself in Lanning's shoes. Ann Twinam read and criticized the chapter on legitimacy and purity of blood and provided me with a new understanding of that issue in its broader dimensions. Also here at Duke University the Reference Department of Perkins Library gave generously of its time and efforts, while the members of the ad hoc seminar in Latin American colonial history made exceedingly useful suggestions on organization of the chapter on obstetrics, one of the most difficult to piece together. Peggy Shell typed the first draft of this manuscript, but as always my friend, Dorothy Sapp, assisted in innumerable ways to get the manuscript into its final form. I have also been privileged to enjoy the support of Duke University, an institution committed to research and scholarship: the Josiah Charles Trent Foundation, Center for International Studies, and the Duke Endowment Faculty Publication and Dissertation Award Fund all provided generous publication subsidies for this book.

As a last word I will not make the usual disclaimer that I am responsible for all the errors that will inevitably appear. The mistakes are not altogether my responsibility: they are the product of the circumstances under which this manuscript was brought together. If Lanning had lived to see the manuscript through to publication, there would have been few errors. I do, however, apologize for those in my human frailty I failed to catch.

THE CRY THAT so often goes up about scholars is that they write for each other, which is supposed to be very witty and penetrating, though after so many repetitions not very fresh. The implication, I suppose, is that, as these abstracted gentlemen are space-borne and out of this world, what they do is lost to men on earth anyway. Simplification, it is safe enough to answer, does not begin before there is anything to simplify. The historian does not set out to write for one limited class of readers; unless the subject matter requires too much technical elaboration, his duty is to make what is said clear to any undergraduate who is both intelligent and, in some degree, alive. After all, can we expect less of him than of Tobias Smollett's weevil-infested bread of New England, "every biscuit of which moved by its own internal impulse . . ."? No one would be more pleased than the historian if he both created and gratified interest. But at the same time it would lessen his pleasure to realize that he was leaving his reader under no obligation to exercise his mind. Besides, if the poor, unintelligible scholar did not turn up something of moment, what would the "popular interpreters" and textbook writers do—go on repeating each other or turn to the scholarship from which most of them have strayed anyway?

Authors undergoing such trials feel, when they begin to put their books together, and always so say in their prefaces, that there is remarkably little written on their subjects. So say I about this one. There is a surfeit of titles on the medical history of the Spanish empire, as anyone can see who consults Francisco Guerra's bibliographies, but of works on the subject of the *protomedicato,* whether preemptions or realizations, the number is strikingly small. There is no history of the protomedicato in the Spanish empire or in Spain either, for that matter, though this institution oversaw and regulated all the medical professions for three-and-a-half centuries. It is true that Dr. Ernst Schäfer published a piece squarely on the subject, called "The *Protomedicatos* in the Indies."[1] It is also true that, being only six pages long, it touches the subject with a feather only. And thereon hangs a lesson. Thus, two things every historian—and I am beginning to believe every novelist—ought to do: set down a title that matches the book he proposes to write and see that the one he does write is as big as the title. Many a sweeping title has served only to spoil and warp, if not steal the title of, the man finally able to fulfill the promise held out on the spine of the other man's book.

For Spain, one might think, there must be a history of so old, so important, and so venerable an institution as the royal protomedicato. Yet, it is not possible to find a single work that gives us a documented account or that really clarifies such essential points as the origin of the tribunal, its functions as an institution, and its ultimate fate. To be sure, in the National Library in Madrid is a manuscript in nineteenth-century handwriting entitled "Historia del Colegio de S. Carlos de Madrid y del Protomedicato," but it offers no clue to its authorship, and because some handler has dropped it and reassembled the pages haphazardly, they come out in an order quite marvelous. Less marvelous, there never has been any training in any language or science to enable all the king's men—or all those of Franco, for that matter—to put them back together again. A little intuition, however, and a moment's collating reveal this to be the same work as D. Pascual Iborra's "Memoria sobre la institución del real protomedicato," *Anales de la Real Academia de Medicina,* VI (Madrid, 1885): 183–592. Unannotated and undocumented, this publication adds little if anything useful to our knowledge of the protomedicato, as the officers and literary judges of the academy admitted, ever so circumspectly, in their prefatory statement.

If we turn back to America, we find books and pamphlets that proclaim themselves comprehensive histories, yet run their unsupported way for a few score pages and expire. Of these sketches, to show the same mercy I should crave for myself, I shall give no examples. In other cases, what the spine heralds as the "history" of the institution in the whole viceroyalty turns out to be only a group of documents on the subject. Juan Ramón Beltrán's *Historia del Protomedicato de Buenos Aires* (Buenos Aires, 1937) is, for example, a collection of documents taken for the most part from a single bundle or file (*legajo*). A model of good editing, though, it contains an excellent general introduction and short connecting passages before each succeeding document. Moreover, it includes a list of papers on the protomedicato in Buenos Aires housed at the Faculty of Medicine of the university in that city. For those with historical leanings, but without access to the Archive of the Indies in Seville, it serves the purpose of a pure monograph.[2] It is not Dr. Beltrán's fault that custom in all Latin countries does not require an index. Dr. Francisco Fernández del Castillo and Alicia Hernández Torres, in their *El Tribunal del Protomedicato en la Nueva España según el Ar-*

chivo Histórico de la Facultad de Medicina (México, 1965), are explicit even in the title. In this little book of sixty-seven pages they briefly explain what the protomedicato was for the sake of people who need elementary information—and that includes nearly everybody—illustrate the chief characteristics of the institution with a single short document, and go on to their main purpose: to present an analytical list of the seventeen slim volumes of the records of the protomedicato in New Spain that they hold in the archives of the Faculty of Medicine of the University of Mexico. It would be hard to imagine a more useful work of such slender proportions, but it is a thoroughly and skillfully prepared archival list, not a history of the protomedicato in Mexico, as the authors themselves are at particular pains to point out. Likewise, Dr. Fernández del Castillo's *La Facultad de Medicina según el Archivo de la Real y Pontificia Universidad de México* (México, 1953) bears an oblique relation to the royal protomedicato and, as in the last case, has the precise virtue of admitting in the title that this work is really a collection of documents only and, I must add, a superbly edited one. On the other hand, Dr. Rómulo Velasco Ceballos, in *La historia de la cirugía mexicana en el siglo XVIII* (México, 1946), though this too is a collection of documents, gives no indication of it in his title, and his citations frequently have no relation to the location of the documents and are accordingly incorrect and misleading. When I have been able to collate them with the original manuscripts, however, his documents are both competently and honestly transcribed.

Since, then, there is no complete history of the protomedicato and the regulation of the medical professions in the Spanish empire, it seemed best to follow the example of Herbert Bolton in *Coronado on the Turquoise Trail* (Albuquerque, 1949) and write my own account simply from the original documents and arrive at my own interpretations before reading the works of others on related subjects. Only then could I detect their leanings, pass on their methods, and critically submit myself to their influence. If this course be a fault, let me suffer for it. After all, any author of a book nowadays is tempted to approve the strategy of Alcibiades, who cut off the tail of his dog, remarked by everybody for its beauty and carriage, especially the carriage of its tail, its chief adornment. When chided, the Greek general, performing as a politician, replied in effect that he would be happy to have his antagonists concentrate upon the amputation of his dog's tail rather than upon the amputation of his political career. In an age, however, when picking up his beagle by the ears may give his enemies a chance to try to drive the president of the United States from office, Alcibiades' system might backfire. So, I have to repeat, broad though my subject is, that I cannot rest upon the authority of works without documentary citation and support, just as I do not and cannot expect my own to stand without such support. Yet, if the authors of unfootnoted works knew it, they do have a case; footnotes horrify readers and put writers in straitjackets.

So, given the penchant of the Spanish for the creation and preservation of documents, the ultimate loss of so many administrative papers of the protomedicato in America makes my burden still heavier. The Spaniards appointed innumerable *protomédicos* in the New World and created over half a dozen protomedicatos—yet the records are not complete for a single one of these tribunals. The surviving papers of the tribunal in Mexico, though the most complete of any in America, are both scattered and scant. The major portion is housed in the Archivo General de la Nación, yet the run of seventeen slender volumes has been preserved by Dr. Francisco Fernández del Castillo and classified, as I have explained, in the archives of the Faculty of Medicine of the University of Mexico. The Archivo Histórico del Instituto Nacional de Antropología e Historia, under the able and amiable management of Antonio Pompa y Pompa, holds four volumes. That the papers of this protomedicato are so dispersed is indication, if the internal evidence were not even stronger, that much else has disappeared also.

In most other places only remnants remain. The archives of the institution in Lima, the only one to start as early and last as long as that of Mexico, can show—not boast of—only a "sole volume" of papers, and these only the ragtag of the last days of the viceroyalty, related principally to a few sporadic inspections of apothecary shops. In Caracas, too, the archivists have been forced to label their Volume I of protomedicato records as *"único"*—the only one. In Guatemala, although the archivists there have scratched together some documents classified under protomedicato, the real archive of this institution went up in flames in 1924. How these things happen it is easy to imagine but hard to explain, yet, as always in Peru, Dr. Juan B. Lastres says[3] that in Lima the loss was owing to the Chilean "sack of 1879"—a charge always received with outrage, when not with apoplexy, in Santiago de Chile. If a man then turns, as he is obliged to do, to records in Spain, town councils (*cabildos*) of the cities, and cloisters (*claustros*) of universities, in America he finds himself doubly foiled, for the claustro minutes of San Marcos have suffered the same fate as the archives of the protomedicato.

Scarcity of archival materials may even be owing to the nature of the subject. Want of systematic papers on midwifery and the practice of obstetrics, for example, is a sure sign of the low status of this science and of the illiteracy of most of its practitioners. Information on the subject, when found at all, is nearly always incidental to something else. Here and there—at rare intervals, indeed—are a notation of the examination and licensing of a midwife, some printed recollection of a difficult if not horrible delivery in a celebrated family, and, toward the end of the colonial period, a few royal orders-in-council (*cédulas*) on radical changes proposed, such as the cesarean operation, a few reports in magazines, a fragment here and a fragment there, and not much more.

Even the Council of the Indies itself was in near total ignorance of the establishment of protomédicos in the Indies at the beginning of the nineteenth century. In 1803 the rising hubbub over the neglect and decay of surgery in America led the council to ask the secretariats of both the northern and southern departments to bring together the background information on the establishment.[4] The secretary of the department of New Spain, Antonio Porcel, could find "only two files": one related to the foundation of the protomedicato in Guatemala that contained a mere handful of documents dated 1792 and 1793, most of them perfunctory; the subject of the other file, also thin, was the petition of Dr. Thomas Travers, physician to the royal hospital of St. Augustine, Florida, that he be made protomédico of that "plaza and province."[5] Such was the extent of the information yielded after more than a month's effort by a secretary with all the archival resources of the government at his command.

Yet the history of the protomedicato is not hopeless. Despite the disappearance of so many archives, and the scattering of all the rest, it is possible to blend the scattered information on the protomedicato into the story of a single institution, bringing in examples from different places. If I had cited every document I could find, or followed out every lead, after I was satisfied that the conclusion drawn from the accumulation I had already made would not be modified, I should have gone on to eternity—as I have in any event.

Because the practice of compiling documents has been going on since the conquest, I have decided that it would be a pedantic waste of time for me to try to cite every place a document might have been printed, especially when it is often far simpler and sometimes far safer to ferret the original out of the archives. I have conscientiously striven, though, to cite the collections to which I am indebted for knowledge of the existence or location of the document in the first place.

Beyond the limitations the documents impose upon me, there are certain others I must impose upon myself. First and emphatically, this is not a history of medicine or of the medical sciences in the Spanish Empire or anywhere else. I make this restriction not because medical history, in both its universal and its national aspects, is relatively well cultivated anyway; I make it because I can think of no historical subject that runs parallel to so many practical problems of government and medicine in

the United States today as does the one I have taken. Even so, I have had
to leave to others the major work still needed on the protomedicato in
the mother country, though the institution there was in some measure
the model for that in America. Other subjects that could very logically
be connected with government and medicine in general or even government and the protomedicato in particular I have been obliged to exclude—in some measure at least. Printer's bills alone are enough to explain why I cannot here undertake a study of Spanish sponsorship of
botanical research in America. In some way the handling of doctors and
surgeons in the Spanish army and navy must be left as a case apart. Nor
could I hope, much less venture, to relate the long-lasting and important
role of the cabildo in medicine in every town and city. What I have done
is just an illustration of what the city did when it assumed all but sole
responsibility for the regulation of the medical professions after the
conquest.

The virtual exclusion of public health from treatment, however,
stands most in need of explanation. If, when they founded the protomedicato, the Spaniards always insisted that they did it in the interest of
public health, why do I not make the relation of the institution to public
health the main theme in this work? The answer lies in the different
concept of public health held by the Spaniards—or any other people in
the times I am writing about—and what the average American understands by the term today. To the Spaniards, nothing was more relevant
to public health than the proper education, examination, and licensing
of doctors, the inspection of apothecary shops, the prevention of false or
dangerous medical publications, the enforcement of medical laws, the
administration of justice in medical cases, and the suppression of quackery—all of these the legitimate work of the protomedicatos. Whether
they always did these things properly and efficiently is another question
that, if not resolved, is certainly faced in this book. The modern American, on the other hand, takes all this as something apart and understands
public health to be the administration and practice of medicine, especially
the enforcement of sanitary standards, the detection of disease, and preventive medicine in general for the populace at large and at no cost to
the individual.

The Spaniards had this conception also, but the state did not supply
money to carry it into practice and merely expected the private doctor to
make up the deficiency by forgoing fees. Only when a dangerous epidemic threatened to sweep the country did the machinery of public
health as Americans understand it actually come into play.[6] By then, the
protomedicato was powerless to grapple with so sweeping an emergency.
Its authority was insufficient, it had no command over army or policy

beyond its own bailiff, and it had no appropriation or budget for this or any other purpose. Only the viceroy—or the king himself—could muster the finances, command the army, and enlist the support of the church. The protomédicos, in such contingencies, issued warnings, supplied technical advice, made reports, rendered administrative service, and served on extraordinary committees set up or sanctioned by the viceroy.

Even if public health in the American sense fell squarely within the limits I have set for myself in this work, there is another justification for not according it major treatment here. Dr. Donald Cooper has published an excellent book, which deals with the handling of a number of critical epidemics in Mexico City during the late colonial period.[7] Moreover, since the official papers on epidemics housed in the national archives of Mexico are by far the best collection on the subject anywhere extant, to duplicate Dr. Cooper's effort for New Spain or any other viceroyalty, much less for a whole empire, would be out of the question. I shall, therefore, deal with the subject only so far as it is necessary to illustrate the bearing of government regulation of the medical professions upon the sad fight to limit epidemic disease. Even the Balmis expedition to disseminate the smallpox vaccine in America, which so surprised Edward Jenner, falls only partially within my bounds. Questions of public health rarely involved sustained change in the manner of regulating the medical professions.

Gradually, almost incidentally, the protomedicato did become involved with public health in the modern sense. If there was recognizable danger of bringing in disease by sea, the doctor was the logical man to meet the ship, and the protomédico as crown physician, law or no law, was bound to be the first man called upon. The task fell first to the local protomédico or, as in the case of Veracruz, the subdelegate of the protomedicato. With the diet unbalanced, the water spoiled, and the ships themselves unsanitary, and sometimes carrying Negro slaves long huddled together and often sick, this was an onerous if not a dangerous chore. Toward the end of the colonial period, when the arrival of ships became so much more frequent, the protomédico could draft all the able-bodied doctors in town. With the increasing danger and discomfort, he not only drafted them but avoided the service himself—a discrimination that the victims in Veracruz carried into the civil courts. The inspection of ships, however, is more an instance of the Spanish genius for keeping the government's hands on everything than an example of a fully developed system of public health.

Just as the beginnings of the protomedicato are remote and hazy, so at the end, in reverse, it once again trails off into obscurity and confusion. Not even the debaters at the Cortes of Cádiz in 1811–12, which revived the institution, nor at that of 1820, which abolished it still another time, give even an acceptable hint of the cause of the antagonism felt for the institution. One is simply left to sense that the public as well as the doctors, especially the surgeons, thought of the protomédicos as a useless clump of men who used their ancient authority merely to collect fees from the good men who came up for examination to practice, to subject the apothecary to a biennial shakedown, and to foil the progress of surgery. In addition, all the healing faculties, save medicine itself, yearned for independence while they developed an inveterate hatred for a tribunal controlled by physicians alone. And to many early national historians of Spanish America, every purely Spanish institution was an incubus; even so sane a man as the Chilean historian Vicuña Mackenna compares the protomedicato to the Inquisition.

In an atmosphere like this, only those with vested interests dared defend the protomedicato. The times were too heated for appreciation of the historical importance of the early enforcement of medical standards with which the protomedicato was linked. Besides, with all the shouts of "down with the Inquisition," and down with this and that, the time was inopportune to begin even a defense of a legitimate institution or of Spain itself for that matter. Yet, the protomedicato showed an unbelievable resiliency; it rose as often as it fell.

The King's Physicians: Spanish Phase

THE historian on this side of the Atlantic Ocean assumes that Spanish history could hardly reach back beyond Ferdinand and Isabella. So, as the development of medical regulations in Spain extends back into Roman times, one should approach them in the mood of Friar Gerund: "First, let me take a pinch of snuff, for this question of yours is a tight one."

Prostitution, abortion, infanticide, and insanity were not problems that could wait for the discovery of America. With these the Romans as well as the medieval Spaniards had had to deal,[1] but they dealt with them, more to control crime than to regulate medicine. The thing that, above all, led to the protomedicato both in Rome and in Spain was the simple axiom that the easier it is to enter medicine, the more doctors there are. Julius Caesar and Augustus extended honors and privileges to these practitioners, but, as might have been expected, the number grew so much that it became necessary to determine which practitioners were in truth doctors and which ignorant and intrusive opportunists. To make this distinction, and to reduce those allowed in each city to a reasonable number, the Romans appointed sixteen archiaters,[2] stationing one at the Temple of the Vestal Virgins, one in the colonnade of the gymnasium where the athletes foregathered, and the other fourteen around the city. These enjoyed a public salary, but at least one oblique reference suggests that they also charged fees—after the cure had been established.[3]

These officers proceeded to purify the practice of medicine in two ways: they subjected every practitioner to an examination and prosecuted those who evaded it.[4] Not even the senate might intervene in the examination or influence the outcome; neither could the praetor nor any other official. Even the emperor deferred to the rulings of the archiaters. In each Roman city one archiater stood above all the other doctors in town, though there is nothing more than a logical presumption that all these practiced only with his approval.[5] It would be folly to suggest that the archiaters were the forebears of the Spanish protomedicato, but given the close tie between Roman and Spanish history, and especially the centuries-long fetish of the Spaniards for Latin letters, to suggest that Roman influence had no bearing at all would be both hasty and rash.

There is an even closer connection in Spanish medieval history between the increase in laws touching medical problems and the rise of the royal protomedicato. To name the kings of Castile and Aragon in whose reigns these laws appeared is calling the roll of Spain's most renowned monarchs. It begins essentially with Alfonso the Learned (1252–84) and comes to a climax, as seems natural to all Americans, in the reign of the Catholic Kings. But in every period of critical administration, notably in the reign of Philip II (1556–98), Spanish medical legislation increased in volume, vitality, and concentration.

From medieval legislation, the investigator can extract, bit by bit, the elements that, when put together, make up the royal protomedicato.[6] Alfonso III of Aragon (1285–91) subjected aspirants to any kind of medical practice to some sort of examination and instructed the "learned and notable" in their "place of residence" to examine them. When John I (1379–90) of Castile a century later took or continued the same step, he named *"alcaldes mayores examinadores"* in conjunction with the *"médico primero"* of the royal household to form the body that examined the aspirants and determined their fitness.[7] A half century before the Catholic Kings, in 1422, John II (1406–54) sanctioned such a board to test and license those wanting to practice medicine.[8] This same king also authorized his physician to assume jurisdiction over medical crimes without allowing any appeal to the king.[9] The essential elements of the protomedicato as it existed in the Indies were, then, reached in this reign and confirmed in the reigns of Henry IV (1454–74) and the Catholic Kings,[10] especially in the pragmatics of 1477, 1491, and 1498.

An institution later taken abroad by the Spaniards was certain to be firmly established at home. Thus, Queen Juana II in 1430 named Dr. Salvador Calenda de Salerno first protomédico of a tribunal at Naples and gave him and his subordinates the privilege of examining and conferring titles upon applicants to practice. That this appointment was preceded by a "Mass of the Holy Spirit" indicates that it was an established and not a casual thing. Other evidence suggests that this was the traditional Spanish medical guild: the protomédico and his associates were free from royal levies and service, such as military service. Besides, a man "supplicating" and getting a license had to be an "old Christian," neither infamous, nor a child of unknown father (*espurio*), nor an illegitimate.[11]

During the whole of the fifteenth century all the elements, if not the precise terms, of the royal protomedicato existed in Spain. On no other ground than the want of the modern name can it be said, as some have said, that Ferdinand and Isabella did not have protomédicos. The truth is that no reign, save that of Philip II, did more to organize the protomedicato as it came into being in America. The very laws of Castile, in their inferences certainly, give clear proof that the Catholic Kings regarded the protomédicos as conventional functionaries.[12] So normal and traditional was the protomedicato that the role of another energetic sovereign, Philip II, was not to create but to vitalize an institution already growing lax and decadent.

Long before there was a body of medical men designated to judge physicians, there were many regulations—some of them not a little hostile in tone holding the physician to a terrifying accountability. The *Fuero juzgo,* the body of laws assembled and perfected under the Visigothic ruler Chindaswinth (642–653) between 642 and 649, was as severe with the derelictions of legitimate physicians as modern law is with those of the pure charlatan. For example, the physician who bled a free man, who should then weaken, had to pay his salary. In case the worst happened and the man died, the kinsmen of the dead man might do with the physician as they thought fit. If, however, a slave or a beast died, the physician or veterinarian might escape by supplying another.[13]

By the time of Alfonso the Learned, the physician's responsibility was such that claiming medical knowledge he did not possess was the most heinous of offenses. If the doctor went ahead knowingly and the patient died, in these circumstances he got the same penalty as men who "kill treacherously," for "it is worse to poison a man than to stab him to death."[14] The excesses feared in the time of Alfonso the Learned reflect the state of medicine as much as they do the cunning and crimes of physicians, surgeons, and empirics. A physician might give medicine so strong or so bad that his patient died. Surgeons might use a knife upon a wounded man, or "saw his head," or "burn his nerves or bones so that he dies because of it." A "man or a woman" might give herbs or medicines to a woman so that she might become pregnant but kill her instead. For all offenses of this kind, the offender could expect banishment to an island for five years and, when he returned, be forbidden to practice the profession he claimed to know.[15]

If we are to trust the contemporary verdict, in Spain medicine suffered decline and decadence before a modern observer would agree that it had achieved much to decline from. Ferdinand and Isabella understood that the art of curing had reached a "lamentable state."[16] The preamble of legislation that followed, as well as the internal evidence of the laws themselves, disclose what they most feared. Ignorant men everywhere were not only practicing but getting licenses to practice. Moreover, the lack of uniformity in medical legislation in the Spanish kingdoms did much to make such evasions possible. The need, then, was to require everybody to submit to a rigorous examination and to make medical laws and practices uniform throughout "these kingdoms and seigniories." Thus Ferdinand and Isabella in 1477 decreed that "the protomédicos and alcaldes examinadores" should examine all who aspired to become physicians, surgeons, bonesetters, apothecaries, dealers in aromatic drugs, herbalists, and any other persons who "in whole or in part" practice these professions—women as well as men. If found to be qualified, they should receive certificates of examination and be allowed to practice "freely and unencumbered, without any penalty or calumny whatsoever." Needless to say, those found unfit were forbidden to practice. Yet the complaints in the preambles of the ordinances of 1491 and 1498 state plainly that because of "laxness" untutored men got letters of examination and licenses to practice in all these categories. So, even if already examined by the alcaldes of previous reigns, practitioners had to submit to reexamination. These laws show two things: that there were royally appointed examiners in the reigns "of our predecessors, the kings of glorious memory," and that the regulation of the medical professions had failed.[17]

The Catholic Kings now took more drastic measures. They empowered the alcaldes examinadores to compel physicians and surgeons, when summoned by letter or by messenger, to appear before them on pain of a fine of six hundred *maravedís* every time they should refuse.[18] What is more, this same legislation gave these examiners jurisdiction over the "crimes, excesses, and derelictions of the said physicians, surgeons, bonesetters, apothecaries, and dealers in aromatic drugs, or any other persons who in whole or in part" engaged in these professions. For the crimes they committed as well as the "false measures" they took, the examiners could have justice on their persons and their properties.[19] Moreover, if any civil or criminal suit should involve these practitioners, whether they were directly or indirectly involved, the senior judges of the protomedicato "shall determine. . . ."[20]

The internal evidence of the legislation of the reigns of Ferdinand and Isabella is of great historical importance. These monarchs not only armed their alcaldes examinadores with the right to examine and reject any candidate for the practice of any kind of medicine, but they likewise gave them the right to try anyone for medical "crimes, excesses, and transgressions." Moreover, they specifically referred to the members of this board as the protomedicato.[21] There should be no doubt not only that the protomedicato was assumed to exist before Ferdinand and Isabella but also that it actually did exist in their day, and that they so labeled it.

One hundred years later, however, in the reign of Philip II, the kingdom was still "full of people who cure without a license." Because the penalty was light and the justices indifferent to enforcement, Philip in a pragmatic of the Armada year established a penalty of 6,000 maravedís for each offense of practicing medicine or surgery without being examined or licensed. As this menace was without result, he fixed a fine of 12,000 maravedís, divided in thirds between the denouncer, the judge, and the chest of the royal protomedicato. For the third offense, the culprit had to accept a fine of 12,000 maravedís and banishment to a place beyond five leagues from the city. This time the money went directly to the chest of the protomedicato. This appeal to the greed of the protomedicato was one of several ways taken to encourage its members to watch for false titles. Hardly a cortes went by that did not devote some attention to these insoluble problems.

The regulation of the medical professions in Spain involved the universities as well as the government. In no nation of Europe was the requirement of a university degree for the practice of medicine more persistent than in Spain. In consequence, many of that host who "intruded" into the practice of medicine sought to protect themselves by a second fraud. The Cortes of Madrid in 1563 took note of the "crafty tricks" to which they had to resort. Since in order to graduate in those days as a bachelor of medicine a person had to show a proper matriculation and then certificates of completion of requirements, many appeared at a university where they were not known, often bearing false documents, yet "supplicating" a degree in medicine. The universities of Salamanca, Valladolid, and Alcalá, with the requisite three professors in the faculty, were alone "certified" in medicine. Hence, to cut down fraud, the Cortes ordered that only in these universities, and after receipt of an authentic certificate from the secretary of the "home" university signed by the student's professors, might a student transfer credits and graduate.[22] When a candidate pretending to have his credits from these three presented himself elsewhere, the presumption was that his documents were false.

For as many as five centuries an even more persistent problem in Spanish universities than presenting false documents for a degree was the practice of exempting students from requirements. Legislation designed to prevent this practice in both Spain and America appeared at frequent intervals for an unconscionable time. After completing the courses for the bachelor's degree in medicine, the candidate under Spanish law had to serve an apprenticeship of two years with a reputable physician before he could get his diploma. If the candidate was poor and there was no doctor in his village or town under whom to serve his apprenticeship, he was under great temptation to begin practicing without a license or to beg the royal protomedicato to exempt him from a part or all of the apprenticeship. Again, Philip II, at the Cortes of Madrid in 1579, forbade the protomedicato to grant such exemptions. At the same time he warned apprentices not to practice. Instead, they now had to present to the chief magistrate (*justicia*) or city council (*ayuntamiento*) their diplomas (*títulos de grados*) and a certificate of having served the full two years' apprenticeship. The penalty was eight years' suspension.[23]

Medical law in the Spanish colonies, and in Spain itself for that matter, was never clear and explicit, if indeed it was ever clear and explicit anywhere. The short section in the laws of the Indies was insufficient in detail to cover many, or even the majority, of questions that arose in the government of medical affairs. Recourse, therefore, had to be made to Spanish law. Toward the end of the colonial period a puzzled lawyer might turn to the *Novísima recopilación de Castilla* (1805), and after this to the earlier *Nueva recopilación* (1640), when medical legislation in metropolitan Spain was about as complete as it was ever going to be in colonial days. When there was nothing in all this to answer his question, then the lawyer might go back to the *Siete partidas* (in force in 1348), and then to the *Fuero real* (1255) or the *Fuero juzgo* (642–49).[24] When all three were silent, as they would be on the details of medical law, he could flounder in an intricate and prolix labyrinth of cédulas, pragmatics, orders, provisions, and local laws that were accumulating long before the discovery of America.[25]

Since medicine had no special guild code, as for example did the University of Salamanca or the University of Mexico, the legal confusion was well-nigh intolerable by the middle of the eighteenth century. Judges were too often confounded and litigation too often unnecessarily instituted and interminably prolonged. In Spain, at this juncture, the Royal Council appointed Miguel Eugenio Muñoz, himself a member of the Royal Council, a judge (*oidor*) of the appeals court (*audiencia*) of Valencia, and a special judge and subdelegate of the protomedicato there, to get together the "laws, decrees, orders, and accords involving the protomedicato after the style of the *Cuaderno* of the Mesta."[26] The plan was to print the collection, distribute it among medical men for their "intelligence," and to "put it on the table" of the protomedicato to determine on the spot what the law was when a question arose. His associates thought, not altogether without reason, that the law should not be concealed or unknown. Published in 1751, Muñoz's work led to the correction of many laws and the abrogation of others in the section of the *Recopilación* dealing with the protomedicato. In some parts it dealt with questions that were still controversial. In one of these Muñoz treated points, for example, where the interests of druggists and physicians were in conflict,[27] or where apothecaries, surgeons, and physicians claimed exemptions of various kinds because of their profession—from military service for example.[28] This work was promptly executed, in part, it seems, because the protomedicato of Valencia had just been annexed to the royal protomedicato. The loyal Valencian was perhaps apprehensive about the centralist tendencies of the tribunal. The extensive commentary throughout this volume makes it the outstanding contribution to the history of the protomedicato in Spain.

One of the most troublesome, and generally the least profitable, of tasks is that of establishing primary local and national pride which insists upon fixing a date that was never fixed in the first place. How can we, then, fix the point at which the protomedicato did indeed arrive? The first criterion is that there should be an official or an official body entitled and required to examine and license all candidates for the medical professions—a very sweeping category in Spain at the end of the Middle Ages. The next test is that this body should have the duty of investigating, prosecuting, judging, and punishing those guilty of "intruding" into the medical professions and those guilty of medical crimes and excesses. The final test is that the members of this body should have guild privileges and enjoy a special mode of address. (No wonder that in an epoch of ceremonies among a ceremonial people the protomédicos should covet the address of your lordship [*su señoría*]!) By all these tests the reign of Ferdinand and Isabella is the unmistakable point at which the Spanish protomedicato became what it remained for three centuries.

The King's Physicians Reach America

If not always in the midst of the Spanish conquest, medicine was never far behind it. In fact, Dr. Diego Alvarez de Chanca, a Seville physician commissioned by the Catholic Kings themselves, sailed with Columbus in 1493. As physician on this second voyage, Chanca might have gained fame of the perfunctory variety, but he was so perceptive of native customs and so engrossed in plant life that, in retrospect, he seems a forerunner worthy of those Spanish physicians who gained fame as botanists in America.[29] Even if he had not written a famous and informative letter to the town council of Seville about the second voyage,[30] either his cunning or his diagnostic skill would have guaranteed him fame, for when the chief Guacamari tried to escape any blame for the slaughter of the Spaniards at Navidad, the first settlement on Española, by feigning a "wounded" foot that laid him up, Dr. Chanca was able to manipulate it and label the claim a "fiction." Chanca, physician of the royal bedchamber, thus began the medical history of America with the penetrating observation and classifying instinct of Francisco Hernández, the first royal protomédico of New Spain.

In those early years, however, medicine came not because everyone appreciated the opportunities for research in medicinal plants but because medicine was to the Spaniards as natural as music—even to those who had never seen a doctor "graduated" from the university. In the instruction to Columbus and Bishop Fonseca, just before the third voyage, Ferdinand and Isabella authorized, if they did not command, the sending "of a physician and an apothecary and a herbalist and some instruments and sheets of music to while away the time of those people who are to be there."[31] In 1511 Ferdinand appointed the Bachiller Gonzalo Velloso, a resident of Santo Domingo, as royal surgeon on the island because he "respected" his "competence" and ability to "cure the slaves and Indians that serve us on it." Accordingly, he instructed Diego Columbus, the son, to see to it that whoever had charge of allotting the Indians on the island should provide one hundred for Velloso, who had the duty to instruct them in religion, provide them with dress, and "whatever else is the custom there."[32] Seven years later the crown instructed Licentiate Rodrigo Figueroa, judge of the judicial review of the official's tenure (*juez de residencia*) in Española, to favor "Licentiate Velosa, physician, inhabitant of the said island for twenty years," because he "is married in the said island and has treated the officials who by our command have gone to the said island as well as Negroes and Indians and, likewise, has been the first to make and invent sugar mills in the said island."[33] The year before in 1517 the Jeronymites,[34] the "commissary judges for the things touching the Indies and Indians in these," got a royal cédula ordering them to give "Licentiate Barreda" 50,000 maravedís, already set aside for the purpose by "our noble parents." The grounds for the order were sound enough. Barreda was already on Española and the island in "dire need of a physician."[35] In this way there began to appear in Española doctors who, after Cortés' heralded triumph, would succumb to the "pull of Mexico" and, supported by the municipal councils, attempt to set up as protomédicos elsewhere. This critical step, however, when there were no other doctors, required the presence of charlatans. Otherwise, as Vicuña Mackenna remarks with cynical wit, the man applying would "have the fancy of making himself protomédico by himself."[36]

The time thus grew ripe for the appointment of officers to keep a watch upon the practice of medicine in the Indies. Since there was no precedent to determine the manner of their appointment, the Spanish protomédicos stepped in, as from time to time they threatened to do for centuries, and made the first appointments. Thus the Bishop of Tuy and Dr. Manuel Liberal[37] appointed and extended their authority to Licentiate Pero López, Licentiate Barreda, and "an apothecary, all living in Española," to assume the office of protomédicos and "to examine the physicians, surgeons, dealers in spices and aromatic drugs [*especieros*], herbalists, bonesetters, oculists, enchanters,[38] the masters of herbs, of breaks, and of those to cure buboes and treat those sick with leprosy in that island." The language of this cédula reflects the categories of medicine that merely needed watching in Spain. In a new country such a document was an invitation to violence if not to rebellion. Teeming with empirics, overwhelmed with unknown and unnamed diseases that ran thoroughly and inexorably through the population, and inhabited by people who were accustomed to get their solace short of university doctors, Española was the last place where self-serving medical officials could expect to go unchecked.

In reality, the protest against protomédicos López and Barreda came not from the people but from the city of Santo Domingo itself. There Antonio Serrano, agent for the city, presented a petition claiming, with supporting arguments, that "great injury" would result if these men went on to carry out their commissions. The king, most likely annoyed that such important commissions did not emanate from the crown, roundly ordered the "said . . . licentiates and apothecary" not to make further use of their power and, in the same breath, revoked their commissions altogether. Upon Figueroa devolved the task of seeing to it, even if punishment were involved, that neither one nor all of these protomédicos assumed jurisdiction in any medical matter whatsoever. The spirited, annoyed tone of this reversal reflects either some surprising revelations in Licentiate Serrano's protest not specified in this cédula, or typical crown jealousy so common later, or as seems likely, both together.[39] The post of protomédico, however, was as likely to be forgotten by physicians as a post office is likely to be overlooked by an American politician. Within nine years, in 1528, Dr. Hernando de Sepúlveda, who was working with Barreda in the hospital founded by Nicolás de Ovando, appealed to Charles V to reestablish the protomedicato—with him, naturally, as protomédico. He pressed his case hard by promising to serve without salary and to serve as inspector of sugar and canafistula (*cassia fistula*). Sepúlveda, certainly recognizing the scarcity of trained physicians, realistically proposed that the planters be allowed freely to treat their Indians, slaves, and their own families, by bleeding them, and by applying salves to their sores (*llagas*).[40] Nothing, however, came of the overture.

One confusing factor in this story of medicine in Española is that the physicians who arrived there, when they reached an impasse, moved on to the mainland in the wake of Cortés and Pizarro. The very year that the king revoked Pero López's commission, Cortés landed on the coast of Montezuma's empire. Before long, López, who had a right to be irate with his summary dismissal as protomédico, appeared in Mexico. There, in 1527,[41] he presented himself to the cabildo of Mexico City, and the aldermen "received him as protomédico in conformity with certain cédulas and powers of His Majesty as a substitute for Licenciado Barreda. . . ." At the same time the cabildo empowered him to fine those "culpable" of illicit practice twenty pesos for the first offense, a mark of gold for the second, and banishment from New Spain for the third.[42] The frustrated Dr. Sepúlveda, who followed the frustrated López out of Española, appeared in Lima in 1537, while the city was still under construction, and the cabildo named him "substitute protomédico."[43]

The Municipal Phase in New Spain

FOR 150 YEARS the royal protomedicato in America was more an idea than an organization, though an idea planted deep in the culture of the conquerors. Except for an occasional, isolated, and casual measure soon itself forgotten, the crown muddled along during all this time. Thus, by default, the protomedicato on the mainland had its immediate origins in the Spanish protomedicato—not in the king. In fact, the appearance of the first protomédico in New Spain in 1527 is a repetition—a literal repetition—of the reception of the first one in Española a decade earlier. In fact, as will soon appear, it was a reenactment down to the same papers, but it was one that the authorities in New Spain never recognized and coped with.

After the crown rescinded the appointments of Pero López and one Fulano Barreda as protomédicos in Española because they had been named by the Spanish protomedicato and not by the crown, Pero López migrated to New Spain, joining the murderous, anticlimactic expedition to Honduras in 1524. Later when Cortés sent him back to Española, on one of those epic voyages for succor, López suffered the classic shipwreck by surviving only on a plank.[1] When he returned to Mexico, he found that his wife, Anna, had salvaged his real property in her own name, on the assumption that he was dead. As a man with a flair for handling money and as a doctor destined for riches, this precaution without doubt stood him in good stead.[2] Typical of his energy, after having cast his lot with Cortés, he appeared before the municipal council of Mexico City in 1527 "with certain cédulas and powers from His Majesty's protomédicos," by which, "in substitution of Licentiate Barreda," "it appears" that he was named "to the said office of protomédico in these parts." His appearance accented the growing realization of the town council that charlatans were popping up on every hand. The councilmen empowered him to impose and enforce penalties against those found guilty, "with neither love nor enmity"[3] at the rate of twenty pesos gold for the first offense, a mark of gold for the second, and disqualification and exile for the third.[4]

The cabildo had worthy aims, as well as perennial problems, in its efforts to contain "the multitudinous seas" of illicit practitioners, yet, in all likelihood, it fell victim to a mild fraud in this its first great effort to resolve the problem. Pero López, the internal evidence tells us, was using exactly the same document that had certified him and Barreda as proto-médicos in Española. He was bound to have known that neither this document nor another like it could be valid. In 1519 the king had canceled his appointment in Española on the specific ground that the proto-médicos had not had the authority to make it—and he had done it in a mood of irritation so pronounced that there is no possibility that the Spanish protomedicato would have returned so soon to repeat its error—name for name if not word for word. Moreover, the movement of this Barreda is an insoluble mystery.[5] What was the sense in making López substitute for Barreda if Barreda was himself in Mexico? But for a single entry in the minutes of the cabildo of Mexico City,[6] there would be no evidence that there was any Barreda moving in Mexican medical circles.[7] Even then, this document on the appointment of López did not set up any regular series of appointments either by the protomedicato or by the crown in Spain. The digest of López's commission—"protomédico in these parts"—as made by the town clerk is just vague enough to make possible the use of the commission designed for Santo Domingo. The logic is that López used a commission that he knew could not legally be put in force. He did not dwell upon the cold fact that at the date of his appointment Mexico had not even been conquered.

If López had had a proper commission from Spain, the future of the protomedicato in Mexico would surely have been far more regular. As it was, the town council took it that it had no protomédicos in 1533,[8] yet in 1536, when it appointed Dr. Cristóbal Méndez and Licentiate Pero López, it recorded that it already "had the use and custom of naming physicians as protomédicos" to enforce the "laws and pragmatics" by observing such duties as the conduct of medical examinations and inspection of apothecary shops.[9] Joaquín García Icazbalceta, a lucid and careful scholar, says he cannot reconcile this appointment of 1536 with the one made in 1527.[10] The quandary is logical when taken on the assumption that Pero López had a valid title, especially a lifetime one, as proto-médico of New Spain. The town council had, therefore, taken the documents he presented more as a suggestion for making an appointment than for confirming a mandate from the mother country. Since López knew the tenuous nature of his original claim, he far preferred to be satisfied with de facto appointment from year to year rather than raise questions about the legality of his invalidated appointment from the Peninsula. In fact, the council in 1528 began the practice of naming López and one other physician as medical officers, usually with the specific obligation to inspect apothecary shops and report back to the council.[11] If they had been the classic Spanish protomédicos, they would have had the authority to initiate their own work. Still, by 1536 these men were being labeled protomédicos, a practice that, as already seen, had congealed into the "usage and custom" of appointing protomédicos that so puzzled García Icazbalceta. Thus, despite long development, in which the cabildo had appointed at least thirteen protomédicos, no notice of it appeared when the king appointed Francisco Hernández as royal protomédico in 1570. The explanation is quite simple: he had no knowledge of this development in the Mexican cabildo. The authority of the cabildo was in lieu of royal appointment and lasted only so long as the king was not interested enough to nullify it.

The town council of Mexico, certainly, felt that in 1585 it had enjoyed "the faculty and preeminence" of appointing two protomédicos for "more than sixty years."[12] This is both loose language and inexact mathematics, but the argument is sound. Between 1536 and 1603 the council made these appointments,[13] usually in pairs, at twenty-one separate times involving only twenty physicians. Since there is a gap of sixty-seven years between these two dates, the city could not have made annual appointments as, under stress, it claimed it had. The understanding was that in those years when no selections were made, those already appointed would go on serving. In fact, now and then appointments were made "for such time as is the pleasure" of the council.[14] Though annual appointment "for the future" was approved in 1563, the cabildo was still divided on the question in 1578.[15]

Disharmony

The work of the municipal protomédicos, if it went on at all, went on with very little friction. That no salary was involved and that the cabildo itself initiated no work of importance largely explain this beautiful harmony. Occasionally, and perhaps for the same reasons, Dr. Pedro López[16] begged to be excused as visitor or inspector of apothecaries and surgeons. In 1579, after his appointment, he appeared and gave his reasons to the cabildo and received his formal release from the obligation.[17] Then, in 1592 the town council had to reprimand a certain Dr. Bravo "for not attending to his office as he should and is obliged to do." The cabildo then ordered him, under threat of naming another man in his place, to cooperate with Dr. Herrera in conducting examinations and inspections.[18]

Eight years later the protomedicato was beginning to have its first faint troubles rising from the almost oppressive sense of place, seniority, and precedence characteristic of colonial society as a whole. When "in accordance with custom" the cabildo named two protomédicos for the year 1600, it issued specific instructions that future examinations and other meetings should be held in the house of the senior protomédico, to which the junior member had to come. There, in this private residence, the two protomédicos would conduct their examinations in the presence of the clerk (*escribano*) of the cabildo.[19] Then, while Dr. Francisco Hernández was in the kingdom, the municipality stepped softly. Instead of grandiloquently naming protomédicos, it toned its terminology down to "medical inspectors [*visitadores médicos*],"[20] and as soon as he was gone it returned with relief and with vigor to the appointment of "protomédicos."[21]

The conflict that spelled the eventual end of the municipal protomedicato in Mexico was the intervention of the proud dyspeptic viceroy, the Marqués de Villamanrique (1585–90).[22] Late in 1585, when the time was nearly at hand for the municipality to appoint protomédicos for 1586, Dr. Luis de Porras presented the cabildo with a "command" from the viceroy making him "protomédico general" of New Spain. His credentials were as imposing as his appointment was alarming. As a mark of royal favor, he had come bearing a royal cédula entitling him to bring four swords, four daggers, and a harquebus to New Spain.[23] He was a graduate of the University of Salamanca, "was a professor there," and physician of the king's bedchamber in Santiago de Compostela in Galicia. The crowning qualification was that the new protomédico had come out in the viceroy's retinue just three months before as his personal physician. Such "letters and experience," the viceroy said in his commission,[24] warranted his appointment as protomédico "for the city and all New Spain"—an extension of jurisdiction to the whole kingdom that nobody in the town council seems to have noticed. The 1,000-peso fine for putting any "impediment" in his way was stiff enough to suggest that the viceroy wished to discourage opposition before it could gain momentum.

The aldermen took a look at the document and forthwith decided not to receive Dr. Porras. To do so would deprive them of the power that they had had from time immemorial to name protomédicos.[25] The high constable and alderman sent to talk with his excellency told him that "for more than sixty years" the council had named two protomédicos at the first meeting every year. Their hope was that, "being well informed," he would suspend his unexpected appointment. What they heard was vastly different, for Villamanrique was not taken unawares. If, he expounded, the city had not had a specific privilege from the king to appoint protomédicos, but had merely done so by custom, "that made little difference to him." He had sent Porras before the cabildo only as a matter of courtesy; he could have made the appointment without any such formality.[26] The city's refusal to receive his choice and recognize his authority immediately was nevertheless "bad." Very well, if the cabildo did not receive Dr. Porras without a word of rebuttal—*"sin réplica"*—at the very next session, he would mete out punishment. He was viceroy.

The councilmen considered downright rejection of the nomination. The plain intimation of the *corregidor,* however, was that in such case the viceroy would order the arrest of the *regidores,* which suggested a more expedient course. The king and the Council of the Indies were far away; the regidores therefore would acquiesce, "solemnly receive" Dr. Porras, swear him in, and protest later that they had acceded under duress. Their final decision was to have Regidor Jerónimo López draw up an appeal to the Council of the Indies, with all the necessary documents, and dispatch it "on this ship" to the city solicitor in Spain. The aldermen were not consoled that the viceregal commission had instructed Porras to get the cabildo to name "an alderman or two"[27] to accompany him in his inspections of titles and licenses as well as in his prosecutions and sentences.[28]

Though the process took nearly twenty years, the viceroy's appointment of his personal doctor as protomédico was the beginning of the collapse of municipal regulation of the medical professions. After one year Philip II merely asked Villamanrique, if he found it necessary to take the appointment of protomédicos out of the hands of the city, to report his reasons.[29] The cabildo waited three years and then resumed its appointments,[30] which continued without serious disturbance until 1602.

The news reaching the cabildo in that year that "some doctors in this city pretend to bring title and appointment from Spain as protomédicos of this city" was upsetting. The cabildo "contradicted" the claim and kept on guard against developments,[31] but the climax came when the viceroy, the Marquis of Monterrey (1595–1603), named Jerónimo de Herrera as protomédico. The hue and cry that went up from the cabildo to protect its immemorial "possession and preeminence of naming two protomédicos every year" was the same as that raised in 1585, except that this time the council added that it had been denied its legal right to be heard. It accordingly authorized Pedro Núñez de Prado, with the advice of the city attorneys, to draw up a petition to the royal audiencia, a copy of which, together with Dr. Herrera's title should immediately be sent Alonso de Valdés to present to the Royal Council in support of a plea not to confirm the appointment. At the same time it asked Alonso Gómez de Cervantes to write two letters, one to the king and the other to Valdés.[32] How the issue went can be deduced from the want of documents; the cabildo of Mexico never appointed another protomédico.

The Municipal Phase: Lima

From the day "of the winning of this land," Lima had the same medical problems as Mexico City, but the history of the protomedicato in the two capitals took different turns. In Lima the first protomédico to appear had a royal title of unquestioned authority to which the city merely gave its exequatur. Whereas Pero López carried his curious assortment of documents before the Mexico City council in 1527, Dr. Hernando de Sepúlveda, also approaching by way of Santo Domingo,[33] presented his to the cabildo of Lima in 1537, but as his commission was in Latin, Sepúlveda had to wait for Licentiate Benito Carvajal to read it. When the learned man had done so, fortunately, he declared that "the writing" gave the bearer powers like those enjoyed by the king's protomédicos in Spain to round up and inspect the papers of physicians, surgeons, and apothecaries "as well as to do the other things his majesty's protomédicos have the power to do." Since the doctor was now conforming to the pragmatic requiring presentation of such authority to the town council, the expert thought your "lordship and your worships" might kindly lend their exequatur.[34]

No doubt the arrival in Lima of a protomédico armed with a royal commission prevented the immediate development of the Mexican system of municipal appointment. Also, in 1569 arrival in Lima of Sánchez Renedo as royal medical officer helped sustain the earlier pattern, eliminating the jurisdictional problems between the cabildo and the viceroy over the appointment process. In fact, the silence of the Lima cabildo records testifies that as the king's protomédico, Sánchez Renedo performed his duties satisfactorily,[35] despite his election as rector of the University of San Marcos in 1573 and 1577. By 1581, however, the city council was again complaining that the city lacked a protomédico. Such laments were always brought on by the spectacle of "so many people" practicing medicine without a license, apothecaries dispensing dangerous drugs without inspection, and others unable to practice for want of any official to examine and certify them. As was characteristic of town councils throughout the empire when faced by a concrete problem, the cabildo without hesitation appointed Licentiate Alvaro de Torres, a physician of "much learning and experience," as protomédico.[36] Recognizing better than did the cabildo the possibility of conflict of authority, Torres told the town clerk that to proceed effectively he needed "full jurisdiction." The council heeded his suggestion that the viceroy be asked to confirm his appointment.[37] Then, before the year was out, Viceroy Martín Enríquez (1581–83), "at the behest of the city," appointed Licentiate Torres and Dr. Fulano Henríquez as protomédicos of Lima.[38]

If these two steps were as far as either the city or the viceroy ever went to assume the royal function of naming medical officers, the crown made more effort in Peru than in Mexico to fulfill this obligation. Nearly a decade elapsed, however, after the appointment of Torres and Henríquez before a protomédico, armed with a royal title, reached Lima. This man, apparently named Dr. Iñigo de Hormero, reached America in the Portobelo fleet of 1589 and proceeded down the South American coast as if in a triumphal procession. His commission was duly set down in the town records of Nombre de Dios, Panama, and at last Lima, for it had been written in precise imitation of the appointment of Dr. Sánchez Renedo, whose jurisdiction extended to all these places.[39] Even the detailed instructions of 1568 were repeated in the commission.[40] In Lima, however, he proceeded immediately to the Audiencia of Lima, where the viceroy, the Marquis of Cañete (1589–96), and the oidores had the authority to name one of their number as judge to sit with the protomédico in judicial proceedings.[41] As the "royal provision and title" Hormero bore required the audiencia to draw up instructions for the conduct of the office, that body very conveniently inserted the instructions issued to Dr. Sánchez Renedo in 1568. In general, however, the audiencia ordered Hormero to follow the royal laws and pragmatics relating to his office "not contrary to this instruction." It then specified that he should come to the audiencia before he assumed jurisdiction and gave sentences so that the oidores could appoint one of their number to sit with him in hearings and in imposing penalties. To guarantee that the decrees of the protomédico would be obeyed and that his indictments resulted in arrests, they instructed all constables (*alguaciles mayores y menores*) to obey his orders. He also got the right to name a clerk to assist in inspections, proceedings, suits, and in examinations and licenses issued by him. The fees he might charge, his only official income, were the same as in Spain.[42] Though the arrival of Hormero stabilized the protomedicato in Peru, when he died some twenty years later, the viceroy, the Marqués de Montesclaros (1607–13), himself appointed Dr. Melchor de Amusgo to take his place.[43] The institution in Peru had not been so much under the domination of the cabildo as in Mexico, but at this stage it also fell under the sway of the viceroy—with consequences that were not sifted and put in order until 1646.

City Medical Service

The king and even the viceroy might ponder and marshal the laws respecting the regulation of medicine, but the city council thought first of relief for those suffering from disease and of security for those well and alive. When the Indians took sick, they called one of their men of medicine if these were close at hand and could be had with little trouble. Otherwise, they lay stoically and either lived or died. On the other hand, the whites struggled against illness to the point of ruin.[44] If one of them died "after twenty days in bed," it took everything that he had accumulated or owned to pay the doctor and the apothecary. For the endless round of responsories, pauses, and vigils in the funeral, the surviving partner had to go so much into debt that Motolinía reported hearing "a learned man" assert that "if husband or wife took sick and death was inevitable," the husband ought immediately to kill the wife or the wife the husband and bury the other in any cemetery; in this way the surviving party would escape poverty, loneliness, and debts.[45]

At this stage, twenty years after the conquest, every Spaniard in Mexico, or someone close to him, suffered from chancres (*llagas*) and then severe skin lesions—all lumped together as the familiar buboes (*bubas*). So universal was this venereal affliction that society could not even work up disdain for its victims. There was, as a result, a curious tolerance for the sufferer, whether he was an aristocrat or the humblest tinker. The aristocrat, though, would have covered the unsightly sores with black patches. If an epidemic was not raging, it was these people under the torment of what the young soldiers of Cortés dubbed the "woman's sickness"[46] who needed the first attention when the conquest was over. Back in Spain, from time immemorial, caring for sores and ulcers had been a separate medical profession.[47] Now, in New Spain, the demand for a professor of this art was so great that he was the first to respond—without a license. And just as soon the town council forbade any man to anoint any person for bubas or llagas before presenting himself for examination.[48]

The Spanish yen to regulate every trade and draw revenue from the process, however, was more persistent than buboes. Thus, on January 24, 1530, the aldermen of Mexico City took up the report that Bartolomé Catalán "was going around treating bubas and other illnesses without a title." For some reason the complaints from the people, who generally tolerated and probably patronized the "intruders," were so wrought up over Catalán that the cabildo now called him in in person to display his license. Since he could not produce such a document, the council ordered him not to practice again until he could and menaced him with a fine of "one hundred pesos and perpetual exile" should he "intrude" a single time more.[49] Reports on the results of this man's treatments must have been alarming to produce such a decisive reaction. The very next year, in fact, Alonso Guisado contested the order that he not practice without a license. His defense, established not just by his own assertion but by witnesses, was the old if not venerable one that he had a record of curing "many people" and had treated the poor free. The town council relented enough to license him "to treat the private parts, sores (*naturas*) and ulcers (*llagas*)"—nothing more.[50]

In 1545 medical care in Mexico City simmered down to the point where there was only one fully active and licensed physician to serve a metropolis that, by modern standards, should have had seventy-five, even without the menace and scourge of epidemics. This was a plight in which the classic Spanish solution—free attention to the poor by doctors who were paid by the rich—had no chance of operating, if indeed it was ever really dependable anywhere. After epidemics of *matlazahuatl* and small-pox had run their course, Dr. Juan de Alcázar, who had been brought to his own bed by overwork, recovered enough not to make good his threat to return to Spain. Besides, the Royal and Pontifical University, inaugurated in 1553, immediately "incorporated" Alcázar as its first doctor of medicine.[51] Since the new doctor's reputation for humanity had sunk to the very bottom during the epidemic eight years before, something would now be required to restore it. Regardless of his motive, Alcázar went before the cabildo and proclaimed his desire to "do something for the city and commonwealth." He was struck with sympathy for the "many sick people, who, because of their poverty, often die because they cannot get a doctor." This time "for God and the commonwealth," and "without salary and without personal interests," he would treat medical cases among the poor free of charge, and, in surgical cases, he would find a surgeon to attend the patients free of charge or he would bear the costs himself. The council promptly received him as "doctor of the poor" and had the news preconized "in order that all might know."[52]

There are no reasons to believe, however, that other doctors in the city hurried to enroll in this generous class. The lot of the indigenes and the poor was not really changed. In fact, it was not until the beginning of the seventeenth century that anything approaching systematic medical care for the poor in Mexico City came into being. Even this, when it did come, was a by-product of the absolute necessity of doing something in the case of overwhelming illness in the public jail. Only then did the city begin a series of medical appointments that, because salaries were attached, induced their holders into treating people outside the jail who could not otherwise afford a doctor. Occasionally, too, the threat of a doctor to leave town brought on the run of all "Spaniards" (whites) who foresaw need for his care or who were already dependent upon the skill of some rare specialist.

Though perhaps not the first municipality to name and pay doctors to serve the public, Mexico City nevertheless did come closest to institutionalizing and perpetuating the practice in the course of the first half of the seventeenth century. Between 1607 and 1643 the city named six different physicians,[53] eight druggists,[54] six surgeons, three bonesetters, one oculist, and three phlebotomists.[55] Though these appointments were either not made or not recorded every year, the appointments according to the holders continued in effect during the intervening years. Occasionally, however, the city steward, especially when hard-pressed for funds, refused to pay salaries when annual appointments had not been made. Though the salaries were not high, even for the seventeenth century, they were much coveted, and the competition was sometimes sharp and the councilmen accordingly divided. Francisco de Urieta, a Mexican-trained doctor, was so intent on replacing Dr. Alonso García as the city physician that he accused him of being grossly out of date. So persistent was he that it must have been a relief to the aldermen as well as to him when, at long last, Dr. García died in 1621.[56] The misery of the people, especially the Indians lying in the hospitals and jails—even in the streets—with broken, unset bones was so deeply affecting that the city readily agreed to retain a bonesetter at three hundred pesos a year for part-time work. When an oculist appeared, the council retained and bound him to the city at the same figure, a decent salary for a university professor. Salaries were not automatically paid, however, and to collect them the holder appealed to the city steward and accompanied his request with a certificate from such officers as the jailer, the chief constable, the *procurador mayor,* and corregidor that he had performed his duties "with punctuality and care."

Bonesetters (*Algebrists*): Mexico City

Mexico City was unique in the appointment of public algebrists and oculists, but, as the Spanish cities in America were in very poor communication with one another, important ad hoc medical developments could occur in one place and never in another. When in 1589 a man appeared in Mexico City who professed to have a record of "great cures" as a bonesetter—the only one in the whole country—the city accepted his offer of service at three hundred pesos a year,[57] and the viceroy concurred. Although some of the aldermen challenged the salary in 1596, claiming that this Martín Sánchez Falcón did not "understand this trade," the council sustained the full salary and required the city steward in 1606 to pay "the algebrist" everything owing him. Three years later, in contrast with its behavior toward other medical officers, the cabildo passed an act notifying Sánchez Falcón that "he was not to enjoy any salary for the three years he was not specifically named," a roundabout and discriminatory way of terminating the appointment.[58] In the meantime the persistent bonesetter appealed to the king for a raise of four hundred pesos a year additional salary, and in 1607 the crown instructed Viceroy Luis de Velasco II (1607–11) to see to it that he got a raise of two hundred pesos "if he seemed to deserve it."[59] Though the viceroy "obeyed" this cédula early in 1609, he noticed over two years later that it had not been put in force.[60] When Sánchez appealed to the cabildo in 1612, however, he had the royal cédula, a favorable decision from the royal audiencia, and a command from the viceroy. There was nothing to do but to bow and "notify Martín Sánchez Falcón in his person" that his salary was now five hundred pesos a year. From the beginning of this crisis the clerk ceased to record any annual appointment for Martín Sánchez Falcón, algebrist.

Such obstructive behavior forced the bonesetter to make such a strong case for his pay that it placed some instructive data into the historical record. Having grown a little too proud to present proof that he had done his work when he asked for pay, he was peculiarly vulnerable to the hostility of the city steward. When his routine request for pay came up early in 1615, the cabildo forced him to produce some specific and, as it turned out, revealing proof of his performance. Saddled with the task of making the investigation and report, a certain Juan Torres de Loranca declared that Sánchez Falcón had treated the poor, and that a nurse of the Franciscans certified that he had successfully treated an unshod friar about to leave for Japan. He had also set the arm of one man, the arm and leg of another, the arm of a "nephew of Sancho López" broken in two places, a broken arm of an Indian, whose name, stout reader, for the sake of the millions of Indians who suffered anonymity in New Spain, was Pedro Jacobo.[61]

Martín Sánchez Falcón always addressed himself to the authorities as "the only algebrist in the land," but when he died in 1620 his son, Bachelor Marcos Falcón, though a priest, appealed to the town council for the post and salary of three hundred pesos that his father had enjoyed since 1589. He brought a license from Dr. Jerónimo de Herrera, the protomédico general,[62] certifying that he had the requisite training and experience, special permission from the archbishop, and several petitions from the convents of the city on behalf of his appointment. The city appointed him for "whatever time it saw fit" on condition that he treat the poor and the religious free of charge and preconize the event.[63]

Far less regular and expected than the naming of a bonesetter, however, was the selection of Francisco Drago, a Genoese, as oculist and specialist "in troubles of the urine." Despite the ever-repeated cédulas against the intrusion of foreigners, physicians and surgeons from outside the empire came to America with about as much regularity as the fleets.[64] So it turned out that in 1616, in one of those recurring campaigns—generally forced upon the viceroys from Madrid—to round these men up and send them to Spain, the net in Mexico City closed about Francisco Drago, known to his patients as Francisco Diego, and his forced departure for Castile seemed imminent.

Thus far the story is the old one, but at this point it takes a unique turn; the culprit so welcomed his arrest and transportation back to Europe that he would not turn a hand on his own behalf. However, there were a lot of people suffering from cataracts, bladder troubles, and "other surgical infirmities" who were greatly perturbed by the news of the impending deportation of Drago. Among these people, he had the stereotyped "many cures" to his credit, and, not at all stereotyped, he had restored the sight of a number of people with cataracts and brought relief to others—most welcome relief—suffering from "stoppages of the urine." Only the humble supplication of these private persons persuaded him to stay at all. In short, sick people as well as those who anticipated that they might need the same care were all so alarmed that the viceregal government was going to deport Drago that they all but stormed the town council, making an appeal so urgent that it demanded the cabildo "take a hand" to try to persuade the viceroy to stop the deportation. If he wished to go voluntarily, as he apparently did, then the viceroy should not allow him to do so; he was the only man who could do these operations in the whole kingdom. In support of this strange petition for the still stranger involuntary servitude proposed, the citizens urged the council to hear the protomédico Dr. Jerónimo de Herrera.[65] When the council accepted the suggestion, Dr. Herrera came before it and testified that "Francisco Drajo" was a "singular and eminent" surgeon of extraordinary skill in removing cataracts by the pressure method,[66] and in curing "any other disease of the eyes." He also mentioned his "efficacious remedies" for urinary troubles and "in spending and extirpating carnosities." Dr. Herrera stated unequivocally that there was no one else in the kingdom equal to Drago and that his deportation would be "a great injury to those suffering from these afflictions." Without more to-do, the city instructed its chief attorney to convey the protomédico's opinion to the viceroy, and "in writing and by spoken word" to petition him and the audiencia not to send Drago back to Castile "except for very grave cause"[67]—such as committing some crime. There can be no doubt that any man with eye trouble and no other doctor in town would be solicitous, but a man unable to urinate without his help would be singularly ardent in his plea that he be allowed to stay in town. He did not leave town.

As Drago certainly knew that the city had been paying a salary since 1589 to the algebrist, Martín Sánchez Falcón, he was bound to get around to asking the city to give him a salary also. He thus appeared in 1621 and, as "the only and singular" oculist in the city, asked to be given a salary for treating those who were too poor to pay him. After all, the art of removing cataracts and relieving urinary attacks was a more difficult one than that of bonesetter. In support of all this, he produced the testimony of Protomédicos Jerónimo Herrera and Diego de los Ríos, and the physicians Alonso García de Tapia and Diego de Cisneros. The city voted to give him two hundred pesos a year.[68] Yet not a year had passed before the city, "without a cause," took away the salary. Drago, who had a genuine grievance, thought that such subsidies "from noble and generous cities" should be permanent and perpetual. Nevertheless, since it was the "agreement for the new year" that naming an oculist be suspended, the city voted to go on making payments on condition that Drago give bond to return the money in case a judge of residencia should so order. As late as 1625 Drago was still drawing the salary. By that time he had become "oculist and hernia surgeon."[69]

City Physicians in Lima and Quito

The case of Lima is further proof that the development of a system of public medical service took a different turn in every city. The reason is that exchange of information between cities was so slight that, for instance, aldermen in Quito could argue against a public health program on the ground there was no city-paid doctor in the City of Kings. The threat of impending disaster in the first stages, however, usually made city councils avidly sympathetic with any search for doctors. Thus, in 1552, when Lima was hardly more than fifteen years old, a certain Doctor de la Cueva appeared before the cabildo, after a full year's service, with a royal cédula commanding that the city should pay him for making the rounds at the Hospital de Españoles. With supporting proof of his work from priests and other dependable witnesses, the cabildo allowed the payment of the salary of two hundred pesos a year.[70] Two years later, at the same salary, Dr. Gaspar Meneses was performing the duties of physician in the same hospital and in the Indian Hospital as well. At this point, however, the city appointed a surgeon for the Spanish Hospital.[71] By 1555, already a popular and busy man destined to become the first rector of the University of San Marcos,[72] Dr. Meneses had resigned his post as physician to the poor in the Spanish Hospital and was succeeded by a certain Licentiate Fulano Aguilar.[73] Still, Dr. Francisco Gutiérrez drew the 150-peso salary for performing this duty.[74] Three years later, when he died, the council, looking around for a person who was not too busy to take care of the duties at the hospital, appointed Licentiate Alonso Gutiérrez at two hundred pesos a year.[75] Less than two years later, however, because he served too many other patients and earned such a high salary, the licentiate had to give up treating the poor in the Spanish Hospital. Thereupon, the cabildo, not to be outdone, named Dr. Enrique Méndez, a doctor "very unengaged."[76]

Licentiate Francisco Franco was one who thought the post of city physician for Lima was most valuable. Most others either threatened to leave the smaller cities, died with alarming frequency in the big ones, or began to get rich so fast that they did not have time to work for the piffling salaries paid for doing the city's charitable work. Franco, who was drawing a salary of two hundred pesos as city physician in the Spanish Hospital in 1566,[77] held tenaciously on until 1580 against a campaign to discontinue the salary. In 1572, remarking that the king had granted the hospital 4,000 pesos a year from "Indian and vacant tributes" and 100,000 maravedís from court fines (*penas de cámara*), the cabildo felt that the hospital could pay its own salaries, especially in view of the income it had quite apart from the royal grant. After devoting the better part of two meetings to the subject, the council voted to inform Franco that it had suspended his salary. He might make his charges and collect his income "to suit himself." When the clerk officially notified the physician, however, he remarked brusquely "that it was not for the city to say" as he served "at the command and by the appointment"[78] of the royal audiencia.[79] Still, in 1573, Viceroy Francisco de Toledo (1569–81) ordered the hospital to pay Franco's salary. However, the matter was still under litigation in 1578, and when the name of Franco disappeared from the record in 1580, the city agreed to pay the salary owing but "without prejudice" to the position it had taken in the salary litigation.[80]

The movement started in the cabildo in 1578 to replace Franco came to fruition with the appointment of Dr. Fulano Vásquez in 1580 by viceregal order, and therefore at the expense of the city. Again the cabildo paid under protest. Licentiate Juan Jiménez, who succeeded Vásquez in 1581, collected the salary from the city, which regularly protested, until 1587 when some councilmen declared that physicians should be told that future appointees need not expect pay from the cabildo.[81] The royal audiencia, however, continued to force the city to pay the hospital to reimburse it for paying the physician tending the poor whites there.[82]

Though Lima was far more reluctant than Mexico City in providing various types of medical care for the poor, in 1625 the aldermen of Lima at last mustered enough sympathy for the prisoners in jail with no separate room for isolation and care of the sick to propose roofing an unfinished room at the hospital for that purpose, but they had to force the commissioners entrusted with the responsibility to proceed with their task.[83] Although the city of Lima earned little credit for the money it so reluctantly supplied to pay the physician for the care of poor whites at the Hospital de San Andrés, it should not be blamed because it did not finance the doctor at the Indian Hospital; that institution was financed by the viceroyalty.

When they came to the appointment of physicians, cities in the sixteenth century were unusually prompt and, given the circumstances, unusually effective. The reason was, of course, that the aldermen themselves knew that their families were just as liable to mortal disease at any moment as were the poor themselves. Thus, when the town council of Quito discovered that the physician it proposed to hire in 1574 would not accept the salary of six hundred pesos, it immediately proposed to petition the royal audiencia to give the city permission to raise the offer to seven hundred pesos. As an indication of the hardships suffered in colonial days for want of money for public uses, the city could think of nothing better to propose than that the cabildo divide the burden between the principal inhabitants, "secular and ecclesiastic," and "anything else it sees fit," without prejudicing the interest of those who did not participate in the allocation.[84] "Because there is nobody else to turn to," the city council nearly two decades later appointed Captains Juan de Logroño and Francisco Proano to canvass the fifty leading houses of the city to raise a salary that would keep Dr. Juan del Castillo from leaving.[85]

If this maneuver was successful, the results were only temporary. In less than five years the cabildo was expounding that "it is fitting that there should be a salaried physician on regular duty because of the many and grave illnesses there ordinarily are. . . ." It noticed that "Dr. Valdés," now residing in the city, presented his diplomas as "bachelor, licentiate, and doctor of medicine. . . ." What made it notice, however, was that the doctor, like those before and after him, "wished to leave the city . . . , an injury in prejudice of both the city and its inhabitants." The solution was neat: give Dr. Valdés 100 pesos salary for treating the poor without fees and forbid him to leave the city.[86] Yet only four years later the same council found itself lamenting that "it has been many years since this city had a physician. . . ."

The observation was provoked by the presence of Dr. Fernando de Meneses, "a physician of great repute, learning and experience. . . ." Since he, like Dr. Valdés, "wants to leave and go to Lima," and "since it is not just that he should leave this city," Quito should give him a salary of 150 pesos for treating the poor—fifty more than the "deceased" Dr. Valdés had received. When summoned and told what action the council had taken, Meneses accepted the salary with such alacrity as to suggest that his move to leave the city was a ruse to get the expanded salary. When the city attorney testified that Meneses was actually the man named in the diplomas he was bearing, the agreement was sealed.[87]

The more efforts the council made, the more the medical problems of Quito remained the same. In 1608 the cabildo learned once again that "the city does not have a salaried doctor," the invariable preface to some kind of an attempt to name one, one who just happened to be at hand. At the moment, Licentiate Jerónimo Leitón, "a doctor of good character and reputation and much learning,"[88] was such a man. True to the old formula, a committee—composed of a general, an accountant, and an alderman—reached an agreement with the itinerant doctor and found the salary among residents and the religious establishment.[89]

Also true to the invariable pattern, the very next year the city was once again entering in its books, with ritualistic repetition, that "for many years there has not been an experienced and trustworthy doctor in whom entire satisfaction can be taken," and "many people die in this city for want of a doctor who understands diseases. . . ." There had come to this city one Dr. Fernando Meneses, who met all these requirements. To reinforce the argument, there was "an alarming mortality reigning. . . ." The rare "unanimous" solution was that the city offer Dr. Meneses three hundred pesos[90] from its own means.[91]

In a plight so critical, quick and determined remedies were highly indicated. Yet the whole business dragged on, without clean and clear resolution, for six full years. To begin with, the royal audiencia took more than a year to ratify the conditions of the appointment.[92] By that time Meneses had once again sung the classic refrain: he would be obliged to leave the city because he was not making an adequate living. The financial conditions were still so stringent that one man willing to vote for an increase nevertheless spoke for cutting the figure by a hundred pesos— still "with the obligation to treat the poor."[93] So slight were the resources, and so tight the purse strings, that it took a second session to decide the momentous matter of whether the doctor's salary should be two, three, or four hundred pesos. At this meeting it came out that the *alférez real* had written to persuade Dr. Meneses to come back to Quito from Guayaquil. Accordingly, to meet the agreement thus reached, the city had provided three hundred pesos of "inducement" while some convents and aldermen privately put up five hundred more for a total of eight hundred. As might have been expected, however, some of the convents and aldermen defaulted. One of these, Pedro Ponce de Castillejo, voted that the city pay Meneses one thousand pesos, but, in view of the shortage—he might have said chronic shortage—of funds, he "conformed" to the vote of the majority for a salary of four hundred. Even so, the *procurador general,* as he had threatened, appealed to the royal audiencia because the city's means were already so "committed and encumbered" that there was nothing with which to pay the increase.[94]

Two years after this prolonged struggle over the increase in salary, Meneses was again threatening to leave Quito. This time certain aldermen now opposed even the original salary. The purpose of it was to secure medical attention for the poor, and "Meneses only treats those who can pay him. . . ." The chief attorney, who always objected to the salary, again did so, because "neither in the City of Kings nor in the most populous cities of this kingdom is any physician paid a salary."[95] The contention, however, that no doctor was paid a salary in Lima was, of course, not strictly correct, for Lima had paid salaries at least since 1552. The issue of the debate was that the corregidor ordered that the city pay Dr. Meneses a salary of four hundred pesos. In some way, however, the salary dropped back to three hundred the next year, and when in 1615 the cabildo proposed to renew that figure for another year, Captain Juan Sánches de Xerez Bohórquez, protesting that there was "a plenitude" of doctors, appealed to the royal audiencia that it was too high.[96]

Such a combination of poverty and stinginess meant the defeat of any medical program in Quito. In 1638 both medicines and doctors were lacking; the doctors who had come "had not persevered." In consequence, there was something grandiloquently called the Royal Hospital, but no doctor to treat patients who poured into it. Such was the distressing plight of a royal audiencia a century after the founding of the city. On the basis of experience in both Spain and the Indies, the city council petitioned the audiencia to authorize bringing in the Order of San Juan de Dios. A member of the order, actually present in the city, had encouraged the move by guaranteeing to bring a physician, a surgeon, and an apothecary if his order was allowed to take over the hospital.[97] Unlike Mexico City, which wanted medical examiners as well as medicines and doctors, the city of Quito was happy to have one legitimate doctor. If there were waves of *curanderos* rushing in to fill such gaps as occurred everywhere else, the cabildo made no effort to restrain them.

City Regulation of the Apothecary and Drugs

The town council in Lima reluctantly recognized that without drugs the city physician was of no avail. And, just as in the case of the doctor, it fell into a bitter dispute with its apothecary over his pay. The first record of the supply of medicines to the Spanish Hospital is a notation dated in 1556 that Francisco Bilbao, apothecary, had a suit pending with both the city and the hospital.[98] The city then entered into a contract with Pedro López de Aguirre to supply drugs to the hospital that required him to submit his accounts every three months. As the business of supplying medicines was still like supplying manufactured goods in a gold rush, López de Aguirre submitted no accounts and refused to render them when so ordered. This behavior came at a time when reports were abroad that for want of medicines "great damage" was being done to the health of the patients. At the same time the assets of the hospital suffered equally from sheer maladministration. The council then named the city hospital superintendent (*mayordomo*) and two deputies to undertake an audit of López de Aguirre's accounts and menaced him with a 500-peso fine for withholding anything asked for.[99] This was urgent business, but it was fourteen months before the apothecary and the chaplain of the hospital appeared before the town council to announce an agreement whereby López de Aguirre would supply the necessary medicines. The apothecary, however, refused to accept the six hundred pesos offered him to lay in a supply of drugs. Thereupon, the cabildo ordered that he either accept or close his shop. Nevertheless, by the next spring the sum advanced him had come to seven hundred pesos.[100] The city, at the time it was squabbling over the sums it advanced for hospital work, had some slight expense in paying for medicine used in the treatment of blacks and other people working in the lime kilns, tile factories, brickworks, and public fountains.[101] One way the city fought the high prices of drugs was to pay, as it did in 1571, only a part of the appraised value of medicines supplied.

Although the city of Lima had advanced sums in the sixteenth century to enable apothecaries to stock their shops, the same problem was considered in Caracas a century later. In 1651 the apothecary Marcos Portero told the cabildo in Caracas that he had remained in that city to serve the commonwealth. After he had accepted the word of the city "to assist him in stocking his shop" and had pledged his word to borrow the money to do it, he appealed to the cabildo to make good its promise. The council merely voted to consider it "without prejudice."[102]

Favors and Concessions

In the Indies, governments, especially city governments, felt that they were entitled to follow the Spanish example and restrain doctors who sought to leave town, but, at the same time they felt under some obligation to offer them a life attractive enough to make them want to stay in the city. Besides, in America for a long time any kind of medical practitioner, whether licensed or not, might expect special treatment at the hands of newly formed cabildos. In 1535, the very year the city of Lima was founded, the barber, Francisco de Cárdenas, successfully petitioned to be received as a legal resident (*vecino*) and given a house lot (*solar*). Then, when little over two years had passed, he asked for and got an allotment of lands.[103] In this way a mere bleeder (*barbero*) who, to be sure did some surgical work beyond mere bleeding, came to anticipate the genuine medical doctors in rewards offered by the city of Lima. In the same manner, the very next spring, Dr. Hernando de Sepúlveda, the protomédico of Peru, and his brother each received a house lot in the same city,[104] while in the very year the king authorized a royal university for the city, Lima accepted Dr. Gaspar Meneses as a vecino with all its privileges. In fact, he got two lots because with his wife and children in the city he needed the additional space for a larger house.

In an environment so favorable, doctors not only collected good fees but also came to enjoy secular office and special business concessions. The cabildo of Lima repeatedly elected the Licentiate Alvaro de Torres as *alcalde ordinario,* beginning in 1561—before he had become a vecino.[105] The viceroy, Count of Nieva (1561–64), however, rectified this want with a royal order establishing him as a citizen and freeholder.[106] For a while, in 1568, Torres even became the chief city attorney, a post more suited to a lawyer.[107] Then, after a while, this same "doctor and alcalde" turned up with a petition to the cabildo of Lima for a building site at the "port of Cupe" to store and secure grain shipped there to await a boat to keep "Indians and others" from stealing it. The cabildo agreed, provided the grant injured "no third party" and that the building "was finished within a year."[108]

In Peru this practice of favoring men in the medical professions with grants of land and public office continued into the seventeenth century. Dr. Hormero, protomédico of Peru, had "a half-straw" of water let into his house on the orders of the viceroy. Though he had paid 150 pesos for this perpetual asset, the cabildo entered a caveat that, since the city fountains should be used, it did not feel obliged to maintain a continuous supply of water from these. At best, Hormero was not happy with this grudging concession; he wanted a full "cane" of water.[109] From such favors, the apothecaries were not excluded. They received town lots and sometimes enjoyed appointment to such active offices as that of familiar of the Inquisition or constable.[110]

Sometimes favors shown those practicing medicine indicate the actual and not the legal public status of practitioners. Before the assassination of Francisco Pizarro, the city of Lima received "La Godíñez," curandera, as a vecina and granted her not a full but half a house lot, fronting, as the record says so revealingly, "that of Juan Hernández, the one-eyed." All this was because she "treated people when they were sick and served the city."[111]

Though no city ever showed a concern with childbirth even remotely matching the appalling importance of the problem, some showed more concern than others, perhaps because they had fewer regular surgeons than did the viceregal capitals. The city of Caracas, for example, in the seventeenth century included midwives among those whom it specially favored in the allotment of house sites. Isabel de Montes, a woman with a large family and "midwife to this whole commonwealth," got a lot at one peso a year! Ana Jiménez, "destitute [*pobre de solemnidad*]" and burdened down with children and a husband "blind in both eyes," yet somehow managed to help many "principal persons" and other women in childbirth. As the truth of her allegations "was notorious," the town council allowed her a lot at a charge of half a peso a year to help her get the house she so sorely needed.[112] Another "midwife to the principal families of this city," in a petition to the town council of Caracas, revealed that, "without contradiction," she had been living with her mother, an interpreter, in a certain house, but that upon the death of the mother she discovered she had no title to the house they jointly occupied. The council acceded to her request for legal possession without charge.[113] In two years (1657–58) the cabildo of Caracas conceded house lots to two other midwives, one of them "examined."[114] By whom she was examined the minutes do not say. In any event, an "examined" midwife was all but nonexistent even at the beginning of the nineteenth century.

Medical and surgical aid to blacks and workers in the tile and brick factories picked up considerably during the time of Viceroy Francisco de Toledo in Peru. In 1572 the cabildo of Lima "agreed" that it was necessary to establish this care for "the Negroes and people" who worked in the tile factory and lime kiln. The physician appointed, Dr. Rego, got thirty pesos a year while the "surgeon and barber Marzillo" received only ten. The druggist set his own prices, but he could not collect until what he had supplied had been appraised.[115] When, very soon, Dr. Rego died, Licentiate Esteban Hidalgo succeeded him. As an indication of the tightness of money, or the stinginess of the government, the cabildo reduced the salary from thirty to twenty-five pesos. When Hidalgo discovered that he had been docked five pesos, he threatened to resign, but his protest was in vain; the city forced him to serve.[116] Ordinary curanderos treated wounds suffered by slaves used in armed bands sent in pursuit of runaways or criminals. "Master Domingo," ordered by Captain Juan de Arreynaga, the alcalde ordinario, to treat Pedro Galán,[117] who had a "great stab" in the chest, received thirty pesos for service spanning more than thirty days.[118]

The City Physician

Though there is much evidence that the algebrist attended the poor at large in the city, there is very little indication that the "physician to the city" was much more than what the records of the town council plainly called him—"the jail doctor."[119] In fact, the main duty of the city apothecary was to supply the drugs prescribed by the physician when he visited the sick in jail. Such practices made it natural, then, for city medical officers to get an official statement that they had rendered the services required of them at the jail.

Every Spanish American city had some kind of public doctor, but as the practice developed to meet the special circumstances of each city, the institution was never precisely the same in any two places. In Mexico City the city doctors examined and treated prisoners in the municipal jail. It was only in the case of some doctor with a unique skill that the city ventured to make free treatment of the poor a condition of voting an annual salary. In Lima, on the other hand, the city physician was merely the attending physician at the Spanish Hospital. In Quito, paying a city doctor was the only way to get any physician to stay in town.

Of course, some people were bound to have had cataracts, urinary stoppages, and hernias, but why the city fathers of Mexico should have considered their people more "peculiarly liable" to these infirmities than to complications of childbirth they do not vouchsafe us. Far more people were bound to get caught in pregnancy, even dangerous pregnancies, than were ever bothered with cataracts, yet the town council never appointed a city midwife nor, so far as the record shows, any surgeon with special qualifications to handle difficult deliveries. The most that can be said in defense of this neglect is that when the cabildo of Mexico City became alarmed at the number of empirics and appointed medical examiners to test them in the fields they had intruded into, it occasionally asked that midwives be examined also. Here and there, in unexpected places and for unexpected reasons, city councils did take a languid interest in the poor midwife who was, generally, no more than a town hanger-on, like a hyena hovering around a pride of lions.

The Municipality and Licensing

An observer from Mars, casting his eyes over the minutes of town councils in the Spanish empire, might very well have gotten the idea that tailors, shoemakers, and carpenters, because they underwent examinations and paid fees,[120] were on the same plane as physicians, apothecaries, and surgeons. Yet such was not the case, for Philip II's statutes remark that doctors who did not know their science "would better sew shoes than practice medicine."[121] The custom of examining and taxing everybody preparing to serve the public in some special art, trade, or profession did actually make the licensing of all the practitioners of medicine that much more certain. The problem was not to overlook anybody who neglected this little preliminary, for the country was broad and towns, not to mention villages and crossroads, were isolated and often far apart. A remote hacienda was all but a sanctuary for a practitioner on the run. Apothecaries, unlike the curandero and the wandering herbalist, because they had stationary shops, could not depend upon their agility and cunning to avoid scrutiny. In the very early days, so great was the yearning of the conquistadores for the amenities and security of the Old World, that an apothecary without a license was allowed two years, while actually practicing, to bring in his certificate.[122] Because they were so few, so prominent in creole society, and so generally clustered in the capitals, genuine physicians had either to present licenses to the town council or manage to falsify their records. Even so, one man with a falsified record did actually become, for a short time, a protomédico of Mexico City.

Romance surgeons, with no university training and highly mobile, practiced illegally in the greatest numbers. They were the ones who disturbed the city councils most often, for finding a surgeon authentically qualified by the standards of Spain in the sixteenth century was no simple matter. For example, in Lima in 1537 Lieutenant Governor Francisco de Godoy put in a special plea for "the surgeon" Francisco Sánchez, who had been forbidden to practice until he presented his certificate of examination to the town council. Yet, running true to the old formula, he had lost his certificate. The cabildo then decreed that "if it is found to be certain that he has lost his certificate," he be allowed in the interest of the public welfare "to cure in matters of surgery," but not in those of medicine. Three violations of the restriction—imposed upon all sur-geons—would make him liable to banishment.[123] The next year Juan de San Pedro presented the cabildo of Lima a certificate of "sufficiency" in surgery "from the protomédicos," but the council qualified his license. As was conventional, it instructed him to observe the laws of Spain and not practice medicine, but it also told him not to undertake surgery of grave importance except in the presence of a physician, "there being one in the town."[124]

Because the preparation of the surgeon was so informal and the range of education so wide, the cabildo of Lima had to keep constant watch to prevent surgery from falling entirely into the hands of intruders or quacks. Despite this precaution, unconditional licenses were rare. The certificate issued to the "barber" Nicolás Martínez apparently carried con-ditions and limitations at the bottom of the page.[125] Just as in Mexico, though the first protomédicos of Lima came with royal commissions, they operated under the final authority of the town council. Licentiate Alvaro de Torres reported to that body in 1552 on four or five surgeons applying for licenses that all but two were satisfactory. Of these two, Francisco Sánchez was plainly not qualified, while Salvador de Figueroa might treat minor cases but he "should not take on major ones accompanied or not accompanied."[126] When he appeared before the council sixteen days later with a certificate of examination, however, the council issued him a license to practice "on the terms relating to surgery with no impediment whatsoever."[127] In the middle of the sixteenth century, in fact, Lima found it necessary to appoint an examiner of barbers and phlebotomists (*examinador y veedor de barbería*). Upon the death of Pedro de Castillo in 1566, Juan Sierra applied for the post. When the city attorney re-ported that his title was in order, the cabildo appointed Sierra to serve "at its will," but with the proviso that he examine no one except in the presence of the inspectors of weights and measures (*fieles executores*) and the notary clerk and that he not bleed, apply the leach or cupping glass, and that he not draw wind without a physician's approval.[128] Despite firm language, sleepy routine tended to take over as long periods went by with no pressure at all put upon the practitioners of surgery to submit to examination and present their certificates to the town council. It was near the end of the century before Lima bestirred itself, "in con-formity with the new law," to call upon the surgeons, barbers, and druggists to present their titles within six days.[129] When a man practiced surgery or phlebotomy without submitting to examination, the presump-tion always was that he was not prepared to take and pass it. Sometimes, however, such an individual, who was likely to be poor, professed not to be able to pay the fees required. On such grounds the cabildo of Mexico allowed Sebastián de Aguilera, when he explained how hard it was to support his children, to go on after giving security for eight months practicing without a license.[130]

In the secondary cities of the empire, often no special machinery for licensing existed in the medical professions. If a man appeared professing to have "examinations and titles," then the city government simply fell back upon its regular formula for passing upon the authenticity of documents. If these were genuine, so great was the need for physicians and surgeons, the city gave its own license without hesitation. As early as 1548, when Maese Martín de Tapia, "surgeon and barber," presented such papers to the cabildo of Quito, the aldermen ordered them scrutinized. When these appeared to prove that he had been accepted for these "offices" in Spain and by the royal audiencia in Panama, the cabildo of Quito admitted him to "the said offices of surgeon and barber." It went a step further; it in effect made him *protocirujano,* for thenceforth nobody, on pain of a fine of two hundred pesos, might practice these occupations without submitting themselves to him for examination.[131]

During the century that followed a man holding a genuine medical degree and license knew enough to present it to the town council for validation. The title presented in 1600 by "Bachelor" Domingo de Almeida aroused enough suspicion for the cabildo to ask its attorney to pass on its authenticity. At the same time, and perhaps for the same reason, the council issued one of those periodic incitations to all physicians and surgeons to present "the titles showing by what right they practiced" according to the order issued by the corregidor of the city.[132] The simple expectation, then, was to submit titles to the town council before beginning to practice anything—down to phlebotomy.[133] Even in the viceregal capitals of Lima and Mexico, where some kind of protomedicato had long been established, it was to the town council that even the most marginal cases came.

The Lament of Illicit Practice

Cortés and Pizarro had not yet finished their work when it became tragically plain that the people would find some solution, however tragic, to the problem of scarcity of drugs, doctors, and surgeons. An incidental complaint to the Lima town council that slaves—even children—were buying bichloride of mercury on the open market will show how calamitous it threatened to be. Probably no gap in the history of man has been more quickly filled than that created by the severe shortage of licensed doctors. When the reconstruction of Mexico City after the conquest was just under way, the aldermen learned that "many persons without being examined doctors and surgeons yet treat people, and because they do not know what they are doing except to relieve them of their goods, they kill some and many times leave others with many injuries and sicknesses. . . ." The invariable answer—for which there was ample precedent in Spanish history before Columbus—was to enact a law requiring valid titles. So it was that in 1528, the year after the city had appointed its first medical officer, the town council passed an ordinance that no person without a certificate of successful examination could practice medicine or surgery on pain of a fine of sixty pesos—one-third for the royal chest, another for the trial judge, and still another for the person making the accusation. The act required all those practicing to appear before the alcalde, Luis de la Torre, and the protomédicos, Bachelor Cristóbal de Hojeda and Licentiate Pero López, to show their titles so that, if these were valid, the city might license them. As an indication of its seriousness, the council ordered the ordinance preconized in order that none could plead ignorance.[134] As busy doctors with lucrative practices and with no legal assistants could not possibly ferret out and prosecute all the quacks and curanderos, Mexico City in 1531 appointed Diego de Pedraza as attorney over "physicians, surgeons, and those who cure by charms and all those who treat sickness and apply ointments" so that he might call them to the cabildo to learn by what right they practiced.[135]

Curing by enchantment was the bane of both the civil and religious courts. In contrast to the case in Mexico, where the Inquisition handled cases of curing by charms, in Peru the city, at first, took cognizance in such cases. In 1538, for example, the cabildo of Lima reported hearing rumors "that some persons in this city cure with charms and other things, without being doctors and without knowing what they are doing, and without a license. . . ." When, as in these cases, the practitioners crossed over into "superstition"—anathema to the colonial churchman—they became dangerous not only to the "commonwealth, freeholders, and inhabitants" but also "were damaging and in prejudice of our holy Catholic faith." In this case, then, the cabildo of Lima confirmed Hernando de Sepúlveda, "the protomédico of His Majesty and judge named by this cabildo," to assume jurisdiction over such violations.[136]

While in the countryside and villages, the poor curandero had a monopoly by default, in the larger cities, which also had these curers, there developed something like the modern quack. After his appointment as protomédico, Melchor Amusco informed the city fathers that "in this court and within five leagues roundabout" there were "many persons who with little fear of God and in contempt of royal justice, freely practice the art of medicine," going so far as to call themselves doctors, licentiates, phlebotomists, surgeons, apothecaries, hernists, herbalists, curers by charms—all with neither license, learning, nor experience. In the same way, he emphasized, many women—whites, *mestizas,* blacks, and mulattas—took over the trade of midwives and everything else that went with it. In view of this sweeping arraignment, protomédico Amusco nominated Alonso Alférez de Jodar as attorney (*promotor fiscal*) to investigate and prosecute these offenders. Alférez de Jodar accepted the appointment, when it was made, to act "without fraud, collusion, fear and . . . without exception of persons."[137]

All these outbursts in the town councils indicate that, even after the appointment of royal protomédicos, the chief prompter of medical regulations remained the city government. If there was a protomédico, the aldermen "appointed" him to keep watch over unlicensed practitioners. If not, they named some doctor "of repute" in the city. Never once did they complain that the duly appointed protomédico lacked initiative to perform his duties without prodding.

After the fairly regular and frequent, if not constant, vigilance of the town councils in the matter of licensing medical practitioners, long periods of quiescence set in toward the end of the sixteenth century that tolerated all kinds of illicit practice. Here and there, someone, generally a legitimate doctor infuriated by his illicit competition, sang the loudest notes of outrage. Whenever he sought appointment as city physician or protomédico, Dr. Francisco Urieta, a resident and a physician who got his doctor's degree in medicine from the University of Mexico in 1615,[138] found himself elbowed aside by other doctors who were, in his view, behind the times. Euripides may have been right when he said that whom the gods would destroy they first make mad, but he could not have been expected to know that in the process they also made history; even more than the madman, the angry one speaks the plain truth when nobody else will speak anything—varnished or unvarnished.

Philip III's (1598–1621) pragmatic in 1617, requiring three examiners to sit in the examination of physicians, barbers, apothecaries, and surgeons, had an immediate echo in the cabildo of Mexico City. When the new decree reached Mexico the next year, Councilman Francisco Escudero Figueroa urged the cabildo to carry out the new decree immediately, but that body merely appointed a committee to draw up the points for discussion—apparently with the viceroy. As nothing followed this slight stir, Dr. Francisco Urieta personally went before the council with a petition to force the protomédico, Dr. Jerónimo Herrera, to sit with other judges while examining candidates for practice. In doing so, he laid bare the "excesses and disorders," and the "everyday and untimely deaths which, without even the sacraments, the sick suffer" because "they are too ignorant to know who is a doctor and who is not." All that was then necessary for a man "unfit for other occupations" was to go into medicine, "put on a doctor's outfit, acquire a horse-cloth," don a cape and cap of the color of his choice, protected by a concession of His Majesty that allows horse-cloths six months of the year. Both in the city and its environs, "as well as in the kingdom at large," hosts of people fell innocently into the hands of these charlatans and died "in such numbers that neither the hospital—where many tragic things can be seen—the church, nor the cemetery can accommodate them." This was merely Urieta's prelude to his request that the city return to its "ancient preeminence of naming two protomédicos," a situation that made his own appointment likely. In reviewing a suit brought by the protomédico, the royal audiencia upheld the Spanish law, but it did not force the protomédico to sit with others in these examinations. Urieta's last chance was to induce the city to assert itself once again and appoint its own protomédicos, without doubt in the hope that he would be one of them.[139]

As in the case of medicine and surgery, concern about the examination and licensing of midwives was an afterthought of some project to inspect drugstores. In this way the cabildo of Mexico in 1538 enjoined the examiners, who had set out to look into apothecary shops, to inspect and examine all those practicing midwifery. After passing this stage, the instructions went on, the examiners should return to the cabildo and give an account of what they had done so that the city could authorize those passing to practice.[140] As an indication of the casual nature of this concern, and the ineffectiveness of the solution proposed, the cabildo in 1540 proposed exactly the same solution.[141] The preoccupation with the correct practice of phlebotomy, as then would have been the case almost anywhere, was infinitely greater.

Since medical inspections during the sixteenth century came as a result of a cumulative process of evils and countercomplaint, they never fell at regular intervals as they did when the tribunals of the protomedicato came to function systematically. At a time when inspections were postponed until agitation forced them, all branches of medicine were more than ready for examination. In such circumstances it is very difficult to separate the history of one branch of medicine from the other. As soon as the apothecary had his shop set up, however, cries of outrage began to appear; he could not conceal his mistakes so well as nature so often did for the doctor. The cabildo of Mexico late in 1529 and early in 1530 ordered the protomédicos Licentiate Pero López and Dr. Cristóbal Hojeda to accompany the alcalde ordinario and the two city inspectors (diputados) to examine apothecary shops and any others that might have "medicine or drugs" and, if they found any the doctors said were not good, to confiscate them.[142] The city gave the same orders in 1538, except that the doctors appointed this time were Dr. Cristóbal Méndez and Licentiate Fulano Ximénez.[143] Yet not two years had passed before the city learned again that "many people complain that the apothecaries trick them, not only because their medicines are spoiled, but that they are not made as required." The reaction of the city was not quite standard; the aldermen and the city inspectors selected physicians and apothecaries to make the rounds with them. Twelve years later the situation was still so out of hand that the alcaldes and city inspectors began visiting drugstores without any physician. Therefore, to supply expert opinion, the city hastily appointed Dr. Juan Vásquez and Licenciate Damián de Torres,[144] a man destined to get the doctor's degree in medicine from the new University of Mexico in 1553.[145]

At almost regular intervals in the sixteenth century the city of Lima grew apprehensive about the quality of drugs dispensed there and followed a course of inspection closely paralleling that of Mexico City. The City of Kings had not been founded five years when the aldermen heard that "the apothecary of this city" carried "spoiled medicines" that were a "danger to the commonweal." The remedy was to instruct the diputados of this city, in company with physician B. Juan de Castro, to inspect the shop, throw out the damaged goods, and present the bill to the apothecary.[146] However, some deliberations on drugs were far from perfunctory. In 1551 the cabildo heard reports that "women and slaves" had taken corrosive sublimate (*solimán*) and had "died of it. . . ." The verdict was that the deaths "might have gone undetected" had it not been "that the said corrosive sublimate and other deadly things" were so openly and freely sold. Then the city enacted an ordinance, preconized in the town square, that no "apothecary-merchant" nor huckster might sell corrosive sublimate, red sulphate of arsenic (*realgar*) (*ocopimente*), "nor any other death-dealing thing" to white men or women or to a slave except to those over fifteen, bearing a prescription by a doctor "with a license to practice." The penalty for violation was drastic: a boarded-up shop and a fine of one hundred pesos.[147]

How low in the scale of importance was the apothecary can be seen from the hubbub around his business in the spring of 1572. In that year the town council suddenly became exercised over the practice of allowing black and Indian employees in apothecary shops to dispense drugs and fill prescriptions. Many times, the complaint ran, "they did the opposite of what the prescriptions called for. . . ." In fact, they had given prohibited medicines containing opium in place of the healthful ones called for and had sold bichloride of mercury. If, "when the very Spaniards trained in the art made mistakes every day," what was to be expected of blacks and Indians? The penalty finally fixed for violation was a fine of two hundred pesos to the proprietor and exile for "the Negroes, Negresses, and Indians."[148] Druggists, to be sure, had to prove their blood purity (*limpieza de sangre*) before they could legally get licenses, but the aldermen of Lima barred Indians and blacks solely on the ground of their lack of training.

Inspections and Coercive Regulations

Establishment of the first royal protomedicatos in America did not have a significant effect upon the regulatory practices of Lima. For many years the Lima town council had had exclusive responsibility for the inspection of drugstores, but upon the arrival in 1569 of Sánchez Renedo the city stepped aside in his favor. This arrangement was not satisfactory, for in 1576 the alcalde ordinario Juan de Arreynaga begged the cabildo to resume the inspections formerly conducted by the city. Without any legal niceties and quibbling, the council authorized Arreynaga and two aldermen to select some physician and make the rounds themselves.[149] Protomédico Sánchez Renedo, however, appears not to have surrendered his prerogatives, for in 1579, three years after the city appointed its own inspectors, the cabildo learned that apothecary shops had not been inspected "on account of the death of Dr. Sánchez Renedo"— which occurred in 1579.[150] Thereupon, the city authorized the inspectors of weights and measures, together with a physician and a druggist, to resume the examination of drug shops and levy the penalties indicated.[151] Two years later the ayuntamiento named the physician, Licentiate Alvaro de Torres, for the same purpose.[152] The city showed how firmly it retained the initiative, or how capable it was of reasserting its customary authority, when it set out in 1598 to enforce "the new law" requiring all phlebotomists, surgeons, and druggists to present their licenses in the ayuntamiento itself. At the same session the council indulged in the usual plaint that "many medicines were spoiled" and the apothecaries were "long unvisited," and ordered the alcalde and the fiel executor, "with the assistance of Dr. Hormero, the protomédico," to close the shops without warning and, if any were found wanting, to close them for good.[153] In 1599, the very next year, Alcalde Joseph de Rivera, together with the inspectors of weights and measures, got orders from the city to take the matter up with the protomédico general, "as you have to deal with him," and then inspect the apothecary shops. At last, in this rather tame fashion, the irritation of the city at having to defer to a man not carrying out his responsibilities on his own breaks through to the surface.[154]

Thus, except where there was a royally established protomedicato under legal obligation to inspect apothecary shops every two years—and with enough shops to make the fees profitable—there were no inspections until the abuses in the shops became so scandalous that some alderman forced the issue still another time. (This process of agitation and collapse went on so long in Lima as to suggest that the protomédico found it more profitable to take bribes than to exact fees.) So, once again, after the lapse of four years the cabildo of Lima returned to the singsong that, as "the apothecary shops have not been inspected for a long time," it was natural to suppose that many medicines were damaged and a menace to health. The remedy proposed was repetitious too: the alcalde and the fieles executores, in company with Dr. Hormero, the protomédico, should inspect them, and on the day when they did so the shops be closed the better to see what was in them and what cried out for remedy. In order to do this work with the greatest brevity and to prevent such frauds as the hiding of spoiled medicines and the transfer of essential drugs from one shop to another just ahead of the inspectors, the cabildo stipulated that all shops should be closed on that day.[155] In far-off Caracas, where, because "medicines were not only excessive in price, but damaged and spoiled and come to be more poisonous than the medicines the people cry out against," the town council instructed the alcaldes and deputies to undertake the inspections.[156] This cry was as monotonous as that of the whippoorwill and the problem was universal; all that was required was a sizable town.

When the Spaniards came to America, they had little time to think of the regular practice of medicine, but when they did so—even before their laws were applied to America in 1535—they expected the laws of Spain requiring a license to practice to be observed. By the time the new cities settled down, however, every aspect of medicine was, in the main, operating illegally. As this was the point when the city governments began to take notice, they rarely took up a problem of crass abuse in one field without attempting to correct abuses in all of them. As taking improper drugs, or not being able to afford proper ones, was something immediately noticeable, efforts to require licenses of those practicing surgery and medicine came as an afterthought in nearly every effort to curb abuses in the compounding and sale of medicines. In 1540, for example, the cabildo of Mexico City, while instructing a commission to inspect drugs, tacked on a rider asking these commissioners to check the licenses of physicians and surgeons and examine their scale of fees.[157]

Since the practice of surgery did not absolutely require academic training, it was far easier to intrude into that specialty. The growing number of reports of disasters to patients at the hands of these intruders led the cabildo of Mexico in 1538 to pass an ordinance requiring all those practicing surgery in Mexico City and the surrounding country to present their licenses or pay a fine of one hundred pesos.[158] In 1554 the same type of complaints resulted in another ordinance requiring both physicians and surgeons to submit their titles to the cabildo within nine days. One of the grounds of concern was not malpractice of medicine or surgery, but loss of revenue that accompanied entrance into the professions. For this reason the councilmen could complain against unexamined notaries and clerks in the same breath with their wails against unexamined doctors and surgeons.[159] How really ineffectual all these appeals to law really were can be seen in the repetition of the ordinances. By 1557 the cabildo of Mexico City was aware of a pragmatic issued by the king of Spain requiring licenses of medical practitioners. It happened that this year was one of those crests of complaint against "the damage and notable prejudice" resulting from illicit practice. The inevitable response was another ordinance: that all those practicing not only had to have a title but also had to register it with the city. The cabildo was specific enough to name some of the intruders, "Cabral, Poza, Segovia, and Espinosa, and others," whom it warned that continued practice without "showing" license would automatically incur the fine of five hundred pesos.[160]

After the appointment of royal protomédicos for all Peru and New Spain with headquarters in Lima and Mexico City, the naming of protomédicos in Mexico fell back into the hands of the municipality. The struggle between the predominant physicians and the less prestigious surgeons for the right to examine and license in their respective fields did not end so easily. When the cabildo of Mexico City appointed two physicians as protomédicos in 1593 and named a surgeon to assist them in examinations and cases involving surgery,[161] there was an immediate outcry from the physicians who begged and got permission to appear before the cabildo.[162] Their plea was that they should go on doing their work, even examining surgeons, without the attendance of a surgeon. The cabildo readily agreed that in the future the protomédicos should perform their duties without the assistance of any surgeon.[163]

Fixing the Prices of Drugs

The idea of fixing drug prices in the sixteenth century was not an alien idea to be imposed upon the public; price-fixing was customary and a constant refuge of the people and municipalities in the fight against inflation in the prices of medicines. The formula for action was the same as in the case of spoiled and dangerous drugs: when the prices went so high that the cabildo could no longer disregard the murmuring, the councilmen would spend a session, or a great part of it, "conversing" about the familiar abuse. In this way in 1537 Mexico City was tied up in a controversy over the price list and the formula for compounding medicines imposed upon apothecaries, who appealed the regulations. At the same time the public protested that the apothecary charged the highest prices without ever compounding the drugs as required. The never-failing answer of the cabildo to both was to call for the alcaldes and deputies to look into the practices of the apothecaries, punish as suitable, and require order.[164] In fact, when another wave of abuse was about ready to break, the apothecaries themselves admitted that the price of medicine was "very dear and excessive." With too much experience to depend upon the tender heart of the apothecary, the municipality appointed a commission to consult as it chose and moderate the official price of drugs.[165] When the new price list was ready six months later, the municipality decided to submit it to the royal audiencia for approval before putting it in force.[166] This course, certainly, was the best hedge against any suits brought by apothecary or merchant. But not even a price list sanctioned by the royal audiencia could stay the rise in prices when the apothecaries, with few imported medicines, found themselves selling drugs to stay an epidemic. In 1547, more than two years after the arrival of the "great sickness which the Lord has seen fit to visit upon this land,"[167] the Mexican town council once again found itself inundated by the vehement complaints of the people against the runaway price of drugs. Once again the answer was a commission to set up and post a new tariff and a charge to the deputies and alcaldes to enforce it.[168]

In their monotonously recurring plaints against the exorbitant prices charged for medicines, Mexico City and Lima were remarkably similar. In 1538, when Lima was just three years old, the town council observed that the "doctors and surgeons of the city" sold medicines at exorbitant prices and, when these were spoiled, used them to treat patients. The city then delegated four men to examine the medicines in the possession of these doctors and surgeons, set a reasonable price, and seize all damaged drugs.[169] Then, later, when the cabildo learned that "the apothecary of the city," being "the only one at present," took advantage of his monopoly to charge "high and excessive prices," it called in Dr. Hernando de Sepúlveda, not so much because he was the royal protomédico but because he was the most learned and conscientious. Sepúlveda was not just invited but ordered to report back to the council when he had done his work.[170] When he presented his inspection report, the council quickly approved the memorial listing the prices he had fixed.[171] Again, in 1553 the corregidor reported that apothecaries sold their goods at outlandish prices to the poor, who came, "silver in hand," with not the slightest prospect of a physician to appraise them. His solution—the customary one—was that two doctors and the deputies should evaluate the drugs on hand and set prices for a year, or, if indicated, for a shorter period. The cabildo responded warmly, appointing Licentiate Alvaro de Torres and Doctor Gaspar de Meneses as the experts, firmly instructing the deputies to draw up a list immediately.[172]

Except in the viceregal capitals, where the Council of the Indies and the viceroys were likely to duplicate Spanish practices, medicines were scarcely under any kind of regulation. In these cases, especially when there were many sick people, the doctors sometimes monopolized the drugs and set the prices at figures the poor could not reach. This situation arose in Caracas, but the town council only got to the point of "discussing" the evil with the inhabitants "without compelling" anybody.[173]

Before the first viceroy of New Spain had been at his post twelve months, in one of those ever-recurring sessions devoted to "conversation" on overcharging, the town council concluded that the doctors exacted excessive fees. The explanation lay in the increase in the number of inhabitants, the ever-rising number of sick people, and the upward trend of wages. In what was, perhaps, their first effort to resist the tide, the aldermen passed an ordinance that no physician charge more than half a peso (tostón) a visit, but that if the patient should send for him to make more than one call, he should charge accordingly. The penalty for disregarding this regulation was a fine of fifty pesos and two months' suspension from practice.[174] How little a solemn and menacing law like this—one confirmed by Viceroy Antonio de Mendoza (1535-50) the same day it was enacted—actually meant in a showdown can be seen when the first epidemics led to spiraling prices.

The cabildo was the institution in the Spanish colonies that most consistently pressed for the interest of the public. The concern of the distant crown with medicine and public health was—as was almost inevitable—historical, customary, and slow. It was the city, not the crown, that had to face whatever struck at the moment, although the government in Spain provided the viceroy with powers that enabled him both to take the initiative and, if necessary, to override the cabildo. Even in the case of epidemics, until they reached proportions taxing the governmental and financial resources of the kingdom, the city council took the action it saw fit, and in minor matters, at least, certainly took it first. If the steward thought that those roaming the streets with contagious diseases should be rounded up, the town council so ordered without more to-do.[175] On the other hand, when smallpox or some other mortal disease began to bring down "whites, Negroes, and Indians" alike, a good viceroy was likely to take notice, call a junta, or act in some other way. In 1620 when both the cabildo of Lima and the viceroy, the Principe de Esquilache (1615-21), decided on a junta of physicians to determine whether they had an epidemic and to decide what to do, the cabildo sent its alcaldes ordinarios to talk with the viceroy and to pledge its support[176]—all without one word from the protomedicato. In Caracas, where there was no tribunal of the protomedicato, rumors of an outbreak in La Guaira led to an offer from an alcalde to investigate. The council decided that the aldermen, by turns, should participate in the investigation. What is more, they summoned Dr. Juan Bautista de Navarro to help them decide whether the "attacks and casualties" in La Guaira were "pestilential" or not.[177]

Wherever it became necessary to mount a campaign to establish universities and, especially, to provide medical education at home, the town council was among the first to move. The cabildo of Lima in 1609, because fathers did not have the means to send their sons to the metropolis, "supplicated" the viceroy, the Marquis of Montesclaros, to order the medical subjects taught in the University of San Marcos "to keep the many good minds in this kingdom in hope."[178] It was characteristic of the seventeenth century and of the chronic lack of public funds that it remained for the viceroy, the Count of Chinchón (1629–39), after a lapse of a quarter of a century, to set up the chair of prima of medicine in 1634. Even then, the best that could be done was to finance the 600-peso salary with money from the monopoly of bichloride of mercury[179]— so deadly because so many ignorant people used mercury as an antisyphilitic.

Organization and Practice

B Y THE TIME the Spaniards came to America, the protomédico—the medical officer—was as much an institution as was the sheriff among the English. The very first moment that the Castilians felt they had subdued the country, almost without pausing for breath, and almost as if they were surprised, they turned to Spain with nostalgia to meet the needs of settled life. Though he had not thought of it, Columbus had to beg for a lawyer to help him out of the morass that desperation, rebellion, titles, and snarls of all kinds were bound to create on that first frontier. Thus, it was not on the first but on the third voyage that the Catholic Kings dispatched a doctor, along with a musician, for the comfort of the little cluster of people on Española. Though well established in Spain, the doctor lacked the prestige to make his presence so necessary as that of the lawyer. When a doctor—even a bachelor of medicine—did appear, however, it was nip and tuck whether his first step would be to begin practice or to run to the town council to get himself named protomédico.

To the government in Spain such a situation cried out for regulation. The misfortune was that the first protomédico general of New Spain was too interested in the field of botany to see to the permanent foundation of the royal protomedicato itself.

The Protomedicato General

The protomedicato in America came in two different stages. In the first, a kind of filling-the-vacuum stage, the towns and cities regulated the practice of medicine—something they never entirely gave up. Between the day of Columbus and that of Cortés, the royal protomedicato in Spain moved on its own authority to appoint protomédicos for America, an ambition foiled by hostile settlers and a jealous crown, and for this reason was ill understood—even by the colonial officials and vecinos themselves. In this way the initial foundation of the royal protomedicato came in response to a vital new interest in New World medical plants that swept through Spain in the mid-sixteenth century. Thus, in 1570 the crown made provision for both botanical research and a protomédico general to regulate the medical professions. Unfortunately for the later administration of medical law, the two types were separated in fact but remained confused in men's minds,[1] a fact that has often tripped not only the reader but the writer of history.

This confusion is compounded by the twofold nature of the instructions issued to Francisco Hernández in 1570.[2] The first part of this significant document dealt with the conduct of Dr. Hernández's proposed botanical research.[3] In it, no doubt at Hernández's own suggestion, the king instructed him to go to America and embark first in New Spain because "the herbs and seeds" reported there were the most impressive. His first duty was to call together all resident "physicians, surgeons, and herbalists" and get their accounts of all "herbs, trees, and medicinal plants" in the kingdom. Thereafter, he could learn their uses and the doses given as medicine. Of course, since the expectation was to cultivate these plants, he also needed to report on the conditions under which they grew and flourished such as in wet or dry places. In view of the repeated fiascos of the eighteenth century, it was almost prescient that he was expected, in case there "were species different from these," to report upon and identify them. As the crown did not foresee the tremendous personal exertions that Hernández was to make roaming the provinces, he was not only allowed but also expected to accept reports from other people, but always with a formal certification. In the end Hernández could send back to Spain any seeds, herbs, or plants not already known there. In the true spirit of individual scholarship, he might write up his findings according to his "good judgment and learning. . . ." Little did the crown foresee the extent or the vicissitudes of this remarkable mission when it instructed Dr. Hernández, "when you have finished what you have to do in New Spain," you may "leave it and go to the provinces of Peru."

This last part of Hernández's orders[4] accounts for the confusion of officials later and, perhaps, historians today. Though Hernández had the title of "protomédico general of all the Indies," he was to reside where there was a royal audiencia with appellate jurisdiction.[5] Despite his sweeping title, however, he had to confine the exercise of his official functions to the seat of the royal audiencia and five leagues round about it. Beyond that limit, he could not even stage inspections of drugstores, bring in practitioners to authenticate titles and licenses, or examine candidates to practice. He might not, however, rescind a license signed in the first place by a person entitled to issue it. If persons beyond five leagues voluntarily presented themselves in the city of his residence, however, he might examine them and, if they passed, grant them licenses.[6]

How little the "protomédico general" enjoyed the powers suggested in his sweeping title unfolds in his instructions. Since the king had already appointed Dr. Antonio Sánchez Renedo as protomédico in "Peru, and Tierra Firme," and since he was sanguine enough to believe that Hernández could finish his researches in Mexico and go on to other "kingdoms," he forbade Hernández to assume jurisdiction in any of those districts unless he actually resided in the seat of the audiencia. Thus, the man with the grandiose title, before he could assume his office in the district of another audiencia, had to present his "Instruction" before the president and oidores of that body. In remote places, such as Nombre de Dios, where there was no audiencia, he nevertheless would have to present his credentials to the mayor (*alcalde mayor*) or chief magistrate (*justicia ordinaria*). The implication in these careful distinctions is that medical credentials were presented to the highest officials present.[7] If he was of a mind, a doctor might travel to the nearest chief magistrate to take the name of the official empowered to accept his papers, but nothing is said of who was to examine candidates to practice medicine, surgery, or pharmacy outside the five-league limit. So, saddled with these sweeping yet restricted responsibilities, Hernández took his commission and 1,000 ducats (350,000 maravedís)[8] and departed on his fateful journey. It was very hard to find evidence that the presence of Hernández in Mexico interfered in the least with the management of medical affairs by the city.

The creation of the protomédico general, then, tended rather to increase than to lessen the confusion in the regulation of medicine in America. Unfortunately, the editor of the *Recopilación de Indias,* using the cédulas that instructed Hernández, tried to combine the concept of the protomédico general with that of the tribunal created in Mexico by the royal cédula in 1646. The result was bewildering jurisdictional confusion in medical litigation. In consequence, the institution of the protomedicato in Peru functioned until the very end through a protomédico general, while that in Mexico stabilized as a tribunal immediately after February 1646.

Organization of the Protomedicato in Spain

This uncertainty arose in part from the lack of clear precedent in Spain. In the interval between the appointment of Francisco Hernández in 1570 as protomédico general and the designation of the professor or *prima* of medicine as president of the protomedicato in New Spain seventy-six years later, a transition was taking place in Spain itself. The history of the organization of the institution in Spain accordingly remains hazy well into the time of Philip II. The laws themselves do not make it positively clear whether there was one or two protomédicos, whether they had permanent examiners (*alcaldes examinadores*) to assist them, or whether the board commissioned subalterns.[9] Neither is it clear whether medicine and surgery were "united" or separated. The series of reforms written into law in 1588 and elaborated in 1593, however, make the structure of the organization clear. In 1588 the law at last stated specifically that there would be only one protomédico who, with three examiners named by the king, would dispatch business and try cases. The protomédico, however, took precedence in seating, or voting, and signed documents first and in the most preferred place.[10]

Five years later the king drastically reorganized the protomedicato into what was, beyond doubt, a serious court of justice in Spain. Since suspicion of fraud and corruption had brought on nearly every change instituted in the protomedicato, the deduction is that, like the chest with three keys, three men would be less likely to agree upon a method for fraud than would one. After 1593, instead of one protomédico, there would be three, all named by the king, all three holding office at his pleasure. In a way the new law[11] continued the appointment of three medical examiners, so that henceforth each of the three protomédicos had an examiner standing by to guarantee a quorum of three, while the senior protomédico had the right to name others from the twelve doctors of the House of Borgoña[12] to represent him in his absence. There was no rank or seniority or special weight in voting in what was now unquestionably a tribunal. Any two of three would always carry. The definite creation of a tribunal, where abuse of privileges and exemptions was less likely, enabled the king to extend certain guild privileges to the protomedicato. Henceforth, its decisions could not be appealed except before the tribunal itself. In appeals to the Council of Castile that did not altogether concern medicine, surgery, or pharmacy, the council decided the proper jurisdiction within thirty days and returned the case to the protomedicato if it still appeared to be medical.[13] The king of Spain, however, never left three professional physicians adrift on the morass of law; he always provided a legal adviser. Philip II not only required that the assessor of the protomedicato establish all proofs and carry through the proceedings as formerly but, before it could be valid, sign the decision with the judges themselves[14]—always on a day of the week set aside for the purpose. In keeping with the classic reluctance of the Spanish crown to incur outright expenses, each protomédico, though his salary was set up at 100,000 maravedís, could collect this sum only from fees collected and penalties levied and deposited in the traditional chest with the keys.[15] The protomedicato in Spain had had the privilege of naming, when

thought necessary, a fiscal, a bailiff (*alguacil*), and a porter.[16] The protomedicato had its own secretary, who collected conventional fees without
drawing upon the chest.[17] Thus, by 1588, with some sharp modifications
in 1593, the protomedicato in Spain had stabilized enough to become a
model for America.

Definitive Organization in the Indies in 1646

In New Spain the viceroy's abuse of his appointive powers led to the
creation of the definitive tribunal of the royal protomedicato. After
Juan de Palafox, the bishop of Puebla de los Angeles, was ordered to
draw up the statutes of the Royal and Pontifical University of Mexico
in 1639, he reported to the king on December 28, 1644, among other
things, concerning the "excesses" in the viceregal appointment of protomédicos in the forty-one years since the viceroy had wrested this power
from the municipal council. The strongest indications are that the abuses
lay in appointing too many men[18] to these posts, particularly the viceroy's
favorites. The king accepted Palafox's proposal, with conditions,[19] and
asked him to incorporate the changes in the statutes he was drawing up
for the university.[20] He then addressed a royal cédula to the viceroy, the
Count of Salvatierra (1642–48), in which he imposed upon the protomedicato the structure it was to hold—until independence.[21]

This critical cédula, particularly in its exordium, is a clear index to
the philosophy behind all regulation of the medical professions. Sound
management of the protomedicato was vitally important to the health of
the king's vassals, not just because the protomedicato inspected drugstores and remedies, but especially because it examined physicians and
surgeons, "masters of the life and death of those sick people who come
into their hands. . . ." This awesome responsibility made it imperative
to get protomédicos of the learning and experience necessary. As in this
case, the government invariably supported the royal protomedicato on
the grounds of public health, a fact that tends to lead the investigator to
assume initially that he is beginning to study some public health organization as distinct from private practice such as that in the United
States today. But no such bureaucracy ever developed. The king's officers
merely meant that the public health could best be preserved by seeing
to it through the protomedicato—that physicians and surgeons be examined and licensed—nothing more.

The king's formula for attaining this end was as good as he could
draw up in the seventeenth century. Henceforth, there would be a tribunal
of three members. The first professor (*prima*) of medicine would be
"perpetual protomédico," preceding all the rest in processions and pre-

siding at meetings. "Annexing" this presidency to an academic chair would lead others to "study and work and try to reach" this honorable post. The senior member of the medical faculty would become the second protomédico, unless the professor of prima was senior, in which case the doctor ranking in seniority next below him would get the second place. The viceroy would appoint the third from among those best-qualified doctors incorporated in the university. He would submit all appointments, however automatic, to the king for his approval. Henceforth, vacancies occurring among the supernumeraries—excess protomédicos already appointed—would go "unfilled until there remain only three." By this slow, natural process of elimination, the protomedicato would eventually become a tribunal of three members. Definite as all this was, the solution accepted by the king left room for the old maneuvering that had tried the skill of Bishop Palafox and the patience of Viceroy Salvatierra. What followed in Mexico exposes the deep-seated feuding over appointments and lays bare the cause of Salvatierra's petulance.

In Salvatierra's time it was already the custom to have three protomédicos in Mexico City, with one of the places going to the senior doctor of the medical faculty. However, when the senior doctor died, Salvatierra departed from custom and appointed his personal physician, Dr. Francisco de Toro Morejón, not Rodrigo Muñoz, the senior doctor of the faculty at the university.[22] The rigid new method of selecting the protomédicos now forced him to supplant Dr. de Toro, his own man, with Dr. Muñoz. As he had the right to appoint the third man on the board, he gave this post to de Toro and not the old incumbent Melgarejo, whose confirmation had not been approved.[23] Then, as soon as he had issued the titles required of him,[24] he turned to complain to the king that the new law was just more fuel for the flaming quarrels over the chair of prima of medicine and another incentive to the "illicit means" certain to be taken to obtain it. In fact, he said, the chair was always obtained by "negotiation," especially when Dr. Alonso Fernández, whom he had just been obliged to honor, had obtained it. When the "bishop visitor" Palafox was "governing" (June 10–November 23, 1664), in order to "carry" the vote, he had "to make his favor public to the point of allowing the *oidores doctores*'[25] to vote." Even after all these maneuvers, Fernández won by only three votes. Salvatierra's view was that these posts ought to be held by the most worthy and highly esteemed figures—men of learning and conscience, "badges that seldom mark the professor" or "the one that time makes senior." "In a country so poor in rewards as this," the viceroy grumbled on, it would be far better to give the few there were to the proper people in order to stimulate others to study.[26] The Council of the Indies decided that in view of the precaution inserted in the law of 1646, the viceroy, when asking for confirmation, should present any objections so that the council could take them into account and correct them at that time.[27] The two men destined to be crowded off the tribunal made a last-minute effort to get their appointments confirmed quickly. Since protomédicos Pedro de los Arcos Monroy from the University of Seville and Dr. Juan de Melgarejo had been appointed by the viceroys in Mexico City before 1646,[28] the fiscal naturally opposed confirmation on the ground that they had been named "before the cédula which set out the practice to be followed in these nominations. . . ."[29]

The tribunal of the protomedicato did not evolve in Lima as it did in New Spain, though four months after the presidency of the protomedicato had been attached to the chair of prima of medicine in Mexico another did the same thing for the first chair in the University of San Marcos de Lima.[30] This particular law, however, though it required the new professor of prima to get his title from the viceroy before he became president of the protomedicato, said nothing about the selection of other personnel in that tribunal. In contrast with Mexico, therefore, the Peruvians followed precedent set in the appointments of Francisco Hernández and Antonio Sánchez Renedo and made their first professor of medicine protomédico general, supporting him in the classic Spanish pattern with examiners instead of second and third protomédicos as in Mexico, a system of organization that endured until the day of independence. Thus, whereas Mexico was overrun with supernumerary protomédicos in 1645, Peru had only one protomédico, who, residing in Lima and drawing fees for examinations and inspections of drugstores, served without salary. He had his court, drew up processes, and passed sentence—all with the assistance of his assessor, the senior oidor of the royal audiencia.[31] Juan de Solórzano reported at that time that "there used to be" a protomédico in Panama, another in New Granada, and another in Mexico. He remarked that these appointments were the prerogative of the Council of the Indies, though actually administered by the executive committee (cámara) of that body. He recognized that in practice the viceroys and presidents presented names to the council, which either "affirmed or denied" them. "Sometimes," he unsmilingly observed, "they have been given or bought for money." When the nineteenth century dawned, all petitioners and litigants in the area of medicine were still addressing themselves to the "Protomédico General."[32]

The atmosphere prevailing in the University of Mexico in 1646, as in the religious orders, was already tense. The very next year after the crown attached the presidency of the tribunal of the protomedicato to the chair of prima of medicine, Viceroy Salvatierra got wind of an impending clash between creoles and peninsulars over the competitions (*oposiciones*) for the second chair (*vísperas*) of medicine. The trouble, he said, was that among the contestants and the examiners with votes were "those born in this City as well as in the kingdoms of Castile." Fearful that instead of "complete calm" there would be "riots and disturbances," Salvatierra warned that if either the judges or the contestants descended "to dispute over nations, the fatherland, and the nature of each," they would be disqualified and not permitted to vote or be voted upon in the oposición and fined five hundred pesos for "the obsequies of the prince our lord." Besides the fine, the penalty for the *opositor* was that, the moment he introduced these forbidden subjects, he would be hauled down from the chair and expelled from the contest. The warning went to the university so that it might not pretend ignorance.[33] The viceroy was now even more testy than when he disputed Palafox's reforms in the protomedicato the year before.

The optimism that foretold a quick reduction of the Mexican protomedicato to three members was wide of the target. The viceroys had already appointed so many "supernumeraries" that two decades later some of them were still holding on.[34] As these supernumeraries cut down on their fees, the regular protomédicos took the occasion of the death of Dr. Juan Mesa, "the last supernumerary protomédico," to ask the viceroy, the Marquis of Mancera (1664–73), to offer complete compliance with the royal will. The fiscal, however, observed that with the death of Mesa, four still remained, and the viceroy accepted his advice to suppress Mesa's post and presumably to do the same for the fourth when it became vacant.[35]

As Salvatierra had foreseen, attaching the presidency of the protomedicato to the professor of prima of medicine accentuated the struggle for the chair itself, but as the chair was "proprietary" and for life, these crises could not arise very often, but when they did, the right to vote and the conduct of the election became a great matter of state. In fact, one year before the end of the century the king had to settle the question of the order of voting. The laws of the Indies provided that in filling a proprietary chair the prima professor and the senior doctor of the faculty could vote as members of the examining board.[36] In case the prima professor died or otherwise vacated his chair, however, the second professor of vespers usually became contestant. This shifting, then, meant that only the senior doctor among these "knowledgeable [*inteligente*]" in a subject could vote. Since the other professors of medicine held temporary chairs (as professors of method and surgery [*método*]), there was some doubt about whether they could be called "in order" from "next below" to vote or enjoy precedence in ceremonies. Because the king felt that two votes from the faculty of the vacant chair were essential, he ruled that the professor of method should vote along with the senior doctor.[37] But even with the voting membership of the board absolutely determined, doubts could arise and petty but implacable squabbles occur.

A prime case of such internecine fighting arose in 1722 when the king called for reports from the archbishop, the viceroy, and the rector of the University of Mexico upon the death of Dr. Juan de Brizuela, professor of prima of medicine.[38] In the election in 1722 Dr. Marcos Salgado, professor of "method," emerged victor by a vote of four to three. After the vote was duly "published," Salgado went, as was the custom, to the rector of the university to ask for possession of his chair, but the rector refused him. Meanwhile, the viceroy, the Marqués de Valero (1716–22), suspended the election while the appeal for a royal ruling was pending. When he appealed directly to the viceroy, Salgado got the same rebuff; the viceroy's only explanation was that one of the judges, Fray Antonio de Córdoba, senior doctor of the faculty of medicine, had entered one vote in the urn as it passed around and then, after being allowed to retrieve it, voted again, thus invalidating the whole procedure. This was the wedge for the charge of "injustice" by Dr. Juan José de Brizuela, another of the contestants for the chair. Because he was professor of vísperas, next in line and "of superior merit," he and his powerful friends felt he should have the chair.[39] Salgado went deeper; he said that Brizuela had appealed to the viceroy with these invalid charges because he counted upon his favoritism. As the voting was legal, Salgado contended, the only possible injustice to Brizuela was that his "merits" were superior. To resolve any doubt on this question, he invited the king's officers to examine the documents submitted. Not only was Brizuela lax in attending where his attendance was called for, but his illnesses were chronic. This was the reasoning on which Salgado based his petition to be given the chair and paid his salary from the day he presented himself to the rector to take possession of it.[40]

Weighing of the evidence in the Council of the Indies was detailed and deliberate. The fiscal noticed[41] particularly that when the archbishop, as chairman of the examining board, asked what should be done, one of the oidores, Dr. Noribe, remarked that "nothing was more contrary to consent than error." The secretary pointed out that the remedy was easy, because as Fray Antonio had handed in his first ballot unfolded, it could be easily identified and withdrawn. When the archbishop allowed the secretary to withdraw the ballot and accept a new one, Fray Antonio, after telling the viceroy that he had voted "according to his conscience," was still heard to mutter "I've also made an error now." There was an unproved suggestion that he had merely folded the original ballot and recast it, but as the fiscal of the Council of the Indies noticed, Fray Antonio himself expressly informed the king that he had voted for the man "with health" so that he could perform the duties of the chair. The rector did actually reconvene the examining board, but it refused to reconsider. The viceregal faction supporting Brizuela had contended that according to the constitutions of the university, the chair should fall to the man who held the senior degree and the chair of vísperas—a false claim. The fiscal said plainly that the viceroy, against express prohibitions, had intervened in matters that were not in his charge. The Council of the Indies accepted the fiscal's advice to ask the archbishop to see to it that the rector give Salgado possession and pay him all back salary.[42] Yet, some quarter of a century later, there was still rancor and room for clarification in procedures for determining the chair of prima of medicine.[43]

Personnel

Despite such contests, the royal cédula of 1646 took the appointment of protomédicos out of the hands of the viceroy,[44] but, equally important, it set up a formal procedure destined to be followed in New Spain to the very end of the Spanish regime. Under this system the professor of prima automatically became first protomédico, the senior doctor of the faculty of medicine the second, and the viceroy appointed the third—all in perpetuity, all subject to royal confirmation. It therefore fell to the viceroy to submit to the king all names for filling these posts. It was not enough to say that a certain man was now professor of prima of medicine, or the senior doctor, or the viceroy's choice. As late as 1799 the Council of the Indies rebuked Viceroy Miguel José de Azanza (1798–1800) for submitting the name of Dr. José Ignacio García Jove as president of the protomedicato without supporting documents on his "learning, quality, and parts." Because the five years since the viceroy submitted the name were about to run out, the government confirmed the title but called upon the viceroy to supply this information in the future.[45] Moreover, a title not confirmed within five years after the viceroy issued it was not valid. On one occasion, for example, the Council of the Indies instructed the crown attorney in Mexico to ask the royal audiencia to recover all emoluments and perquisites received by Dr. Juan de Brizuela as first protomédico and remit them to Spain because his viceregal title had not been confirmed after a decade. Then, before the order could go into operation, the council confirmed Brizuela's title.[46]

As soon as the cédula of 1646 outlined the organization and makeup of the tribunal del protomedicato in Mexico, the effects of royal intervention began to be felt. Instead of many members in the protomedicato, some of whom at least had bought their posts, the crown insisted upon confirming every viceregal appointment and strictly limited the membership to three. Moreover, the need of royal confirmation was not forgotten and remained the regular formula until the end of the colonial period. In 1647, for example, the Council of the Indies rejected the confirmation of the viceroy's appointment of Dr. Juan de Melgarejo, substitute professor of prima of medicine, as protomédico because his appointment antedated the cédula of 1646.[47] Thus, when a man won the chair of prima of medicine, though he was sure of the chair,[48] he could not count on confirmation in Spain.

Confirmation of titles, from first to third seats, was still being practiced with regularity as the eighteenth century ended.[49] After the first protomédico, who was invariably the prima professor of medicine, the membership of the Mexican protomedicato is more difficult to trace, for there is no reasonable way, if any way at all, to tell who held the senior degree in the medical faculty, and it was the senior man who became second protomédico.[50] The same procedure prevailed in the appointment, in perpetuity, of protomédicos to the third seat in the tribunal. Sometimes getting confirmations of titles from the king, for which the law allowed five years, was so protracted that it was necessary to appoint somebody else. The same punctilio that marked the titles of first and second protomédicos marked the third.[51] These seats were "proprietary" or in perpetuity and often fell vacant because the incumbent, if he did not die, "rose" to a higher post—quite possibly while spending four years waiting for confirmation from Spain.[52]

In time the tribunal of the protomedicato in Mexico came to have three extra or "supernumerary" permanent examiners—one in medicine, one in surgery, and the last in botany. The examiners in surgery and botany appeared in examinations with the regular protomédicos to supply technical information in their own fields that a man in medicine alone could not be expected to have. Moreover, they were not, as in the case of an inspection (*visita*) in pharmacy, appointed for a single assignment; their appointments were "perpetual." As logical as it was for the physicians on the protomedicato to have specialists sit with them when they examined surgeons and druggists, not until late in the eighteenth century did they accept—and only then when they were forced—specialists on the panel with them. From the first they recognized, probably because the law required it in Spain, that an apothecary should accompany the protomédicos when inspecting drugstores, but even in such cases they sometimes sought to do the work themselves in order to avoid allowing the apothecary his fees. Surgery did not assume a place in New Spain dignified enough to allow a surgeon to sit permanently with the proto-medicato in the examination of surgeons until after the establishment of the College of Surgery in the Royal Indian Hospital in 1770—and even then it required a royal order to force the tribunal to accede to this very natural demand. Moreover, not until the botanists came into their own in the late eighteenth century and claimed a great importance in medi-cine, perhaps more than was their due, did they finally win a place beside the protomédicos in the examination of physicians and apothecaries. Both the surgeon and the botanist, though they were anxious after the fashion of the time to piece out their incomes, saw a place on the protomedicato as recognition of their "faculty" and for their own personal prestige.[53]

Retirees and Fringe Benefits

While these petty struggles went on, the chair of prima of medicine continued to obtain more side benefits in addition to the presidency of the protomedicato. As proprietary holder, after twenty years of continuous service he was entitled to apply for exemption from the duties of his chair without losing the salary, "privileges, honors, exemptions," as well as the gratuities (*propinas*) attached to it. The original statute, however, en-titled him to receive gratuities from the candidate in examinations, in-vestitures, and other acts only when he was personally in attendance. Another statute actually ordered the rector of the university to restore any gratuity accidentally paid to a master or doctor not in a "parade or accompaniment."[54]

These provisions greatly curtailed the value of a proprietary pro-fessorship when a man was superannuated and, presumably, with ailments enough to keep him away from many ceremonies. Therefore, in 1698 the University of Mexico petitioned the king to permit lifetime professors, after legally retiring from the duties of the chair, to receive the gratuities whether they were actually present or not. After all, in the licentiate and doctors' degrees, the fees were paid more for the honor than mere physi-cal presence. But operating on the thesis that fees were paid to get the largest assemblage (*concurso*) of persons possible to dignify the occa-sion, the Council of the Indies brusquely ruled that any fees, even when paid accidentally, to a retired proprietary professor be "in conscience" returned.[55] Thus, it appears, there was no legal restraint upon the chief protomédico when he wished to perform his official duties, including those that entitled him to collect fees. However, since there were no statutes for the protomedicato to go by until 1751, and since these were prepared for Spain and rarely seen in America, it is more than reasonable to assume that the protomédicos themselves determined when fees were payable.

Distinct Organization of the Lima Protomedicato

The protomedicato in Lima did not evolve in precisely the same way as in Mexico. When the Council of the Indies asked Juan de Solór-zano in the mid-seventeenth century about the protomedicato of Lima, he replied that there was only one protomedicato there[56]—just as there was in Spain, with its functions identical to those of the tribunal in Mexico.[57] The assessor in Lima, however, was the senior oidor of the audiencia, while in Mexico the oidores served the protomedicato by turns of one year each. Though the laws of the Indies stated that the office of proto-médico general in Peru was to be held by whatever doctor won the first chair of medicine, as was the case in Mexico, Peruvian viceroys in the eighteenth century, at least occasionally, were still appointing proto-médicos generales from men of their own preference regardless of who was professor of prima of medicine.[58]

When, at the death of Dr. Isidro Pimentel, Viceroy Agustín Jáure-gui (1780–84) appointed Dr. Juan José de Iturrizarra to succeed Pimen-tel as protomédico general, without waiting to see who won the chair of prima in the oposición, he precipitated an instructive controversy.[59] His first step was to lay out Iturrizarra's "merits and good qualities"—he was an outstanding physician of Lima and, most useful as a protomédico, instructed in pharmacy. This Jáuregui put before the Minister of the In-dies, José de Gálvez, with the design of persuading that renowned figure to overlook the cold fact that his candidate could not legally qualify.[60] Seen by the doctors and professors of the jealous university cloister, this was an outrageous threat to their guild "privileges and exemptions." As was natural, their address to the king urged that the law making the first professor of medicine protomédico general be observed.[61] The fiscal of the Council of the Indies said, as in good conscience a legalistic crown attorney had to say, there was not sufficient justification for stripping the first professor of medicine of the presidency of the protomedicato. He crowned his rebuttal of Jáuregui's case by asking that the trial lectures be staged in Lima with all due speed to select the prima professor of medicine.[62] A royal cédula to that effect went out thirteen days later, ordering strict observance of the law.

But the very prospect of the trial lectures brought on such "vio-lence" that Dr. Juan José de Aguirre, who was offering himself as a con-tender for the chair, protested to the king that his opponents proposed that no one who could not establish quality and birth in legitimate matrimony could enter the oposición, although he was a graduate and even a professor. He asked that no graduate be excluded either as a voting judge or as an opositor because of origin or birth.[63] The Council of the Indies took the position that graduates and professors could not be excluded from oposiciones on these grounds. It was too late to demand proofs that should have been produced, if they were going to be produced, before the university conferred degrees upon the candidates.[64] The secretaries of American universities from time immemorial, as one of them candidly put it, had simply ceased to demand proof of legitimacy as a prerequisite to registration in universities.[65]

Dr. Aguirre, who was not barred from the oposición because he was illegitimate, won the chair in Lima. Moreover, Viceroy Conde de Croix (1784–89) succeeded Jáuregui on April 3, 1784, and Dr. Iturrizarra at last in the role of supplicant himself, asked that he be allowed to continue as protomédico,[66] though Aguirre had been installed in the chair of prima on December 15, 1784.[67] Viceroy de Croix gave Aguirre title a week after he occupied the chair of prima, and royal confirmation followed.[68]

The protomedicato in Lima, then, had an entirely different organization from that of Mexico. First, the protomédico general was much more independent and sometimes more powerful than the chairman of the tribunal in Mexico. He, and not the viceroy, appointed his two associates permanent examiners and sometimes a supernumerary. He also enjoyed the privilege of appointing lieutenant protomédicos in the principal cities of the viceroyalty of Peru. Moreover, in cases of examination in special subjects such as surgery or pharmacy, he appointed experts from these fields to assist him.[69] In judicial matters he handled cases of first instance with his own legal assistant, but in cases of second instance he sat with a member of the royal audiencia. The viceroy, who had reported these extensions of power, did not mention the two permanent examiners, but these were nevertheless an established part of the protomedicato in Lima. In 1807, for example, Dr. Juan José de Aguirre was operating with a supernumerary,[70] a custom that had overloaded the Mexican protomedicato in the seventeenth century and led to its reorganization in 1646. The practice of appointing supernumeraries, however, was both hoary with age and blessed by the precedent of appointing extra judges to the royal audiencia itself.

In Peru, the protomédico general had the power to name an inspector for his immediate district. As substitute, this man enjoyed the same authority as the protomédico himself. In distant places, if provision were so made in the letter of appointment, he actually conducted examinations, but he remitted the official papers of the examination together with the proper fees to the protomedicato in Lima. If these were in order, the protomedicato issued the license. On a more permanent basis than that of inspector, who might also be itinerant, the protomédico general named lieutenant protomédicos.[71] These, first of all, had a task impossible to fulfill—that of "watching out and preventing people from beginning the practice of any branch of medicine without licenses." The lieutenant had the same authority as the protomédico general himself "to repress quacks [intrusos], conduct examinations in all [medical] faculties, inspect drugstores, prosecute and sentence—subject to review in Lima—in both civil and criminal cases."[72] In fact, when their letters of appointment allowed, three lieutenant protomédicos could set up a tribunal by joining together and naming a fiscal, a clerk, and a porter.[73]

Examinations: The Spanish Model

The prerequisites for examination in medicine that prevailed until the day of Bolívar were determined in Spain, for the most part while the conquest of America was still under way. Though the Spaniards at home took some fundamental steps in the epoch of Ferdinand and Isabella (1477) and Charles V,[74] the most sweeping as well as the most minute regulations came in the time of Philip II (1563, 1588, and 1593). In fact, seven years before the establishment of the protomedicato in Mexico and Peru, the requirements for practicing medicine were specifically established. To be licensed, a man had to study medicine for four full years after the baccalaureate in arts, fulfill all requirements for the bachelor's degree in medicine,[75] serve an apprenticeship of two years under a man who was himself a university graduate and "examined" physician, and finally undergo an examination by the royal protomedicato.[76] The candidate could not receive his bachelor's degree until after he passed this scrutiny, served his two years' apprenticeship, and passed the examination by the protomedicato. Those graduated and licensed outside "these kingdoms" of Spain also had to undergo reexamination.

Philip II appeared to be in a constant state of ferment lest candidates evade some "part" of the law and, especially, substitute one thing for another. Following the Cortes of Córdoba in 1588, he repeated an injunction to this effect.[77] This same suspicion forced a system of accreditation of Spanish universities in medicine. Such suspicion was justified. Some Spanish universities without chairs of medicine—such as Irache, Santo Tomás de Avila, Osma, and others—gave bachelors' degrees in medicine with which students went on to get licenses "to sally forth to cure, without science and without experience. . . ." The remedy was that none but the three principal universities of Salamanca, Alcalá de Henares, and Valladolid, or those with the three required chairs of vísperas, anatomy, and surgery, might give medical degrees in the future.[78] Interestingly, 163 years later an oidor of the royal audiencia in Valencia observed plaintively that as the university had three chairs and Valencia postdated the law, this school should be put in this class with the three "principal ones." Seven medical doctors, or, if there were not that many in the cloister, seven doctors and licentiates, together with the professor of philosophy "who taught physics," examined the candidate and voted to pass or fail him. Then, when the candidate presented himself for examination by the royal protomedicato, he had to present notarized proof that he had graduated, that his university had the required three chairs of medicine, and that his professor taught—or read them—the old masters during his courses.

In that day before experimental techniques, Spaniards wondered why their medicine always stood still or atrophied, and as it was the intellectual vogue to have clean-cut answers, even if they were subtly arrived at, they answered their own puzzlement with the declaration that medicine shriveled up because of the neglect of the old masters and old methods—rote memory, for example. Thus, in 1593 when the king learned that there was "a great shortage of physicians in whom satisfaction can be taken" and that it might come to the point where royalty itself could not avail itself of the best, he added protomédicos (there had been a protomédico and the examiners) and specified more rigorous conditions for examinations. Upon the advice of the Council of Castile, the king determined that the medical faculties of the three principal universities, the protomédicos, and the physicians of the king's bedchamber "(*de cámara, y los de mi casa*)" should render their opinions. The upshot of this high consultation was the considered judgment that the evil sprang from the droning, moribund presentation of medicine in the universities, where time was wasted "in disputes and trifling questions which had to do with neither the understanding of diseases nor their causes, nor their prognosis and cure." In the old days, when there were "great physicians," they used to read the "doctrines" of Hippocrates, Galen, and Avicenna out loud. When the students "raised doubts," the professors "satisfied" them succinctly. Now, on the other hand, they read rancid notebooks from the chair—something that any student who knew Latin could do for himself. Instead, trusting in their notebooks (*cartapacios*), the students did not pay attention, nor did they take the trouble to come to class as they could copy somebody else's notebook.

Another fruit of all this consultation was that the other principal cause of the decadence in medicine or decline in the quality of doctors (*médicos*) lay in the faulty examination of candidates before the proto-médicos. For one thing, as they had to come with Dr. Luis Mercado's *Institutiones*[79] by heart, they spent so much time memorizing these that they neglected other things and ended up forgetting what they had acquired so painfully. Even if they had retained what they once had known by heart, they would not have had enough, for Mercado did not treat "fevers, pulses, purges [*purgas*]," things necessary to know.

The solution hit upon was to issue another "pragmatic sanction" to amend the laws in force. First, of course, the universities would now teach the doctrines of Hippocrates, Galen, and Avicenna "as they did in olden times." The professor would read the text literally for one hour, repeat it once or twice, and then resolve the questions raised by the students "and run from irrelevant questions in order not to spend time for nothing." The last half hour should then be spent in dictating and writing down summaries of what had been read.[80] The penalties clearly indicate the cause of the trouble. The rector would order university bedels to report professors not meeting their classes, and the rector would deduct the corresponding part of his salary for the first offense, double it for the second, and for the third, report him to the Council of Castile so that he might be deprived of his chair and barred from holding others.[81]

The laws of 1588 also required the bachelor of medicine to submit a certificate of two years' practice with a licensed physician "as specified by law" before admission to examination and set out the method of proving that the candidate had undergone this internship.[82] For this purpose the graduate went before the magistrate of the town where he had practiced and established proof through witnesses, one of them the man with whom he had practiced, or, if he were dead, obtain a sworn deposition from a reliable witness.

The appointments and conduct of a medical examination were no trivial matter. In Spain the protomédico convened the three examiners—who had a status comparable to that of second and third protomédicos in New Spain—in his own house or some other place of his choice. The protomédico took the preferred seat, under the canopy when there was one, and signed and voted first; among the examiners seniority determined preference and precedence. The vote of the protomédico was only equal to that of an examiner except that, in the case of a tie, the side of the protomédico was adjudged the winner. Thus assembled and arranged, with all the "laws, pragmatics, and institutions of the tribunal" at hand, the examiners were ready for business. The four of them then examined all the legal instruments, and if they were all in order, the examination proceeded very solemnly and formally.

This examination, fundamentally, was based on a thesis that still holds: that the candidate should have a complete grasp of theory and the literature of medicine and demonstrate clinical competence. The examination was therefore broken into two parts. Under the heading of theory, the examiners, after determining that the candidate had learned by heart the digests of all the remedies currently in vogue,[83] proceeded to put into his hands one of the medical authors he was supposed to know. After 1593 the law exempted the candidate from committing "the institutions" of medicine to memory and stressed the need to vary the questions put from examination to examination.[84] The examiners then ordered the quaking candidate to open up a chosen medical book, state what he found, and elaborate upon the subject. The examiners did not question the candidate for a certain number of hours and then vote to pass or fail, but kept examining him until they were satisfied of his "learning and sufficiency" or until they were sure he was not competent. If he passed, the protomédico set a time for examination in the general hospital or the court hospital and nowhere else. In the hospital the examiners directed him to "take the pulse" of four or five sick people and as many more as they thought proper. In each instance the examiner asked the candidate the nature of the sickness, and whether it was light, dangerous, or mortal. They then inquired into the causes, medicines, and treatment indicated for a cure. After all this, the board of examiners reassembled and the poor candidate, just as if the protomédico and examiners had not accompanied him in the ward, gave account of what he had done. They then either passed him or, if he were salvageable, imposed the necessary additional tasks.[85]

Examinations in America

The display of the medical examination did not match that of the joust in the Middle Ages, but it owed something to the pomp of those days. It took place in the separate room allotted to the royal protomedicato in the Royal Audiencia of Mexico. Under a canopy stood a large table covered with an expensive cloth, neatly arranged and reaching to the floor, on which were "silver ink-wells," quills, a seal for official papers, and a bell that, as is the custom of the Spanish, always did service as a gavel. Three imposing chairs stood at the head, the center one occupied by the protomédico general, with the senior examiner on his right and the junior on his left—all in the attire of office. On the right side was the fiscal's chair. Directly in the front of the presiding protomédico and examiners, on a bench with a back, sat the clerk. When the examination was in medicine, the candidate entered wearing the dress of a Spanish university student (*manteista*) and took his seat on the bench beside the clerk where he was examined on theory by the proto-médico and the other two examiners in order. When they desisted, the candidate withdrew, and the examiners, now turned judges, sealed the fate of the candidate. Taking one of the big brass A's for "approved [*aprobado*]" or R's for "failed [*reprobado*]," they proceeded to vote by placing their letter in the urn provided. If the vote was favorable, the candidate was called back into the room to take the customary oath and then sent to the hospital for an examination in clinical techniques. If certified as competent by the chief physician in the hospital, the proto-medicato issued the license to practice.

The formalities varied with the dignity of the profession involved. The examination of Latin surgeons and pharmacists took place with the same seats, dress, and etiquette as in that of a Latin physician, though it was necessary to call in an expert in pharmacy (*protofarmacéutico*) to assist the tribunal. In the same way, in "minor" examinations the proto-médico general had to appoint experts to assist in the examination of candidates to practice phlebotomy (*protoflebotomiano*), rupture-surgery (*cirujano hernista*), algebra (bonesetting), and midwifery. When exam-ining a romance surgeon or phlebotomist, less rigor prevailed. Whereas the candidates in "major" fields—medicine and Latin surgery—sat down during the examination, those in "minor" ones stood at attention, though they must have felt naked already from their position, exposed and apart as their bench was from the examining table with nothing before it to give them cover from the examining fire. The *"protos"* entered and took their seats on a bench with a back on the left side of the president and opposite the fiscal. After the examiner, the three officials questioned the applicant in order and voted just as they did in the case of medicine, except that this time the "proto" also had a vote.

The Spaniards in America could resist neither the custom nor the temptation to have a celebration at the expense of the fellow reaching an academic crisis such as a doctoral investiture or the passing of an examination for a license before the royal protomedicato. It was there-fore an "inviolable" practice for the successful candidate on the night of the examination to offer the "gratification" of ices and sweets "to make the function staged for his benefit less tedious." At the same time he offered a more concrete "gratification"; he distributed money—four pesos to each permanent examiner, the same to the fiscal, ten to the spe-cial examiner, ten to the clerk, four to the soldier-porter, and "the rest"[86] to the protomédico general.[87]

The all but perennial preoccupation of the Spaniards both at home and in America with the integrity of their academic degrees and pro-fessional licenses gives decisive indication of the size and persistence of the problem itself. Thus, under no circumstances were gifts—big or little—to be received from a man being examined by the protomedicato or engaged in litigation before it on pain of returning the gift with a fourth part going to the treasure chest. At the same time the intervention of persons of power and influence was prohibited.[88] In America, where a salary was set with compensation derived only from fees, there were still other areas of danger. In Havana, for example, some members of the protomedicato in the eighteenth century took it upon themselves to issue licenses "to practice medicine and botany" without the prerequisite examination.[89]

Fees and Salaries

One may puzzle at the hesitation in this country over the setting of fees and prices in the medical professions, but there never was a moment in Spanish history in America when set fees were not taken for granted. To begin with, the law in Spain set fees that the protomedicato might charge a candidate for the practice of medicine, all laid down in details of Philip II's ordinances published in the year of the famous Armada. Not only did these laws set out what the aspiring physician or surgeon must pay for his examination, but they specified the examination fee for those practitioners who treated "cataracts, ring-worm of the scalp or scaled-head [and] carbuncles, for bonesetters, for the surgeon who cared for ruptures [*hernista*], and for those who extracted stones." The applicant paid the fees when admitted to examination without any expectation of getting back the deposit in case of failure. Those who graduated from an *estudio general* (a university that offered degrees in the "major faculties" of theology, law, canon law, and medicine), however, and those who had to take the examination a second time paid nothing, though this provision was later modified.[90]

The ordinance of Philip II, promulgated in 1593, set the practice for charges in all Spanish protomedicatos for a century and a half.[91] As was too often the case, the fees then established[92] remained unchanged until 1740 when, because of the complaints of the protomédicos, the crown at long last made upward adjustments. But, since the salaries of medical officers were still paid from the fees they collected, and though these were raised, in years when there were few candidates to examine the deposits in the money chest of the protomedicato were sometimes still not enough to pay the stipulated salaries—an issue unsatisfactorily resolved by distributing proportionally what was actually in hand.[93]

In America salaries established exactly equaled those in Spain, but as the only source of funds to pay them came from fees—and these did not amount to the salary—the stipulation was superfluous. To the last day of the colonial protomedicato, scrounging for fees, more than the quality of medicine, remained the major preoccupation of medical officers. The protomedicato in America, however, did begin with a provision that should have made the income of the protomedicato flexible enough to support medical examination, inspection, and prosecution. The instructions to Francisco Hernández, for example, made it the duty of the royal audiencia, when there was one, to set the fees levied by the protomédico. When there was no such tribunal, as in Nombre de Dios, the mayor took this responsibility. In places too small to have even this officer, the magistrate assumed this task.[94] As the institution evolved in America, there was extreme rigidity in the charges made by the protomedicato for its services. Not even the religious, who, outside the great cities and sometimes in them, found themselves playing the role of apothecary were exempt. When a man in the habit of a religious order and professing poverty found himself obliged to pay the fees for inspecting his drugs, he was, surely, not a little resentful.[95] When no budget was provided for the salaries of doctors serving civilians, physicians who rushed off under compulsion to cope with epidemics in towns and villages often had a hard time getting their pay,[96] and when they did it required a viceregal order. Moreover, officers did not escape the detested salary tax (*media anata*).[97] The crown, however, was very solicitous, and generally prompt, in providing pay for army doctors and surgeons.[98]

In imitation of Spanish practice institutions like the protomedicato had a way of evolving quietly and reporting vaguely. In 1789, to get information for a report requested by the Council of the Indies, Viceroy Manuel Antonio Flórez (1787–89) got two reports (*informes*) on fees and tariffs in Mexico City—one from the regent of the audiencia and the other from the rector of the university.[99] Typical of the history of the protomedicato is that, though the government had in 1738 ordered that a tariff for all governmental tribunals and departments be drawn up, this compilation, though the lists were ready by 1746, did not appear until 1759.[100] Also, the four pages of the tariff for the royal protomedicato were not available thirty years later.[101] One of the viceroy's investigators, Dr. Francisco Baso Ibáñez, then reported that the fees for an examination of a prospective physician came to sixty pesos, but he could not learn whether the fee for examining barbers and, presumably, all those examined in "minor" branches of medicine, was forty or fifty. The viceroy, however, said he was able "with vigilance" to "satisfy himself" that druggists paid twenty-five pesos for each biennial visit and that the protomedicato exacted one hundred pesos from those they named inspectors. Though there were ten more drugstores paying fees in Mexico City than in Lima, the president of the protomedicato, with a salary of five hundred pesos a year, fell about 280 pesos short of matching that of his counterpart in Lima. Other medical salaries in Mexico were, even for those days, very low. Although a salary of 100,000 maravedís was assigned protomédicos in Mexico, they never did collect it.[102]

The critical fact in the financial history of the protomedicato, and the chief reason for the self-centered approach and weakness of the tribunal in relation to the civil government, was that the protomedicato had no endowment and no salaries. The salary that the protomédico in Lima enjoyed as professor of prima of medicine amounted "with difficulty" to eight hundred pesos in 1789.[103] These conditions forced everybody connected with the tribunal to rely entirely upon fees as compensation, and chiefly from fees exacted from druggists upon the occasion of the biennial inspections. Examinations in medicine even at the end of the eighteenth century were very few, and those of surgeons did not amount to more than three or four a year. At that time in Lima the protomédico staged about twenty inspections of drugstores every biennium, exacting fifty-four pesos each from these. When he had paid the examining pharmacists accompanying him, the fiscal, the clerk, and the porter, the protomédico could retain about thirty pesos for himself. The seventy-peso fee in an examination of an aspiring physician was distributed in the same way, except the assessor and the two examiners got their portion too. The fee charged an Indian was ten pesos less than that charged a white man.[104] The perquisites of the protomedicato then "hardly reach two thousand pesos a year."[105] In all such affairs, fiscal or not, the protomedicato made no attempt to assume power over medical publishing.

Exemptions and Dispensations

As the Spaniards in America ruled more with psychology than with force, they never really faced the problems of military draft and exemptions until the wars of independence (1810–24). In Spain itself, when that great disruption began, 278 years had gone by without any new light on the conscription of doctors in time of war. In the fifteenth century, though, King John II had found it necessary to go beyond "common law" in determining exemption from "going to war" on account of occupation. While excusing various types of government officials and "scribes who show lads how to read and write in the cities . . . ," he also exempted physicians and surgeons, "except when we need them"[106]— a situation very comparable to modern regulations in military draft. Surgeons, especially, might expect to be called when the demand was great. Physicians, apparently, enjoyed the same exemptions and privileges as freemen (*vecinos*),[107] but there was no specific statute to that effect in Spain. Since freemen enjoyed exemption from such onerous things as the lodging of troops in their houses and municipal contributions, inclusion in this class of citizens was a boon to them. Physicians, surgeons, and druggists, however, were excused from all types of royal duties that hindered the practice of their professions.[108] In keeping with this principle, medical men who served with the army had a special call upon the crown when they retired. Félix Chazary, for example, after serving as surgeon of the Mexican garrison regiment, retired at half pay with a prior claim on any vacancy in surgery occurring in any hospital in New Spain.[109] Noting that during the Morelos campaigns, many men died in besieged places—a fate to which military surgeons were uniquely liable— the Cortes of Cádiz decreed that soldiers who died in these besieged places were to be considered "killed in action" for the purposes of military pensions (*montepío militar*).[110] By the time of the wars of independence there was no serious question of exemption for physicians, surgeons, and druggists; only on the margins of the medical professions was clarification necessary.

The protomedicato, however, was too occupied with its mundane affairs and fees to make any concerted effort on behalf of any medical profession except that of the physician. At the time that San Martín was liquidating Spanish military power in Chile, the viceregal government in Lima, virtually cut off from the mother country, found itself so hard put to raise troops that marginal medical men felt the pinch. In consequence, phlebotomists, who had never before had occasion to ask whether they enjoyed exemption as practitioners of medicine, now had need to clarify their standing. In Lima, Luis Ratera, a "master and graduate phlebotomist" with a "public shop" who could hardly scrawl his name, petitioned Protomédico José Pezet for exemption from enrollment in the mulatto battalion (*Batallón de Pardos*).[111] Proceeding almost as if he had authority to grant exemptions, Dr. Pezet certified this one as supported "not only by the statutes [*constituciones*] of our tribunal[112] but by the ordinances of [military] levy." Supported by Dr. Miguel Tafur the very next day, this petition apparently resulted in release from this duty.[113]

Viceregal Intervention and Decline of Standards

No doubt what actually troubled the viceroy was irritation at being crossed in the infractions of university statutes that had become habitual. Though the fact does not often emerge in the minutes of the cloister of the University of Mexico, a year scarcely passed that the viceroy did not excuse some medical student from courses, internship, or other pre-requisites for a medical degree and license to practice. A half century before the Salgado case, the king got word that in the University of Mexico "the number of doctors outshone that of students," and that for this reason the University was "in a sad state and that the complete ruin of so useful an institution springs from the orders of the viceroys in violation of the ratified statutes of the University and of the bulls of His Holiness. . . ." The plaint continued that by special charges and com-mands—*"ruego y encargo"*—to the *maestrescuela,* with two courses, they graduated anybody they chose and made substitutions in chairs for what-ever time they saw fit, exempting the candidates from everything with-out any hope of rectification. So urgently protested by Visitador Palafox y Mendoza, this corrupt practice led the king, just two days after Palafox became viceroy in 1642, to forbid the viceroys in Mexico to make any exemptions whatsoever from courses or to fill chairs, as one was in violation of the rights of the university and the other of the royal pre-rogatives. Every instance of "dispensations" thereafter would be reserved to the Council of the Indies.[114] In 1692, when the criminal judge of the audiencia got the rare assignment of advising the viceroy on exempting a candidate from half his residence (*pasantia*) for the degrees of licen-tiate and doctor in canon law, he displayed an impatience that clearly shows that exemption, though common, was even then distinctly malodor-ous. Though he deviated from what he knew was expected of him, he flatly stated that such "dispensations" would not be made in the best universities of Spain "and should be denied in this one, as its cloister is so crowded with doctors and masters in all faculties."[115] Against such a backdrop Bernardo de Balbuena's famous line that doctors in Mexico were more numerous than "grains of sand in Ganges mighty flow"[116] may appear a little less than a boast.

Overplaying his role as vice-patron and guardian of the university in the course of the second half of the eighteenth century, the viceroy made exemptions in every faculty and with every degree—baccalaureate, licentiate, and doctorate. Occasionally, a candidate for the bachelor's de-gree bothered the highest official in the land simply because he had not known that he had to register. Still another failed to get the required statement from his professors attesting to his having taken this or that course, particularly in another institution.[117] And there were others who found acceptable excuses for exemption from a whole year or even two.

The handling of appeals for exemption from the prerequisites of degrees degenerated into mere ritual. It began with a "memorial" from the student to the viceroy, who passed it along first to the rector and then to the fiscal [*de lo civil*] for their official opinions. The rector, the guardian of the guild privileges of the university, who drew no salary to make him subservient, was nevertheless always malleable. Even fiscals, as able and incorruptible a body of men as ever served the king, invariably advised in favor of the petitioner—generally with the same facts and claims. If nothing else, the fiscal could, and generally did, say to the viceroy that as "vice-patron" and protector of the university he had the power to override its statutes. With the "memorial" back in the viceroy's hands, bolstered by the two opinions attached, the viceroy issued a writ of mandamus (*ruego y encargo*) to the rector and cloister in the case of bachelors' degrees and to the maestrescuela[118] in the case of the licentiate, doctor's, and master's. Running through all this compromising of standards and statutes was the sanctimonious agreement that the student would prove his "sufficiency" in a "rigorous" examination.

Whoever tries to understand the exemptions from the requirements for the licentiate and doctorate must know what the hurdles were.[119] First of all, after getting a bachelor's degree in one of the five faculties a candidate for the next degree, the licentiate, had to pass a certain period of time—generally four years—in residence, performing certain acts and duties but taking no further courses before submitting to a terrifying examination called the "funeral night [*noche fúnebre*]." Because it was largely ceremonial and financial, the doctorate could come immediately after the licentiate. Thus, for all it contributed to the candidate's education, the doctorate itself might have been dispensed with. However, because the ceremonies attendant upon the investiture forced the candidate to pass fees to the members of the cloister, and because of the proud ostentation for the family and entertainment for the public in the "pomp and parades," this degree was as persistent as beggar's lice. Thus, since no one had the effrontery to petition for exemption from examinations, the candidate could seek to escape a part of the time in residence (*pasantía*) for the licentiate and all the extremely expensive "pomp and parades" for the doctorate.

Though instances in medicine were less numerous, perhaps because there were fewer students in the faculty, medical students did win exemptions—all without any comment that medicine was peculiarly unsuited to this relaxation. Even the scrupulous Viceroy Payo Enríquez de Rivera (1673–80) of New Spain, without flurry or to-do, exempted Bachelor Juan Marroquín from ten months of pasantía in the medical faculty.[120] When another student could not finish his courses and graduate in medicine because the professor was cutting his classes, the viceroy interposed to order the professor to appear and discharge his responsibilities.[121] At the beginning of the third of four years required for the degree of bachelor of medicine,[122] Juan Giginio Godíñez returned to his home in Puebla for the Christmas vacations in 1691 and nearly died of small-pox and typhoid (*tabardillo*) fever. He also found himself the sole support of a "widowed mother" and a sister, and without the means to return to the University of Mexico in the capital. He therefore implored the viceroy, on the basis of "notorious precedents," to exempt him from the nine-months of courses and "acts" he lacked. In his advice to the viceroy on this case, the rector of the university cited previous exemptions in medicine. The viceroy made the concession on the usual condition: that the candidate undergo a "rigorous" examination—this time by the royal protomedicato.[123] Francisco Acevedo even petitioned Viceroy Monclova (1686–88) to overlook his failure, because he was out of town or sick, to get his courses confirmed—"to swear them," in the Spanish idiom.[124] To support his case, he fell back upon his "great poverty," his "notorious sufficiency," and two precedents, Dr. Pedro de Villafranca and Dr. Joseph de Campos. The fiscal thought that if the candidate could produce the certificates from the professors, he might be heard—"otherwise what is the use of having universities and professors paid by his majesty?" On this footing, the viceroy acceded to the request.[125]

Various if not devious were the justifications for exemptions. In contrast to an age when the appearance, at least, of the use of influence to gain personal favors is frowned upon, Mexicans in the seventeenth century played this harp proudly. The father of one candidate, exempted from the residence requirements for the licentiate and doctorate in canon law, had been an official (*oficial mayor*) in the Secretariat of Government and War of New Spain for thirty-three years.[126] Another granted the same favor was the son of the reporter (*realtor*) of the royal audiencia with thirty-one years' service and the nephew of a "gentleman of the Order of Calatrava, viceroy of the Canaries, and afterwards counselor of the Council of the Indies."[127] Some students actually invoked "the title of nobility" that, by the statutes of Salamanca and by pontifical decree, permitted exemption from the fourth year of residence.[128] An invariable argument for exemptions was the abundance of precedents. In the field of medicine, because of these "many precedents," five of which he cited, the Count of Galve (1688–96) exempted Bachelor Joseph Díaz from eight months toward the licentiate.[129] The Marqués of Mancera forgave Bachelor Alonso Menéndez, from Havana, a half year's time for the licentiate in canon law on the ground that the viceroys "used to exempt" those who came "great distances."[130] Later the Count of Galve excused Bachelor Matías Joseph González Maya from all except a year and a half of his four years of residence for the licentiate in canon law and six months' internship before taking the bar examinations because he had to accompany Bishop García de Legaspi y Velasco to Nueva Viscaya—a distance making it impossible for him to graduate.[131] And, by Salamancan precedent, it was legal to overlook all requirements remaining when a man won a proprietary chair so that he could immediately take the doctor's degree—itself a prerequisite.[132]

The viceroys could and did cite the precedents of their predecessors.[133] Since the precedent of exemption from residence time thus fed upon itself, the longer the violation went on the more normal it became. Some candidates for all classes of degrees claimed that the traveling imposed unbearable hardships. One of these, Joseph Monzón, a candidate for the degree of bachelor of arts, won exemption for a whole course (year) because, as a native of poverty-stricken "St. Augustine in Florida," he could no longer bear the high cost of living in Mexico City.[134]

As in nearly all American administration, where there was a good human reason for an exception, and sometimes when there was not, the viceroys never quite ceased to suspend the requirements for academic degrees—not even in medicine. On the other hand, it was in keeping with the best tradition of the Spaniards in America that they were inclined to bend the law in the cases of poverty and sickness, especially in the case of candidates from overseas outposts such as Florida and Cuba who did not have the means to sustain themselves in Mexico City. Even the protomedicato, which, be it noted, had something to lose in fees, and that hard-biting "mouthpiece" of the king, the crown attorney, were known to develop soft hearts. Viceroy Sarmiento de Valladares (1697–1701) exempted Bachelor Marcos Antonio de Gamboa from four months' internship. In addition to everything else, the good bachelor needed to return to his native Havana to "sustain a poor family." In recommending favorable action the protomedicato cited just "precedents in the archives," and the fiscal thought that testimony of the royal protomedicato on his excellent qualifications was still necessary. That the candidate's academic mentor was well known in medicine and influential as well did not hurt Gamboa's case. Typically, though he had petitioned for exemption from eight months' internship when Viceroy Sarmiento de Valladares (Count of Moctezuma) intervened, only half of that time remained to be overlooked.[135]

The Licentiate Nicolás Altamirano y Castilla, because he was "sickly" and it was Lent, won a viceregal exemption from "pomp and parades" when the maestrescuela, that watchdog of higher degrees in the colonial universities, recommended it.[136] Though it is difficult to see how exemption from the expense of "pomp and parades" had any adverse effect upon a candidate's medical knowledge, it is barely short of a miracle that those who stood to collect fees at the investiture accepted the idea of dispensation of requirements for the doctor's degree. Nevertheless, Licentiate Ignacio Calderón, quick on the heels of Gamboa Alta-mirano, got a similar concession from the Count of Moctezuma when he alleged "poverty, sickness, and precedents." Having gone blind, how-ever, he was unable to take advantage of it, but when the maestrescuela concurred, the archbishop-viceroy renewed the exemption.[137] In view of the Salamancan precedent allowing a waiver of all requirements when a man obtained a permanent chair[138] and because of the doctor's degree needed for that chair, the exemptions granted are not too surprising.

At a time when some professors did not get more than a hundred pesos a year and nobody got more than seven hundred, numbers of candidates sought to escape the costs of "pomp and parades," which, when combined with the fees to the cloister, could amount to 15,000–16,000 pesos and never be less than two hundred. Whatever involved money, however, was a much touchier matter than what involved time. Never-theless, the viceroy did intrude into university affairs to exempt an oc-casional candidate from staging the "pomp and parades." In consequence, within weeks of getting exemption from residence time, the candidate professing to be poor and unfortunate, and probably was both, made an appeal for exemption from ceremonial costs and sometimes got it.[139]

Much risk is involved in the assumption that the viceroys who granted such "dispensations" to students were corrupt. In fact, the names that stand out in the seventeenth century—the Duke of Albuquerque (1653–60), the Marquis of Mancera, the Count of Monclova, and the Count of Galve—could stand the test of vigilance, uprightness, and competence better than most. Instead of reflecting corruption and mal-feasance, these exemptions, more likely than not, indicated a certain im-patience with the rigidity of the "eternalized" statutes and, possibly, the decadence of the university itself. After all, the university cloister itself, after calling for "volunteers," exempted Joseph de Herrera y Regil from his time as pasante and from the costs and trouble of the "pomp and parades" when, as a donation for the king, he put up 1,600 pesos that, otherwise, the cloister itself would have needed to raise.[140] This gift was enough to pay the professor of surgery for sixteen years. Such trafficking in degrees to avoid expense to the cloister was a common resort.

Encouraged by the ease with which the civil authorities had illegally exempted candidates from the prerequisites for degrees, students also found ways to exempt themselves from courses.[141] The statutes of the university[142] required the student at the end of the academic year to pre-sent a certificate from his professor that he had had the course. However, the professor became lax, and the secretary of the university began to accept solely the deposition of two fellow students, "most of the time just as trifling as he is. . . ." To meet the requirement that the student submit his own written record of the lectures bearing his own initials (*rúbrica*), he merely presented somebody else's notes. Such a practice enabled a student to get credit for a course "even though he has not attended class a single day. . . ." When the cloister voted in 1742[143] to require all professors to state in their certificates that the students' papers were of the exact material presented and that "John Doe" had heard the entire course, some professors opposed this simple revitalization. The rector then had to appeal to the king to approve what the cloister had resolved and, if necessary, to give him the authority to compel all involved to comply with the statute. The royal government acceded to the petition and set up a fifty-peso fine for the secretary who should accept documents improperly drawn up; it also enjoined the professors to adapt themselves to the statute and not only to make out the certificates but to make them out "without alteration or addition. . . ."[144]

Thus, the cédula of 1642, for all the effect it had, might as well have invited the dispensations it forbade. Yet, because a more "senior" academic degree was more valuable, the holders of legitimate degrees, especially of licentiate and doctor, writhed at the prospect of a man whose academic obligations and requirements had been waived actually taking precedence over them and entering the oposiciones for chairs. The matter reached the crisis stage again in 1695 when the Dominican Maestro Fray Diego de la Maza complained to the Council of the Indies that, all laws to the contrary,[145] the viceroy had not only waived requirements for many licentiates and doctorates, but had also exempted many students from the course requirements for the bachelor's, many of them "not with the consent of the cloister, but freely and arbitrarily in gravest prejudice of legitimate graduates. . . ." In a sharp reaction the king ordered the viceroy to follow the laws exactly and to make no exemptions without first reporting the circumstances. At the same time he enjoined the cloister not to accept such dispensations. The penalty was loss of professorship or any other academic post for any employee of the university who should admit such dispensations. If he had no post in the university, he thus disqualified himself for entrance into any trial lecture in an oposición for a chair. The new law, as a fitting climax, nullified all these dispensations made by the viceroys.[146]

At the same time that the viceroy was "arbitrarily" making dispensations from the requirements for academic degrees, the viceregal government was also intruding upon the selection of professors. The same indefatigable Fray Diego de la Maza, who had provoked the cédula forbidding exemptions from degree requirements with certified documents, had also sharply drawn the king's attention to the "political" handling of the trial lectures, or competitions for chairs. When the rectors and councilors of the university, after a vacancy, had actually gazetted a competition to take place in a period of time specified in the statutes and, with the expiration of the specified time,[147] had actually closed the entrances, the audiencia had accepted appeals and extended the time to allow favored candidates to enter the contest. And, said the complaint, as the "opositores enjoy enough favor to reopen the contest, they also have enough to win the chairs" to the exclusion of those entering the oposición legally. The Council of the Indies accepted the arrangement and demanded full compliance with the law, allowing only the postponement of the deadline for two days, provided there was unanimous agreement among all opositores. All chairs won after the deadline set by the university according to statute would be invalid as well as all those already won after the illegal extension of the time limit by the audiencia.[148] Despite all these solemn orders and decrees, however, the king, beset by pleas from the university, interposed his authority time after time.[149] At last, in 1739, the royal government repeated every cédula on the subject of dispensation except the first one and enjoined the royal audiencia of Mexico to enforce them. Moreover, it canceled all bachelor's degrees that depended upon exemptions from courses,[150] though those students who had received their degrees with exemptions prior to the date of the cédula might retain their seniority.[151] This perennial problem, of course, affected all faculties—not just medicine.

The tribunal of the protomedicato was adamantly against exemptions from prerequisites for medical diplomas in those cases where the dispensation meant that the protomédicos could not collect their fees— the only pay for their official duties. José Fulgencio de Araujo, six months short of the legal requirement of two years' practice with a licensed physician, appealed to the viceroy for exemption from this half year. He wanted "to cure publicly"—tacit acknowledgement that he was already in practice. His excuse is representative: he was in debt, his father was old and worn out, his sister sick, and all his kinsmen were "in the greatest misery." Besides, the royal protomedicato had entrusted him with the 554 inoculations on the haciendas of Pate, Camalco, Cerillo, Majadas, and Solís during the last smallpox epidemic of 1797. Of the 554 inoculated, he said, "only three perished." When asked for the university's position, the rector of the university responded that, counting the time from the end of the candidate's last course, two years had elapsed. When the protomedicato, unaware of this technicality, interposed no objection, the viceroy granted the exemption.[152]

Even more striking than exempting a student from time in the university was the persistent danger of dispensing the statute that, after finishing all requirements for the degree of bachelor of medicine, he

spend two years as an apprentice of an "examined" and licensed physician. The laws of Castile, specifically extended to America, forbade universities or protomédicos to exempt candidates from any part of this two
years' practice.[153] To practice surgery, the same laws required that a man
should have four years' practice with a physician or surgeon graduated
from a university and himself duly licensed.[154] The two-year requirement,
however, applied only to university men. Since candidates in other medical professions, except occasionally in surgery, underwent no training at
all except as apprentices, it was very dangerous to exempt them from the
time prescribed. In 1688 Viceroy Monclova, however, exempted Jerónimo
Díaz from a one-year internship in surgery and bonesetting when he
represented that he had actually practiced.[155] As all the medical laws in
the next decade indicate, the royal protomedicato had been improperly
bypassed.

The same compulsion that led the viceroy to breach the statutes by
exempting students from requirements for degrees led him to fill academic chairs that were legally obtainable only through oposiciones duly
conducted by the university. In New Spain Viceroy Luis Enríquez de
Guzmán (1650–53), in disregard of the protest of the maestrescuela,
in 1651 went so far as to give the temporal[156] chair of vísperas of medicine for life to Joseph de Prado, merely because the holders of proprietary
or lifetime chairs lived forever (*por eternizarse*) and left no opportunity
for others to advance. The only arguments in Prado's favor were that he
had befriended poor students, that he had contended for the chair of
prima of medicine on two occasions, and that this chair was proprietary
in Salamanca.[157] After 1653 the Duke of Albuquerque appointed the
professors of prima of medicine and thereby automatically controlled
the presidency of the royal protomedicato.[158]

Seven years later, when they protested that the delay was retarding
their education, the students and pasantes won the right to select the
professor of vísperas of medicine "by vote," but since all doctors and
licentiates in medicine in the city also had a right to vote,[159] Viceroy
Mancera named Dr. Juan Manuel de Sotomayor, oidor of the royal audiencia, "to regularize" the procedure.[160] He simply appointed Juan Germán
Quiroz to the chair of surgery and anatomy when the incumbent "went
up" to the chair of vísperas of medicine.[161] So customary was appeal to
the viceroy in academic appointments that Dr. Juan de Brizuela, professor of vísperas of medicine, appealed to Viceroy the Count of Galve
in 1694 to give him this temporal (four-year) chair for life. He had
served twenty years—the minimum time for retirement with pay—in
different chairs and represented that this service entitled him to be made
proprietary professor of vísperas. Far from objecting to his irregularity,

the university cited precedent, showing that the Marquis of Mancera had granted proprietary privileges in this chair on two occasions. The Count of Galve acceded to Brizuela's petition[162] on condition that the university consult the king who, in turn, approved this lifetime arrangement[163] but did not make the chair a proprietary one for future holders.

The Protomedicato and the Wars of Independence

The protomedicato in the peninsula was so often abolished, disunited, reunited, and reestablished that it is not easy to fathom the reasons for these vicissitudes in Spain, much less understand their effects upon the tribunals in America. Thus, on July 22, 1811, the cortes suddenly "reestablished" the tribunal del protomedicato in Spain as a supreme tribunal of public health and simultaneously invalidated all the powers of those corporations holding interim authority. The jurisdiction of the reestablished body, however, extended "to the whole peninsula and adjacent islands," with its residence ordinarily at court. As another example of the strange oscillations in the late history of the tribunal, the cortes decreed that, once again, the faculties and obligations of the body would be those prescribed for it in the laws of Castile before 1780, "when its attributes began to vary with grave damage to the public good." This time, the personnel of the tribunal would consist of five faculty members (*facultativos*) of "established probity, patriotism, learning, and experience," but with the condition that there be two in medicine, two in surgery, and one in chemistry—all on an absolutely equal footing, except that the senior man, counting from the date of his appointment, would preside at meetings. As was natural in those days of nearly impossible financing, the cortes limited the salary of each to 12,000 reales annually. It demanded that as soon as the Council of Regency named its members, the new tribunal should submit the rules of its internal organization to the cortes, emphasizing economic factors in the vain hope that there might be a surplus to revert to the "general treasury." In each epoch of debate, reform, and counter-reform, the cortes proposed that the new five-man tribunal immediately propose to the cortes "all the plans, reforms, and improvements" necessary in the teaching of all the "diverse branches of the art of healing and in their auxiliary sciences, . . . the establishment and direction of hospitals, especially military hospitals. . . ."[164] It was the first time, apparently, that the obvious union between the protomedicato and hospitals had so plainly surfaced, perhaps caused by a crescendo of murmuring by wounded soldiers suffering in a time of prolonged war. Even before this cédula was dispatched to New Spain, the cortes enlarged the membership of the tribunal from five to seven in order to include two pharmacists. Thus was corrected a patent error that should have been ferreted out in the first place, for the proto-médicos, at least in America, held on tenaciously to their right to examine pharmacists and surgeons.[165]

But this legislation—legislation that should have been critical to America—went out belatedly to the viceroy of New Spain, merely "for his information."[166] With a war raging, the viceroy, even if he had had the authority, was not likely to follow this example in New Spain. More-over, if he had been so disposed, the protomédicos—frozen to their not very lucrative fees and alert to their dignity as members of a high tri-bunal—would have fought such action, just as they actually did far less serious infringements upon their jurisdiction and their precious "prece-dence." The news of this step—among the many drastic and sometimes ill-considered ones taken by the Cortes of Cádiz—had just had time to circulate freely when in 1814 the *Gazeta de Madrid* announced that the protomedicato "stood abolished." In its stead, the cortes created juntas of surgery, medicine, and pharmacy to examine its own practitioners, con-duct its own inspections, and try its own malefactors.[167]

This news from Spain did little more than sow confusion in Mexico. Half a dozen pharmacists, headed by the botanist Vicente Cervantes, "supposing" the tribunal del protomedicato "suppressed," made an effort to get the inspection of the empty drugstores out of the hands of the protomédicos, who were so blithely ignorant of chemistry and botany, and never had enough interest to master these subjects, and had to depend upon a commissioned druggist to collect their inspection fees. The peti-tion is shot through with so many assumptions concerning "suppression" of the protomedicato that it leaves one believing that the apothecaries thought it necessary to persuade the authorities that the tribunal actually had been abolished.[168] In fact, there does not appear to have been any more specific extension of the new law abolishing the protomedicato to America than there had been in 1811 when it was "reestablished."[169] In fact, in 1815 Dr. García Jove treated the very royal audiencia as if its powers were no more dignified or firm than those of the royal proto-medicato. When in 1820 the crown decided to reestablish the tribunal in Spain—in exactly the same language used for the same purpose in 1811—it was to be "composed of the same" seven individuals who com-posed it in 1814. And the new creation was confined to "all the peninsula and islands adjacent."[170] After the reestablishment of the Constitution of 1812, however, with the colonies ordered to observe this fundamental law once again, the viceroys had to abolish or modify all tribunals in ac-cordance with it. In July 1821, though, the Peruvian protomedicato, still holding on, had the vitality to take the oath to support the declaration of independence.[171]

The old protomedicatos in America, with their long-established usages and vested interests, simply took the route of inertia when the tribunal was abolished in Spain. Before their enemies could force the issue, the protomédicos waved in their faces the recent news that the tribunal at home was restored. Although a tribunal in process of establishment was more likely to suffer, Miguel Gorman, who became provisional protomédico of Buenos Aires three years before this process of abolition,[172] proved as adept at survival in Buenos Aires as was "Doctor and Master" García Jove in Mexico.

Problems of Jurisdiction

I F THE MORTAL feud between the judicial tribunals in the Spanish empire had been a disease, as it very nearly was, it would have been endemic. Two conflicting conceptions of the administration of justice had been allowed long historical development, and by the eighteenth century were everywhere in collision. Medieval privileges allowed many guilds to assume jurisdiction over their internal conflicts and, short of "drawing of blood and mutilation of member," over the criminal offenses of their members as well. Moreover, none of the jurisdictional acts of the tribunal of the royal protomedicato admitted of appeal to the Royal Council except in the case of the rejection of proof of blood purity (*información de limpieza*) from an applicant to practice medicine, pharmacy, or surgery.[1] On the other hand, the ideal of absolute royal authority in all spheres came into full flower in the sixteenth century. From then until the end of the colonial period the professional courts waged a remorseless verbal and legal war to retain their privileges and exemptions against the growing power of the state. In the New World, where the very earth was the king's personal property, the crown did not have to uproot deeply intrenched corporate privileges. In fact, these were allowed only for the convenience of the government. Thus, with the increased emphasis on regalism that marked the time of Charles III (1759–88), the royal patience with any kind of guild justice grew very thin.

The Laws of the Protomedicato

The want of a set of statutes then common to all governmental agencies and professional corporations was very damaging to the right of the medical profession to control its own affairs. One of the first steps in the history of a new university, for example, was to get a draft of these precious statutes or "constitutions" approved by royal cédula and papal bull. Despite this practice, the royal protomedicato in America never had a set of statutes to go by. The viceroy of New Spain had to order that the protomedicato itself should draw up the by-laws of its own internal functioning.[2] At the end of the eighteenth century Dr. Vicente Sonogastua y Carranza thought that the protomedicato in Guatemala should have statutes based upon those of Castile. Instead, he wrote, they applied the Mexican statutes in the mistaken belief that the Mexicans had such laws published.[3] As late as 1815 the legal adviser (*juez en turno*) of the royal protomedicato in New Spain demanded that protomédicos, who were contesting his jurisdiction, know what their "ordinances" were. The implication in this supercilious request was that any corporation fit to demand rights would have its own statutes. When the chief protomédico replied that it was the compilation by Eugenio Muñoz published in Spain sixty-four years before, the judge replied that he had never heard of it— an utterly astounding admission for a Spanish judge. A good way to make a point, this admission means something more. A prolonged search in the records of Spanish colonial medical history has turned up only two references to the Muñoz work. One of these—in 1758—referred to the author as "a so-and-so [*un tal fulano*]" Muñoz,[4] and in this case Dr. García Jove of the Mexican protomedicato apparently did not have a copy, or else he would have produced it. The only other tenable hypothesis is that Dr. García Jove was afraid that, if he did, the judge could see for himself that the compilation was drawn up for the protomedicatos in the peninsula.[5]

Insofar as they were affected by the laws, protomédicos in America had to turn to the general compilation of the Indies, which, because the laws were few and the editor confused, simply did not cover the innumerable contingencies arising. Thereafter, they could resort to the slightly fuller compilation of the laws of Castile, from which they had been drawn in the first place, but always with the uneasy sense that nobody would agree that the law was applicable in America except as an arguable but convenient hypothesis.

Territorial Jurisdiction

In the early stages the protomedicato in Spain might not exercise authority beyond five leagues from the city in which it had its seat. If after 1539 it conducted or sponsored examinations outside this circle, the local justices had authority to arrest the examiners and send them to the court jail for punishment.[6] Historically, this limitation on jurisdiction, apparently, sprang from the inclination of the protomédicos to extend their reach for money so far as to pass candidates in remote areas merely for the fees collected.[7]

Incredible though it seems, the viceregal authorities in New Spain still did not know in 1791 whether the royal protomedicato had jurisdiction throughout the whole kingdom or was limited to the city and the district within five leagues surrounding it. At that time Viceroy Revilla Gigedo (1789–94) wrote the king, in a plaintive if not a despairing mood. He had in hand an "overblown file [*cumuloso expediente*]," which, because of its want of system and clarity, was almost impossible to reduce to any kind of summary.[8] The problem of jurisdiction treated in the file, in fact, sprang from another: the right of the protomedicato to sentence a doctor for administering lethal drugs.

In this case the Bachelor Miguel Mariano Rojano, an examined and licensed physician in Puebla, found himself in dire straits when the druggist, José Francisco Cruzado, noticed that his prescriptions were reckless and dangerous. Supported by his fellow druggists, he sounded the alarm. This was followed by a consultation—an academy—of doctors. The druggists, thus fortified, refused to fill Rojano's prescriptions and notified the royal protomedicato in Mexico City, sending eighteen prescriptions to prove their charge—tacit proof that the druggists at least acknowledged the authority of that distant body. Thereupon, the royal protomedicato wrote Rojano, asking him "in soft words" to modify his practices or, in case of a recurrence, to expect punishment.

As was natural, the culprit sought to avoid correction by appealing to the Superior Government. Advising the viceroy with an ineptitude rare for a crown attorney, the fiscal cited, among others, a law[9] drawn up in 1570 for the guidance of a "protomédico general" to show that the jurisdiction of the tribunal in 1791 extended for five leagues beyond the city "but no more." He was, however, orthodox enough to suggest that the viceroy ask the protomedicato for its opinion—a defense it was bound to be. That body easily showed[10] that the law of 1646—only one page removed from the one the fiscal relied on—extended the jurisdiction of the tribunal not only to Veracruz and Puebla but also to "all the rest embraced under the name New Spain."[11] Such a law, they said, far from conflicting with the earlier law, only amplified it. Besides, under the authority of this law, they had often asked for and received the exequatur of the viceroy. However, as the fiscal professed that he did not know whether this extension authorized the tribunal to do anything but inspect drugstores, a notary clerk, in a review of its papers, proved that the protomedicato had prosecuted purely medical offenders. For example, in 1724 it had fined Nicolás Ruiz de Calera 6,000 maravedís and forbidden him to practice either medicine or surgery because he had given a girl a purgative from which she died.[12]

Any fiscal in the Indies who found grounds for extending the jurisdiction of the crown, viceroy, and audiencia at the expense of the "privileged justice" of such guilds and corporations as the royal protomedicato could normally expect approval in Spain. In this case, nevertheless, the fiscal of the Council of the Indies held the appeal to the Superior Government illegal and slashed the opinion of Fiscal Posada in Mexico for not recognizing the obvious: that the law of 1646 extending the jurisdiction of the protomedicato to Puebla amplified and, where indicated, took precedence over prior laws when the two were in conflict.[13] Thus the king notified both the viceroy and the royal protomedicato that the laws of the Indies (Libro V, Título VI) left no doubt that the protomedicato had jurisdiction and ordered both of them to see that the laws were carried out.[14]

Other clashes of jurisdiction arose because of uncertainty about whether protomedicatos in areas that were politically dependent upon the viceregal government had to operate through the royal protomedicato in the seat of the viceroyalty. The protomedicato in Santiago de Chile, "seven hundred leagues" from Lima, thus felt terribly abused. A principal complaint was that the protomédicos could not, for example, "extirpate" the curanderos, as they were required to do by the fundamental law, because they faced reversal by the tribunal in Lima.[15] Moreover, they faced a reduction in their pride if not in their fees—both of which had a profound hold upon them. The creation of a university with enough faculties to include medicine was a good point at which to break off from the tribunal in the capital, because the first professor of medicine was automatically the chief protomédico. Thus, when the University of San Felipe got under way in Chile during the mid-eighteenth century, the time was ripe for the professor of prima of medicine not only to claim the post of chief protomédico but to break off from the authority of the tribunal in Lima. Then in 1786 a royal cédula of July 22, 1786, made the Chilean protomedicato independent of that of Lima and annexed it to the chair of prima of medicine in the university. For some years, though, Dr. José Antonio de los Ríos, the protomédico, had to put the coat of arms of the tribunal of the protomedicato of Lima on all the certificates and licenses that he issued to physicians, surgeons, bleeders, and apothecaries. The Audiencia of Santiago, however, ruled that instead of putting the royal arms and, around an ornamental border, the words "The Royal Protomedicato of Lima," Dr. Ríos might put "Real Protomedicato del Reino de Chile." These titles, of course, had first to be issued on stamped paper (*papel sellado*) for purposes of the royal revenues.[16]

Subdelegaciones

The tendency throughout the Indies, if the distance was great enough, was to create protomedicatos independent of each other. However, precedent had developed for centralization in Spain, where subdelegations (*subdelegaciones*) in Valencia and La Coruña were dependent upon the royal protomedicato in Madrid. Stimulated, perhaps, by the radical changes that had been made to increase the centralization and efficiency of government in America, the tribunal of the protomedicato in Madrid proposed that, as in the case of Valencia, the crown set up medical subdelegations in Mexico, Lima, Santa Fe de Bogotá, Buenos Aires, and other places and even offered to draw up the plans. The preface to this piece was a devastating condemnation of the state of medicine in the Indies. There, it coldly stated, the public health of the "Americans" was generally in the hands of "charlatans, mulattoes," and other "most inept" fellows. The conduct of the "professors," whom "greed more than capacity" lured to those dominions, was intolerable, as repeated suits and reports proved. In an iconoclastic mood, the Madrid tribunal just as openly charged that this evil sprang principally from the bad teaching of medicine in American universities. The crowning defeat, as the Madrid protomédicos saw it, was that the "three tribunales" in America were independent of the Castile body and should accordingly be put under it and reorganized. Still others might be created if necessary. The chief argument in favor of this innovation was that Ferdinand and Isabella had decreed that the protomedicato of Castile should also be the protomedicato in all the "kingdoms and seignories" that "then were or ever should be" under the crown of Castile. This paper had the earmarks of a legal document prepared by overconfident doctors. Still the private property of the king, America was not "incorporated" as a part of Spain. Moreover, as a note to this report made clear, the law of Ferdinand and Isabella referred to had been nullified by the creation of protomedicatos in America independent of that of Castile.[17] Thus, the king did not agree to the proposal.[18]

Jurisdiction Over Examinations

Highly centralized medical control was, of course, subject to the same and sometimes more drastic criticism than concentration of civil power in the viceregal capital. Even before the middle of the eighteenth century, in the time of Philip V (1700–1746), the royal protomedicato in Madrid underlined the force of this argument by proposing to delegate the examination of aspiring physicians to "the most accredited physicians of the provinces and cities," too far from the court to permit all acceptable candidates to appear in person. In fact, the argument ran, experience had taught that not only the "distance from court" but "the shortness of means" and "attacks" of illness that "others" underwent often made a trip to the capital altogether impossible. Of course, candidates appearing before the proposed "subtribunals" would have to present the same certificates of baptism, legal proof of blood purity, internship (*pasantia*), and academic degrees, and "the proper deposit." The royal government in Madrid then agreed (1741) to permit the royal protomedicato to delegate its jurisdiction, if its laws and formalities were rigorously observed. It even agreed to allow the delegation the right to try medical cases, but required the provincial judges to remit the sentences to the protomedicato in Madrid for final determination.[19]

By the last decade of the eighteenth century the protomédicos in Mexico City were at long last in possession of the medical laws of Spain, which showed that examinations there might be delegated to physicians in distant cities.[20] The Mexican tribunal, accordingly, asked the king for the same privileges.[21] The Mexican protomédicos, however, brought it out into the open that some with the proper qualifications had to practice without a license while many "whose insufficiency made them unworthy of approval" practiced with equal legality. The Council of the Indies had no objections, though it accepted the recommendation of the fiscal of New Spain to ask for the opinion of the royal protomedicato in the Spanish court.[22] The petition apparently never finished the circle it started.

Away from the capitals where there were tribunals of a protomedicato, practices developed that invariably led the ambitious local doctor either to assume or to secure the position of protomédico. If no one objected and some governor could be induced to make a vague appointment, a man might spend an entire life enjoying the prestige and even collecting the fees and emoluments attached to this office. When, however, such men, grown confident in their isolated freedom from competition, went to the crown for greater leverage to pry out money or to secure another miserable sinecure, they ran the great risk of being reminded of the jurisdiction of some remote tribunal. In 1714 Bachelor Juan José López, by gubernatorial appointment, fell heir to the place of protomédico of Portobelo and physician to the garrisons there. When, however, he tried to get the crown to send him a diploma not only confirming him in this post but also specifying that, as the law stipulated, he might inspect drugstores and regulate the price of drugs, he was asking for a review of his pretensions. He lessened his chances of success by asking that the surgeon of infantry be Spanish (that is, white) and be examined and approved by him. Because of his work attending the sick in the Presidio de San Jerónimo and those who came on his majesty's ships, he asked for "two simple posts" in the fortresses there.

This request for means to live "respectably [*con decencia*]" only led to a study of his case. The Council of the Indies advised the crown that

López's father, Miguel, had served for thirty years and that, with the salaries of his various posts, and one real a day from every soldier, he had actually made more than a thousand pesos a year—twice as much, be it said, as that enjoyed by university professors in the capital cities. The most that the crown attorney could sanction and the Council recommend, then, was that—most unlikely—if the Bachelor Juan José López, "poor man [*pobre*]," was approved by the protomedicato of Lima, he might go on enjoying his post and emoluments but might not have the two posts requested nor the title of protomédico he sought. He might inspect drugs and regulate prices, when these were excessive, but only by agreement with the tribunal in Lima. With respect to the request that the surgeon should be Spanish and not a foreigner and that he, López, might conduct the examination, the Council of the Indies felt that if the incumbent had been duly examined and approved by a tribunal of the protomedicato, he should not be interfered with.[23] That his education had ever gone beyond apprenticeship under his father, however, made it doubtful that he would ever make the arduous trip to stand at attention before the protomedicato. Yet others bolder than he were to come. The Caribbean area was highly suited to their plucking.

One day in 1760, for example, Francisco Ventivoglio de la Case, setting himself up as a graduate in medicine from the University of Anjou, prima professor from the University of Quito, and protomédico géneral of Panama and all the province of Tierra Firme, confidently and on his own authority "gazetted" an edict calling upon all the druggists of the city of Panama to stand ready to lay out their stocks for his inspection. The need was more than ripe. Twenty or thirty years had passed since any apothecary of that town had felt the fear of a visitor with an ominous tipstaff standing by their doors to announce to the gawking passersby that the apothecary's training, his honesty, and his goods were in the balance. When, one by one, he had probed, questioned, and listened in all the shops of the white druggists, Ventivoglio turned to those run by black druggists, some he observed "are perhaps not even druggists." Just then, Pharmacist Manuel Maitin, who had been in the country "taking some baths," returned to the city and reacted as if a catastrophe impended. Perhaps it did, for he had not been paying the rather heavy inspection fees that could have fallen upon him every two years, and, perchance, his shop had "spoiled" drugs or, even more likely, lacked half the drugs required by an unbribed inspector.

Maitin's nervous and, in the circumstances, curiously arrogant petition to Antonio Guill y Gonzaga, governor of Panama (1758–61), challenged Ventivoglio's jurisdiction.[24] The protomédico was not of that class called "general," as those in the viceregal capital. Otherwise only viceroys, presidents, and governors could order visits, set the time for them, and order spoiled and inert medicines thrown out. Thus, according to challenger Maitin, Ventivoglio had no authorization from the governor because he was a lieutenant protomédico and not of that "general class" authorized to make inspections on their own authority. Moreover, as the inspector had worked alone, and not accompanied by the governor, corregidor, mayor, or, for want of these, by the chief magistrate, everything he had done was null and void. Governor Guill ordered the inspections suspended and turned the petition over to his assessor and asked Dr. Ventivoglio to state his case.[25] Within three days, that outraged disciple of Hippocrates made an informed if interested rejoinder.[26]

Ventivoglio began by expounding his view of the types of protomédicos existing in the Indies. The first of these were inspectors (*visitadores*) bearing the title protomédicos generales, named by the king alone and dispatched upon rare occasions.[27] The laws did require these visitadores—he was good enough to admit—when they made inspections more than five leagues away from town to go accompanied by the governor, corregidor, or magistrate in order to pass sentences. In practice, this stipulation had been disregarded. In the second category were the protomédicos generales resident in the capitals of the chief kingdoms and provinces and appointed by the viceroys and governors. In the third were the lieutenants designated by these protomédicos generales of the second class. The men of this third type, resident in the little towns that were not seats of government, were subject to the jurisdiction of the protomédicos generales under the terms set out by a recent royal decree of April 19, 1741, in Aranjuez. His illustrations of such appointments in Peru, Cuba, and Panama were prolix; he even showed that his predecessors had their own lieutenants in such towns as Portobelo.

Ventivoglio's claim to being a protomédico general of the second class rested upon some fairly solid ground. He was not among those in the first class, for he had not been named by the king and did not have jurisdiction over protomédicos who were "judges and alcaldes mayores." Moreover, he had not only enjoyed the appointment of the local governor, but he had a title from Viceroy José de Solís Folch (1753–61)[28] for which, he never dreamed of mentioning, he had been obliged to pay fifty pesos. Ventivoglio denied being a lieutenant of the protomedicato in Lima, as his accuser had said he was; he owed his place to appointment by the governor and then by the viceroy. His motive in this stance was plain: he wanted the independence enjoyed by the class of protomédicos he claimed to be in.

Though he would argue, if necessary, that lieutenant protomédicos might inspect drugstores by "delegated" authority, he spent his main effort on the contention that protomédicos of his type had such authority. For this purpose he paraded the *"primeras ordenanzas"* of Castile[29] that commanded the protomédicos to inspect drugstores in person. Beyond five leagues it was necessary for corregidores, magistrates, and two aldermen and an "approved physician" of the place involved to make the inspection—and that only because in those days they did not have lieutenant protomédicos. Moreover, the laws of the Indies, he insisted, required the American protomédicos of his class to obey the "royal laws" governing the inspection of drugstores.[30] Ventivoglio did admit, though, that the laws entitled viceroys, presidents, and governors to have drugs inspected in their districts when they thought necessary. He denied the contention of his accuser that there was any law requiring the protomédico making an inspection to accept any "accompaniment" beyond the necessary clerk and professional druggist examiner.

Ventivoglio took the position that his diploma entitled him to conduct the inspections without being accompanied by any person save these two humble functionaries. His title from the viceroy gave him jurisdiction as set out in the laws of Castile for protomédicos of his class. No tribunal might dispute this power, and much less "this druggist, if he is one." So, did the viceroy in Bogotá have the right to issue his title? If the governor had made such appointments, how could the same power be denied the viceroy in the new viceroyalty? With the governor's appointment and no confirmation from the viceroy, his predecessors had exercised the right to name lieutenant protomédicos, a fact that made him writhe at the druggist's trick of calling him "interim lieutenant." Ventivoglio even insisted that, on the grounds that the position of chief protomédico was annexed to the chair of medicine as in Lima, he could qualify because he was the professor of medicine in Quito.

Two weeks after "rendering" his report, Ventivoglio was still awaiting a resolution of the case from the governor. In a most impolitic way the angry protomédico petitioned the governor to reach a decision, telling him that his decision was damaging to the public health and an indignity to the protomedicato. Moreover, his mission was terminated just after he had inspected the drugstores of the whites and was about to inspect those of the Negroes—"who are perhaps not druggists." Was this not enough to suggest, he told the governor in his teeth, that he favored the blacks and was hostile to him?[31]

But Ventivoglio's case was not altogether bereft of friends. Bartolomé Pinto de Rivera, the city attorney, remarked in his report to the governor that Ventivoglio's "laudable" effort was at least a start at the inspection the laws demanded. He too was aware that the drugstores had not been inspected for many years. In fact, he himself had requested the

Superior Government "the year before last" to get such inspection under way, to see to it that the drugs dispensed were not inert, and to guarantee the assortment required by law. He thought it a pity that such a beneficial step should be held up because of a dispute over whether the protomédico should institute these inspections or whether they should be undertaken at the instance of the Superior Government, there being no doubt that viceroys and governors had the legal authority to do this.[32] The governor thus accepted his advice to issue such a decree,[33] but after Ventivoglio had asked for a permit to go on managing the inspection himself, the governor elaborated his instruction by confirming the inspections already made, though the rest would have to be done in the company of the magistrate Mateo de Izaguirre. There was even more of a sting in the governor's final requirement that Ventivoglio should neither post nor put into effect any legal papers without first allowing him to review them. The governor put enough stock in Manuel Maitin's charge that Ventivoglio had it in for him to ask the alcalde to accompany the protomédico to his shop.[34]

These do not seem harsh or unbearable conditions, even if this protomédico had the power to undertake them on his own authority and without the company of any governmental functionary. Yet so great was the need to keep face in the Spanish colonies, and so pressing the need for fees in the many posts where salaries were not paid, that Ventivoglio refused to begin the inspections and declared his intention of appealing to the viceroy.[35]

At this impasse, the frustrated Ventivoglio could get no lawyer with the temerity to draw up his papers or a scribe to notarize them. When he did it himself, these "writings" were adjudged legally faulty and the appeal rejected at its source. Copies of documents that he needed to go before the viceroy no notary would dare prepare for him. Any supporting documentation that he might send, he admitted, was "furtively" copied. So he fired off a series of letters to the viceroy that were revealing if not legally drawn up.[36]

These letters had the cunning design of convincing the viceroy that it was his authority, not the person of Ventivoglio, that was being outraged. On every hand the scheme to frustrate his mission was visible. He was not allowed to function as protomédico nor assume his post as médico at the hospital. Everybody said in the streets that he would not be accepted for these posts even if "orders to that effect should come from Your Excellency," the viceroy. Instead, it was bruited about that the government in Panama would do as it pleased and report to the king with the assertion that the appointment of Ventivoglio had been accomplished as an unfortunate act. Rumor also had it that "Your Excellency has stuck your hand into the naming of the protomédico" here.[37] Pups, Ventivoglio reminded the viceroy, often bit and savaged the walking stick parrying them because they could not get to the man carrying it. The curanderos, therefore, "made a mockery" of his authority, for "wherever there were two charlatans yesterday there are now twelve or fifteen who pass me every day in the streets with disdain and with a smile." Indeed, there was no "miserable barber" not called "doctor." Even the suspension of his inspection, he said, was a part of a plot to prove that the viceroy would not help him but, instead, leave him at the mercy of the Superior Government.

Ventivoglio had very concrete ideas about how to counter the sinister moves foiling him at every turn. First, he needed a soldier to accompany him for the "honor" of it—a satisfaction that other protomédicos in Panama had enjoyed and that, in Quito, he had too, "without the need for one that I have here." They had even accepted the half year's salary as physician of the hospital without allowing him to assume the post—a clear case of fraud.

For all these troubles, Ventivoglio blamed the governor's assessor, Jerónimo Macías de Sandoval. Without his bad advice, the governor would never have accepted Maitin's "writing" and that would have been the end of it. Because the "governor was influenced by his assessor who blindly patronizes the colored curanderos," these and self-licensed druggists triumph, "taking lives and laughing at my authority"—authority flowing from "the most excellent" viceroys themselves. He wanted, first, a new appointment, but, now "disposed to give up medicine for the moment," he besought the new viceroy to name him to any government post falling "vacant in Portobelo, Cartagena, or in any place in Your Excellency's viceroyalty." While it was natural for Ventivoglio to think of giving up medicine—"briefly"—as the want of records from this point indicates, the issue of jurisdiction remained unresolved.

Role of the Royal Audiencia

Professions and guilds in the Spanish world had their own courts, but in America, at least, they operated under the close scrutiny of some agency of the civil government representing the royal person alone. Selected by the viceroy and rotated every year, one civil judge of the royal audiencia always sat with the tribunal of the royal protomedicato.[38] Yet at the beginning of the nineteenth century, when the practice was already hoary, a quarrel was still raging between the protomédicos and this "accompanying" judge over their respective functions and, hard as it is to believe, over still unsettled questions of etiquette.

The crown, of course, had long been moving to dampen ardor and restrict the jurisdiction of such special tribunals, but in Peru Viceroy de Croix stated unequivocally in 1789 that, among his obligations, the protomédico in Lima, not the audiencia, had exclusive jurisdiction over physicians, surgeons, and bleeders for the crimes committed in the exercise of their professions.[39] By 1800 the question should have been settled. In fact, when the royal protomedicato of Mexico was prosecuting him in 1792 as a curandero intruso, Dr. Narciso Alemán appealed to the criminal *sala* of the audiencia where a dispute arose as to whether the case was appealable.[40] Viceroy Revilla Gigedo, as arbiter, ruled in favor of the audiencia, but the viceroy, the Marqués de Branciforte (1794–98), later put the question to the Council of the Indies, which clearly took the position that the law plainly required the protomédico "to be accompanied" by a judge, and not the physicians on the board, who legally sentenced. Otherwise, citizens in the Indies, where access to the person of the king was not possible, might suffer "in their property, in their honor, and in their lives" without ever being heard by a tribunal representing the person of the king. The royal government had already upheld the view that practicing without a license fell within the jurisdiction of the royal audiencia and was not a medical issue (*"caso o cosa de medicina"*).[41] Now, in a decision that did little to allay feeling, or even to clarify the matter, the crown broadcast in a printed cédula that in all preliminary procedures "of those that precede admission to examinations," litigants should present their appeals to viceroys, presidents, and independent governors to the end that, by consultative vote of the audiencia, they might be decided.[42] And, in contentious suits concerning excesses committed by medical men in the practice of their professions, they should appeal to the criminal section of the same audiencias.[43] The meaning of the Alemán case of 1798, then, was that judgment of the protomedicato was an advisory opinion—an expert one, to be sure—but merely advisory nonetheless. If it had not been that so many cédulas fell stillborn only to be dropped again and again, one might wonder why the exact authority of the juez en turno should ever have been questioned after 1798. Yet questioned it was to the dawn of independence.

In 1805, for example, the matter had reached one of its periodic boiling points. Going to the house of the senior protomédico to sit with the protomedicato when it had meetings outraged the pride of the judges and violated the spirit of the Alemán cédula.[44] So, when Viceroy José de Iturrigaray y Aróstegui (1803–8) appointed the oidor Ciriaco González Carvajal as juez en turno of the protomedicato, he told the judges of the audiencia that "it was not fitting" that the juez en turno should go on meeting days to the house of the chief protomédico.

Thus, after 1798, it was not a question of the jurisdiction of the audiencia but of the indignity of a judge in the highest tribunal—and the one representing the king's sovereignty—having to attend an official meeting in a private house where the head of another tribunal presided. The physical setup that would have met the ceremonial demands would have been a salon in the viceregal palace—a kind of Canossa for the protomedicato. Wanting such a place in the royal palace, Iturrigaray ordered the dosel[45] and other symbolic adornments moved to the house of the juez en turno and commanded that the meetings be held there and that the protomédicos, as experts only, attend "in accordance with the sovereign dispositions in the matter." He also agreed to rebuke the protomédico Dr. García Jove for the terms in which he said that the juez should consult the tribunal of the protomedicato, in the case of the penalty assessed against Buenaventura Godall for illicit practice of medicine.[46]

That González Carvajal was behind the move to shear the prerogatives of the protomedicato is shown by the vigorous moves that followed his appointment. First, he prepared a peremptory summons to Dr. García Jove and his colleagues, ordering them to convene "tomorrow afternoon" at four in "this house," bearing an inventory of the "ornaments and utensils" of the protomedicato. The meeting would take up "pending matters," especially the incorporation of Dr. Buenaventura Godall. When the notary delivered the summons—imagine the indignity of this!—he found Dr. García Jove and his colleagues, Dr. Vicuña y Mendoza and Dr. Eguía y Muro, waiting for him. They told the notary they would come but that they protested his "despoiling" their legal privileges and exemptions.[47] Six weeks later, saying that Dr. García Jove had disregarded the first summons, González Carvajal had the notary serve still another upon the proud and irascible but shrewd protomédico.[48] The fiscal advised the viceroy that not only were the protomédicos forbidden by the cédula of 1798 to "sentence" in "contentious suits," but also they might not "sentence" at all unless accompanied by the oidor named for that purpose. The assessor went beyond this opinion to say that the royal protomedicato was wrong even in doubting the spirit of their superiors.[49] Meanwhile, Dr. García Jove had not complied with either summons. When, in the middle of March 1806, Judge González Carvajal issued still another decree ordering García Jove to obey without reply or excuse, that stubborn man explained that he had not obeyed because his "uninterrupted occupations" had not permitted him to do so.[50] The strategy of the chief protomédico worked; González Carvajal's terms expired, and the protomedicato had not had to budge a centimeter.

A full nine years later, another conscientious juez en turno, Manuel del Campo y Rivas, complained that García Jove had not complied with the 1806 decree ordering removal of the canopy and ornaments of the protomedicato to the house of the tribunal's juez en turno. It astonished him also that the royal protomedicato had no intention of putting itself in accord with anything he did. Worse yet was the injury the rotating judges suffered because the tribunal still sat in Dr. García Jove's private house. Since Campo did not want the meetings in his private house, which could explain why nothing was done after the time of González Carvajal, he asked the viceroy to provide a small room in the viceregal palace in imitation of that provided for other tribunals. Yet this was not done and—worse injury—the tribunal went on blithely meeting in Dr. García Jove's house,[51] and the viceroy still disregarded the old plea to provide suitable neutral quarters, probably because he had none to provide.

When García Jove felt Campo's new pressure, he meekly conceded that the protomedicato should comply with the cédula of 1798 but maintained that the cédula showed plainly the intent of the Council of the Indies that in the cases heard by virtue of their profession they could pass valid sentence when the oidor appointed to sit with them was present. Plainly, he went on, Campo's assumption of jurisdiction in the case of the curandera Manuela Morgado had deprived the protomédicos of the jurisdiction they had by virtue of their office (*de oficio*).[52]

In response to such overtures, Campo challenged García Jove to supply him with an "authorized copy" of the regulations or ordinances under which his tribunal functioned.[53] The chief protomédico then named—so inexplicitly as to suggest that he himself did not have a copy—the compilation made by "Señor Muñoz in a printed volume." To these he added the various laws in the title of protomédicos in the laws of the Indies and variations contained in cédulas issued by the crown from time to time.[54] Campo admitted that he "had no notice" of the Muñoz work, but even supposing that it conformed to the laws of Spain and the Indies and knowing that the "protomedicato had no special ordinances," the judge felt quite capable of substantiating his own position. He was clearly irked that García Jove "supposed" the protomedicato "despoiled" of its authority, preeminence, and judicial faculties by the rotating judge.

The basic disagreement between the judge and the medical members of the protomedicato was over the manner of legally drawing up a case and then of the method of rendering the judgment on it. Oidor Campo felt he was entrapped when García Jove sent him two petitions or complaints requesting him to meet with the protomedicato to pass sentence and to submit this opinion in the matter. The tacit basis of this request was that Campo alone, as juez en turno, did not have the authority to process and dispose of any medical case—not even in the "contentious" category. Yet that was precisely what Campo was accused of doing in the case of Rafaela Morgado, indicted as a curandera. Though, Campo said, this was not the first time the protomedicato had complained of being "despoiled" of its faculties, it was, on the contrary, the "judge-assessor who had been deprived of his prerogatives by the protomedicato."

The only new thing was the sinister charge that Campo wished to prepare medical cases and make the final disposition of them without taking the protomedicato into account. The answer lay in an analysis of the case against Rafaela Morgado as a curandera. Campo simply could not understand what was dangerous when, in the eight months or so he had been juez en turno, this was the only case that had arisen. The charge against Rafaela was the "supposition" that she illegally practiced medicine by treating Joaquín Felpi. At the insistence of García Jove, the woman had been arrested by the constable, and her case turned over to Campo to dispose as he saw fit. So, "why complain?"

At any rate, Campo continued, the complaint was groundless; he had neither sentenced the woman nor put her at large. It was the royal ministers who, in the form of a tribunal, made inspection of jails who had turned her loose for want of just motive for holding her.[55] They had found that the patient Felpi testified that José Pérez had treated him, not Rafaela, but because he was a bachelor, she had nursed him. The evidence is clear, as this irritated lawyer was very ready to emphasize, that the indictment did not contain acceptable preliminary information to justify the long stay in jail already suffered "by this unhappy woman." With such sloppy preparation of an indictment, any parent, servant, or charitable person willing to turn a hand at nursing a sick person could end up in jail. Campo could not leave the point without asserting that one case would not be considered adequate business for any other Mexican tribunal. Most of all, though he had not taken the action in this case, he was not the prosecuting attorney but judge and president of the protomedicato in contentious cases and also in the informative ones that required an assessor's opinion. Thus, anything done in a serious matter without consulting him not only did violence to his authority but was null and void besides.

Even the old bone of bringing the canopy of the royal protomedicato to the house of the juez en turno was dug up and gnawed again. Campo reminded García Jove that he not only had been rebuked by Viceroy Iturrigaray for the "manner and terms" he used in suspending Buenaventura Godall but also had been ordered to send the canopy and adornments to the house of the oidor, where the protomédicos would come only as experts (*péritos*) to act in accordance with the "sovereign dispositions in the matter." Despite the repeated commands (1806–15), this order had not been complied with. Though the last thing Campo wanted was to have the physical apparatus of the protomedicato dumped in his private house, he resented, after he had made every conciliatory effort, the refusal of the protomédicos to join him in overtures to the viceroy for a suitable place in the palace. Since this behavior indicated that the protomedicato wished to reduce the juez en turno to a mere assessor, Campo told García Jove that he could not meet with his tribunal until he had delivered the canopy to his house. To go to the house of the protomedicato would make the judge a party to this disobedience and anger his colleagues.

Campo weakened a very cogent document by arguing his case from peninsular law and precedent. In Spain over fifteen years many innovations in regulation of the medical professions had taken place that were almost unheard of in America. His statement that the punishment of "medical offenders" was the function of the civil officers of the crown left only public health matters to the protomedicato, which despite early hopes, had always lacked the authority and financing to endure as a public health agency. Protomédicos, of course, had administrative functions and were responsible for the licensing of men in the medical professions, but otherwise they might serve only as experts or consultants to the government as was done in other arts and sciences. Campo followed with a barrage of citations from peninsular law that the civil justices had jurisdiction in medical offenses and that the medical board or protomedicato could only come to the crown in case the civil judges dissembled or failed to punish practitioners as intrusos.[56] Campo sought to close the gap in his argument by stating that the laws of the Indies and those of the Peninsula declared that the royal laws of Spain pertaining to protomédicos should be obeyed in America.[57] Besides, the laws in America were explicit on the point that the royal judges took cognizance in trying and punishing those venturing to practice without a license.[58] In this case the protomedicato did not even obey the Superior Government's declaration. After this long if not prolix argument,[59] the harried judge broke out: "You have no idea of the work this answer has cost me!" Unique confession! Here was an able Spanish official extremely annoyed at having to go to the trouble of composing such a long document by García Jove's adroit inaction. While the two stood on their dignity, quarreling over whose house they would meet in, José María Morelos, the second and greatest of the Mexican revolutionary leaders, awaited his doom. Could it be that the viceregal government was loath to close with a recalcitrant chief protomédico because its prestige was declining or because more important things than where a canopy should be hung engrossed its thoughts?

Blaming his delay upon his information, the contentious García Jove rejoined in an elevated fury that interlaced wrath with argument for forty-eight pages.[60] The Alemán cédula of 1798, he said, was so clear, so final, and so decisive that to dispute it was to dispute that the sun shines. Trust, this was not the first time he had litigated nor would it be the last, for he would elevate his suits to the very throne if necessary. And it did seem, when he had finished, that the medical laws of the Indies needed clarification if not codification. One by one the chief protomédico put the complexion of his own views on the high points of his antagonist's argument. He did, he said, send the Morgado case to Campo so that he "could set out what he thought justice called for," but this was no ground for Campo's assuming the role of "the only and absolute judge" in "scorn of the actual protomédicos" whose duty it was in company with his excellency to pass sentences according to the Alemán cédula of 1798 that established joint authority over such cases. So, instead of getting the case returned to pass sentence, the protomedicato had to stand aside and see the prisoner released. Though Campo now disclaimed this act and said that the royal visitation took the step, had he not told Dr. Luis Montaña that he had the right to do it? If no other case had gone to the judge, it was not because the protomédicos sentenced without him but because there had been no other "contentious" case. As "I am gentleman, . . . you should take my word for that." In all other matters the protomédicos needed to check out only with their assessor.

As there was no copy of the *Novísima recopilación* (1805–7) in Mexico—strange revelation!—he could only ask whether it was applicable to the Indies. Though Manuel del Campo had cited one law of the Indies to prove this claim,[61] Dr. García Jove cited another to prove that royal laws were not applicable in the Indies unless there was a specific cédula ordering "that they be observed in those provinces."[62] Patently, the authors of either law, so casually drawn and so forcefully cited, could not have foreseen their application to the contingency of 1815.

Above all, García Jove was resolved not to budge that precious canopy—the symbol of authority now hanging in his own house for sixteen years. His explanations were of a more expedient tenor. González Carvajal had not wanted it in his house. Though the protomédicos were willing to send it to his house and have it returned whenever a "contentious" case arose, such a course involved such high costs that the protomédicos went there many times without these symbols. "Why do you think, then, it was my arrogance?" To shift the canopy and adornments now would "be costly and damaging." Though García Jove could cite the law to show that the tribunal should meet in his house or at some other place of his selection, he countered the charge that he rejected all peaceful proposals. He claimed to have gone to the palace to look for a place to hear "contentious" cases and professed his willingness to go anywhere else, even to move the precious fittings on those occasions, but to leave it in his house at all other times. The enraged chief protomédico also refused to give ground on the contention that his tribunal was composed of mere experts and could not pass sentence. The tribunal had always sentenced, and, besides, the Alemán cédula of 1798 only forbade its passing sentence when not accompanied by the juez en turno. Accompanied, it could pass sentence.[63]

Yet as the oidor was not likely to overlook, the viceroy and the audiencia had ordered the furnishing and canopy transferred to González Carvajal's house in 1805. When appealed to the next year, the Superior Government had maintained this decision. González Carvajal had even ordered the transfer made within five days, "without reply" yet "you excused yourself on the ground that you were too busy." In conclusion, Campo made it clear that his statement to Dr. Montaña that he had turned Rafaela Morgado loose did not mean that this had not been done in agreement with the proper legal officials and Fiscal Oces. Campo concluded by saying that the method of the protomedicato in substantiating its cases was not in keeping with the practice in the merchant and mining guilds and other tribunals.[64]

At long last, ten years after the impasse was reached, the viceroy summarily ordered the dosel and other furnishings transferred either to the probate court rooms or the criminal court in the viceregal palace.[65] García Jove, in an effort to counter the juez en turno, had written the viceroy of his willingness to transfer to a room in the palace.[66] Now he was caught. And the sudden cessation in this interminable wrangling indicates that he acquiesced.

Other Jurisdictional Problems

The process of weakening the professional tribunals, begun in the time of Charles III, reached a peak with the Constitution of 1812. During all this time, however, no one seemed to know for sure whether the laws enacted for this purpose in Spain were applicable in America. The Constitution of 1812 was most certainly formulated for both the kingdoms of Spain and those of America. Yet so great was the distance between Spain and America, political events in both worlds shifted too fast for the measured thread of putting new legislation in force. Three or four major changes in the tribunals regulating the medical professions in Spain were made and discarded before their advocates could get them applied to America. A law governing appeals from the sentences "given in the last instance" by special tribunals was enacted in 1812 and put in force in America by a decree of the cortes.[67] At the same time class cases involving jurisdiction in America drew out endlessly with only an occasional vague reference to the "law of tribunals." Apparently the glee that the enemies of the protomedicato got from the prospect of the overhauling of such tribunals turned sour when the old tribunals, after a moment's suspended animation, came back to life in the old form—just a little more decrepit, dyspeptic, and ineffective than before.

When read by a layman, Spanish law seems quite explicit on jurisdiction. In the first place, any plaintiff had to demand justice before someone who had authority to compel the attendance of a person summoned. Any outsider challenging a doctor in a medical case would expect to prove his charges before the protomedicato;[68] or, as another example, anyone seeking redress from a student might expect to make his case before the rector of the university.

There is nothing here, however, that covers the complaint of one protomédico against the other in the conduct of their business. When three members of the tribunal of the protomedicato in Mexico City in 1688 undertook an examination in the Hospital del Espiritu Santo, the second protomédico, Dr. Félix Vela del Castillo, refused to go on with the examination. The law, he said, was that they examine four or five patients, and there was only one in the hospital. Thereupon, the first and third protomédicos ordered him to join them in this task on pain of a 200-peso fine. Claiming that the jurisdiction of "each was equal," Dr. Vela del Castillo appealed to the viceroy to keep the other two within their limits. The viceroy's assessor advised him that the cédula of 1646 making the first professor of medicine the president of the protomedicato did not give him the authority to proceed against other members. The presiding officer's vote thus had no greater weight than the other two, but, as president, he could determine whether the tribunal was in agreement. And, in case they were quarreling, he could have recourse to the viceroy, who could ask the protomedicato to defer to the laws of Castile governing protomédicos. As for the recalcitrant protomédico, the viceroy might inform Dr. Vela del Castillo that he should participate in the examinations, because examinations and inspections were of such seriousness as not to admit delay. As for all three members, there was nothing to do but urge them in strong language to live in peace and concord on the supposition—a natural one for a Spaniard—that there were "laws governing the style, custom, and form" of the protomedicato. The viceroy, the Count of Monclova, accepted this advice in detail.[69] Years later the viceroy, the Conde de Galve, added that the full protomedicato should examine the documents and decide whether Dr. Vela del Castillo had been right.[70]

Though the royal protomedicato in America had been enjoined in the reign of Charles II (1665–1700) to go by the laws of Spain in examinations, inspections of drugstores, and everything else,[71] Mexican protomédicos soon found that the viceroy had inserted himself, by taking cognizance and carrying on judicial processes in matters in which the protomedicato had jurisdiction, even admitting challenges of the competence of the medical judges. By Spanish law, those sentenced by the protomedicato for practicing without a license might appeal to the Council of Castile, but no one else might appeal at all for any reason, including criminal violence. Thus, it was not hard for the Council of the Indies to reach a decision. The king ordered the protomedicato in Mexico City to follow—for "all the provinces of New Spain"—the style, practice, usage, and custom of "these" kingdoms. Specifically, he forbade the viceroy and audiencia of Mexico to take cognizance or proceed in cases involving examinations or inspections of drugstores and, in fact, allowed only this: that the audiencia might hear the appeals of those sentenced by the protomedicato for practicing without a license "in case the sentence might be unjust or if there should be some particular defect in legal matters," as the audiencia "knew not a single thing about medicine."[72]

The laws of Castile forbidding any appeal from a decision of the protomedicato except before that tribunal itself were not likely to pass unchallenged in the growing regalism of the first half-century of the Bourbon dynasty. The tendency of the regular courts to assume jurisdiction, especially in areas where there was no protomedicato, was a natural one. Sometimes, too, the protomedicato behaved in a way that, if not whimsical, was at least a departure from correct legal procedure. For example, in Spain the royal protomedicato refused to examine Manuel de Castro, a physician who had practiced successfully for twenty-six years in the town of Mondonedo, because of some unproven private quibbling about his bachelor's degree, his internship, and his purity of blood. Though he was able to establish legally that he had lost the papers establishing these points through a fire in 1713, the protomédicos and their confederates remained so inveterately hostile as to suggest personal rivalry as a motive. The victim of this adamant stand appealed, and the Council of Castile duly ruled that the protomedicato give Castro an examination.

Thereupon, the protomedicato asked the crown to enforce the law requiring all appeals from the decisions of the protomedicato to be heard before that tribunal itself. At the same time it petitioned to be excused from obeying the decision while the case was pending and even asked that the Council of Castile be required to return the papers of all indictments pending before it or already decided that related to the medical professions. Instead, the council advised the king to order the royal protomedicato to examine the unjustly "oppressed and afflicted" Castro without "the slightest delay," to turn down the appeal of the protomedicato for the delivery of all medical cases to it, and to see to it that the "established practice" for cognizance in such cases be followed. Thus, in the legal process, the council did advise overriding the protomedicato, though it did not pretend to pass on the qualifications of "those who licensed physicians, nor on the methods of curing diseases, nor on whether the doctors had erred or not in the treatment of some patients and diseases, which is the forte of the protomedicato, and in which very little punishment is meted out, though many tragic occurrences painful to see are undergone every day because of the inexpertness of licensed doctors, as other scientists proclaim."[73]

Intrusions of Civil Governors

On the face of the law the royal protomedicato not only heard all medical cases but all appeals from its own decisions; still the final judge of conflicts was the colonial official who really determined jurisdiction in close matters or contested cases. In fact, a viceroy or governor found infinite ways to control both the personnel and the decisions of the tribunal. For example, when the first protomédico of Havana refused to seat the second and third after they had been appointed by Governor Juan Manuel Cagigal (1781–82), the governor charged him with stubbornness and pride, and threw him into the castle prison "where he remains until he purges himself of his contumacy."[74]

A civil governor simply had the power, at least until checkmated by the Council of the Indies, to deal with medical men without reference to the royal protomedicato, especially if these practitioners, departing from their specialties, were witless enough to criticize his administration or to stir up trouble. When the Cuban surgeon José Rodríguez had the bad judgment to read a letter in the presence of three persons only—stating that the new tax of 3 percent on fincas had been paid by only two or three subjects—he brought down on himself a wrath that he should have expected from a governor who was a Knight of the Order of Malta. In his confrontation with the governor, he heard himself addressed as a "rogue [pícaro]," "false witness," and, until the clamor of the public came to his rescue, found himself barred from practice. The Council of the Indies took no worse view of this offense than that Rodríguez was indiscreet, yet, without complaint from the protomédicos, Rodríguez had had his license taken up by the civil government as punishment for a nonmedical offense.[75]

A little while later the surgeon Andrés Fons, in collusion with a ship's mate, smuggled over 3,300 pesos from Veracruz to Havana. Thereupon, the intendant of Havana confiscated the money, sentenced Fons to two years in prison, and dispatched him with the fleet to Seville. When the case came up for review in Madrid, the Council of the Indies decided that the long imprisonment Fons had already endured was sufficient punishment and ordered him "put at liberty immediately."[76] This, too, did not fall within the purview of the royal protomedicato.

A governor might intrude upon the medical profession, or upon the protomedicato itself, but he dare not intrude upon the royal authority in doing so. In 1682 the governor of Venezuela took a rebuke, more suited for a lackey than for a Knight of the Order of St. James, when he ventured to appoint Bernardo Francisco Marín protomédico "without either jurisdiction or authority" to do so. Though his "supposed" motive in making the appointment was to drive unprepared and unlicensed persons out of the practice of medicine, the governor soon learned that the only way he could remedy this situation was to punish those who practiced without examination and licenses.[77]

Infringements on the Protomedicato by the Government in Spain

The royal protomedicato in Madrid also attempted to intrude upon the jurisdiction of the protomedicato in America. In 1778 the fiscal of that body asked the king to give him exequatur to its appointment of Cristóbal Tamariz, a physician of Veracruz, to examine the licenses of physicians, surgeons, and druggists going from Spain to America and seize all those that might be false, suspected, or illegitimate. However, when this request was submitted to the Council of the Indies for its approval (*despacho auxiliatorio*), it ran afoul of insignificant clerical procedures. When it did reach the fiscal for his opinion, that official reminded the overeager protomédicos of Madrid that the tribunals in Mexico and Lima enjoyed all the privileges, honors, and faculties of the protomedicato of Castile.[78] In that case, of course, the request for an exequatur involved "a notoriously excessive usurpation" of jurisdiction. The fiscal even thought that the council should inform the protomedicato in Mexico of its reasons for refusing to enable Dr. Tamariz to carry out his assignment.[79] The council agreed in every particular.[80]

Appeals to Spain for preference in the medical professions in America were, it is natural to suppose, mere efforts to gain what an appeal to American tribunals would have rejected out of hand because, for one thing, they would have understood American law better. In 1790, for example, the Council of the Indies received an appeal from Mariano Aznares, a Spanish physician living in Mexico, asking to be named lieutenant protomédico of the army in New Spain, with the same powers as the protomédico of the army in Spain itself.[81] Though Aznares had a medical degree from the University of Zaragoza and could show an extensive record in Spanish military hospitals,[82] the Council of the Indies turned him down because he did not establish that the new post was needed, though it did approve authorizing Viceroy Revilla Gigedo to determine whether such an appointment would prejudice anyone else and to ask for the opinion of the protomedicato in Mexico City.[83] Such a disposition, in all likelihood, meant the end of Aznares's scheme.

Manipulating the Chair of Prima of Medicine

Since the first professor of medicine automatically became the presiding officer of the protomedicato, an adroit manipulation of his election in the university had a bearing upon the management of the medical professions. In 1776, when the protomédico in Chile died, two aspirants came forward for the oposición. The first of these, the friar of the Order of San Juan de Dios, Dr. Pedro Manuel Chaparro, of well-known nobility and of "proven service to the public and his profession," challenged the other, the Bachelor D. José Antonio de los Ríos, "son of unknown parents, and without the least practice in his profession," to establish his legitimacy. In addition, he requested that the theologians not be excluded from the voting. The rector, however, disregarded this petition, and with the support of the president of the audiencia, qualified the voters, and in a proceeding that might have been drawn out into months, conducted the oposición, voting de los Ríos possession of the chair—all within the forty hours' time. Even "the hours of the night" and a Sunday were used as if they were regular work hours in Chile.[84] When Chaparro appealed to the audiencia, the president ruled that this was a matter "of government" and thus a matter of his jurisdiction alone. While the fiscal wasted five or six days on matters calling for less than an hour, and while clerks and notaries very efficiently mislaid papers, the president "ordered perpetual silence." The audiencia, not wishing a frontal conflict with the president, resignedly acquiesced, but, realizing that the rules of legal procedure were being violated, began to dispatch papers to Spain in bundles.

In Spain the fiscal of the Council of the Indies[85] could not have thought such precipitation possible had the documents from Chile not proved it. Nor could he believe that the urgent demands of public health and the efficacy of medicine justified ramrodding the selection of this professor of medicine. Though the audiencia might bow to the president to avoid quarrels, his imposition of "perpetual silence" on the oidores was not permissible. A royal cédula thus sweepingly disapproved everything done in this oposición and ordered a restaging of the trial lectures according to law. The president in Santiago, however, did not execute the cédula, asserting that it was obtained by "obreption and subreption [*obrección y subrección*]." Outraged at the legal irregularities, the fiscal of the Council of the Indies could find no evidence of such "vices" and advised the council to approve repeating the first cédula. As the president had disregarded specific laws—laws that his foes were quick to cite—this case illustrates the old device of "obeying but not executing" as well as another means of taking the management of medicine out of the hands of medical men.[86]

Even the university, in some cases, might exercise jurisdiction over the president of the protomedicato. In 1697 in Mexico a man to stir up such trouble thrust himself forward: Dr. Antonio Jiménez, professor of prima of medicine in the University of Mexico and first protomédico, had an obsession, aggravated by a quick and terrible temper, to hold his doctor's degree up to scorn. For such reasons the irascible doctor had found himself bidden adieu in Antequera and Michoacán. Then in Mexico City he dumbfounded the cloister of the Royal and Pontifical University with a series of slights to its dignity and high sense of protocol: he refused to march with the cloister in the reception of the viceroy the Count of Moctezuma. At another time, in a full cloister meeting at the university when asked for a monetary contribution, he replied that he would give fifty pesos as Francisco Jiménez, but as a doctor only "two bits."[87] Again, when he went to join the university cloister at the ceremonies of doctoral investiture in the cathedral choir, the master of ceremonies asked him to give way so that a more senior doctor of the faculty might take his rightful place. Thereupon, he rushed down the aisle, screaming and shouting as he tore off and flung away his hood (*borla*) and other insignia. A murder could scarcely have caused more outrage to this decorous if not pompous body than did this amazing act—so foreign was it to the solemn dignity that marked all ceremonial in the Spanish colonies. With the moral support of the full cloister, the rector responded with a 100-peso fine and two months' exclusion from university employment.

Dr. Jiménez, however, was physician to the tribunal of the Inquisition and sharp enough to take advantage of it. Instead of accepting the jurisdiction of the university, he claimed immunity because of his capacity as physician to the Inquisition. That tribunal even summoned the secretary of the university before it for a full report, an arrogant step which suggested that it had authority over the rector and cloister. Then, without reaching any decision, the Holy Tribunal asked the rector of the university not to execute the sentence, and, surprisingly, to this irregular overture, he acquiesced. Meanwhile, Dr. Juan de Brizuela petitioned the cloister to make him "judge of the protomedicato," a post automatically lost to Jiménez with his chair. Without the benefit of any law or precedent, the cloister approved him as substitute.

After more than a year the university got off a letter to the king stressing the scene in the cathedral choir. The Council of the Indies was outraged both at the rector for making no effort to defend his jurisdiction and at Dr. Jiménez for fostering conflict. The fruit of this imbroglio was a royal order to the rector of the University of Mexico to warn Dr. Jiménez not to obstruct jurisdiction. Even the audiencia received instructions to summon and warn Dr. Jiménez that if these excesses and disturbances continued, the audiencia would use its "political and economic faculty" to send him back to Spain.[88]

The Surgeons Challenge the Protomedicato

Though the protomedicato in Spain was divided into three separate tribunals in 1780—medicine, surgery, and pharmacy—the Council of the Indies did not transfer this innovation to America. But since the feeling between surgery and medicine was almost innately hostile, occasions were not lacking for conflicts between surgeons and the protomedicato. For one thing, the establishment of the surgical colleges in Spain so picked up the confidence of surgeons, especially the surgeons from Spain, that they themselves began to feel superior to physicians. When the viceroy of New Spain, the Marqués de Cruillas (1761–66), proposed to Charles III the creation of an "academy of anatomy," soon stretched into "school of surgery," he unwittingly precipitated an open and running fight between the royal protomedicato on the one hand and the successive professors of surgery on the other that did not cease until the Spanish regime itself ceased.

This harmful, and yet illuminating, controversy came in part from the vicissitudes of Spanish history in the Napoleonic epoch. From 1780 to 1822, the Spanish protomedicato was first divided into the separate agencies of medicine, surgery, and pharmacy, then "reunited," then abolished, then reestablished, and then abolished. Given the uncertainty about whether these inexplicable shifts—the reasons for them are hard to discern in the cold and literal legislation that produced them—were applicable to America, and with the consequent fumbling, no one could expect the laws and tribunals to reflect adequately the modest scientific possibilities of that generation.

As was natural with the inheritor of traditional privileges, the royal protomedicato wished neither to surrender its exclusive jurisdiction and privileges nor to give up its control over fees from every branch of the medical professions. Occurring soon after the establishment of anatomical instruction under Spanish surgeons in the Indian Hospital in 1770,[89] this atmosphere was bound to explode. Licentiate Manuel Antonio Moreno, a professor of anatomy, first accused the royal protomedicato of examining the barber Mariano Vera in surgery without his having the certificate in the subject, required by a decree[90] of Viceroy de Croix (1766–71) in 1770. When the viceroy turned to the protomedicato for its reaction, that body declared that under authorization from the Council of the Indies candidates prepared before the decree were not obliged to produce the certificate from the professor of surgery. Moreno was one.[91] The evidence indicated that Vera had registered in surgery in 1777 without finishing. Viceroy Martín de Mayorga (1779–83) then required the protomedicato to produce a certified copy of the order from the Council of the Indies.[92]

There the matter must have dropped, for nearly ten years later Moreno renewed the complaint, charging this time that the protomedicato had examined and approved Rafael Hernández and José Esquivel in surgery, though, as he had failed them in the college, they could not possibly produce the requisite certificates.[93] This time the protomedicato, swelling with pride and bursting with indignation, could hardly keep calm. In fact, the retort that the charge was a "calumny, a fraud, and a false charge" was scarcely a sign of calm at this "opening of wounds nearly healed." Moreover, said the protomedicato,[94] if it could not so sweep away these calumnies, it "would be covered with horror and shame at finding itself remiss and infringing the superior orders of Your Excellency, losing at a stroke the good name and luster of Your Excellency's patronage gained by dint of hard work, zeal, and sleeplessness." They cited an order of the interim judge Villarrutia, now of twenty years' standing, authorizing the protomedicato to rule and suspending the decree of 1770. Since Moreno had the file in hand that contained the proof that the protomedicato had been left in charge as well as two royal cédulas to the same effect, the protomédicos repeated that his charge was sinister, fraudulent, and false. Now they sought to prove that Moreno had never legally established "either with sworn proofs, or on stamped paper," that he had been duly installed. The last part of this bitter reaction was an assertion that if Moreno got by with denying the authority of the protomedicato, he would be joined by "countless others" just waiting for such an opportunity. The result, evidently, would be a rise in quackery and a continuation of the disorders—horrible word—of which Moreno had already and for so long been guilty.

The arrival of Antonio Serrano in the Royal School of Surgery in 1794 offered only a respite in the fight of the surgeons with the royal protomedicato. The antipathy this man inherited from Moreno and the stifling containment that the royal protomedicato imposed upon him disposed his attack on the first good occasion. This opportunity came in 1804, the year after he had become director and professor of the School of Surgery.

Provoked by intermittent reports on the decadence of surgery and pharmacy in America, a junta of royal officials (*Junta Superior Gubernativa*) in Spain took advantage of the separation of medicine, surgery, and pharmacy to maneuver the protomedicato's loss of its ancient and onerous control of medicine. This junta of scornful peninsulars, professing alarm that surgery was "completely abandoned" in America, called for a complete separation of surgery and medicine and recommended that the protomedicatos of the Indies cease to take cognizance of the "things and cases [*cosas y casos*]" of surgery there. Instead, the junta called for the creation of subcommissions (*subdelegaciones*) to conduct examinations and see to the enforcement of the laws governing surgery. Its scale of fines for those practicing surgery without a license, if these did not present themselves within two years with documents qualifying them for examination by the subcommission, was more than drastic. If there had been any prospect of enforcement, it might have had some bearing on the innumerable offenders, for it proposed a fine of fifty pesos for the first offense, one hundred pesos and exile at least beyond twenty-five leagues for the second, and six years' banishment and a fine of two hundred pesos for the third.

The crown, however, after "hearing the Council of the Indies," could only propose a junta[95] to study the question as well as the plight of pharmacy. After hearing the protomedicato, and any other experts it thought fit, it might then proceed to draw up regulations adapted to the peculiar circumstances of each country and send to the crown a complete record of everything done.[96]

In Mexico, Viceroy Iturrigaray asked for the opinions of Antonio Serrano and Vicente Cervantes, a professor of botany—the closest thing there was then to a chair of pharmacy. Though it is not necessary always to believe the documents from disaffected persons, without them the truth about the decadence or progress of the medical sciences would never emerge clearly. Thus, when Serrano and Cervantes turned in their reports, lights of truth and frankness though they may have been, the heat of passion, too, certainly glowed. Serrano, who evidently felt that there were many horrors in the practice of surgery and obstetrics, did not hesitate to give examples. He took it for granted that the faculties of medicine, surgery, and pharmacy had been separate since 1801 and considered the only point at issue to be whether the protomedicato should retain its jurisdiction over surgeons.

The worst, perhaps, that he could argue was that the regulation of surgery by the protomedicato was the primary evil. Though the protomedicato examined surgeons, phlebotomists, and dentists and was supposed to keep each within limits, the result was a "plague of quacks." In the first place, physicians were not qualified to pass on the training of a surgeon. Hence, they called in a "romance surgeon" to assist them, and what was more, they generally called in the last, and therefore the most pliable, of those they had admitted. "How," Serrano wanted to know, could an examiner whose "theory and practice are limited" and who is a fellow student or a kinsman of the candidate examined be an upright and impartial judge? It is not hard to see why Serrano asked if there were no respected, "properly certified [*condecorated*]" surgeons who could serve all the time and prevent these "variations" and "bad results"? But, no! The protomédicos wanted some hireling examiner whom they could pay a couple of pesos while they kept all the rest of the 108 pesos deposited by the applicant before examination. How, then, could the protomédicos protect the public in a specialty they themselves did not understand? And in dentistry and phlebotomy, where the applicants deposited eighty-four pesos, the protomédicos kept all the rest.[97] The fees paid for incorporations also went to the members of the tribunal. Serrano made it clear that, after the fees of twenty pesos were deducted, everything else should fall into a fund to finance the School of Surgery. In the present circumstances the very men who already held posts as the physicians of the viceroy's and the bishop's bedchamber fell into this extra money.

The whole system, Serrano argued, aided and abetted the "plague" of healers and curers while discouraging the properly trained and legally qualified physician. Fees that fell to the protomédicos as manna might have been used to finance a chair of obstetrics, then entirely lacking. Though most commentators on "the horrors" unfortunately avoided examples, Serrano brought them into the open. "Right here in this capital" women, with no more knowledge than some smattering picked up from a mother or relative, to the "horror of the true professors," practiced as "destroyers of humanity." One of these, with a difficult case, instead of delivering the baby, delivered the mother's intestines. In another birth, when an arm presented itself and the professor, who should have inserted his hand to take the infant by the feet, "tried to pull it out by the arm, but seeing that his efforts were in vain, he cut it off." Yet there was no school of obstetrics in the whole kingdom, and those trained abroad, of whom there were a few in Mexico City, were ruined by the competition of these quacks. The fees deposited for examinations that fell to the protomédicos should go toward financing a school, and, in case of objections to this outlay, the school proposed would increase the number of fee-paying graduates examined. In effect, Serrano made a plea for the School of Surgery as the only legal and qualified examining tribunal in the kingdom and named—outside Mexico City, where there was a school of surgery—the subcommissioners called for by the Junta Superior Gubernativa de Cirujía in Spain.[98]

The year 1804 saw the culmination of a renewed agitation to correct the neglect of surgery in America, but every push toward improvement quickened the hopes of professors in the School of Surgery that they might be free of what they thought of as the incubus of the royal protomedicato. Nothing was more natural, then, than that Antonio Serrano, recently made "director-professor" in the school, should use his new broom to sweep away this hoary mortification. The drastic separation of medical faculties in Spain would have made this independence inevitable, but a tendency to reunite them even more rapidly left the controversy in America, as the Spaniards sometimes said, "suspended in the air."

But Serrano could not rest. Within three months, his adrenaline still up, he fired still another missive at the viceroy.[99] First, he said, the School of Surgery was founded in imitation of those of Cádiz and Barcelona,[100] which did have the rights of a tribunal with judicial power (*tribunal facultativo*). Moreover, the ordinances of the colleges and schools of surgery, printed in Mexico in 1799,[101] made the School of Surgery a tribunal facultativo, which meant that it and not the protomedicato had the exclusive right to examine applicants for licenses to practice surgery, phlebotomy, dentistry, and midwifery.[102] His position, then, was that he expected the protomedicato to stop conducting these examinations. He did not, however, explain how a surgeon could understand dentistry any better than a protomédico could understand surgery.

The independence of surgery was bolstered by the official separation of medicine from surgery by a royal cédula of September 28, 1801, and, of course, Serrano elected to think the protomedicatos would no longer take jurisdiction, "direct or indirect," over matters of surgery. Such legislation in Spain, however, only served to handicap the official medical machinery in America until it was too late to set up new. In this case, before it was clear whether separation of the facilities in Spain applied to America, the whole issue underwent still another diversion. The governing body for surgery in Spain, the Real Junta Superior Gubernativa de Cirujía, appealed to the king in 1802 to allow it to take over the government of surgery in America through subdelegates. Since the junta based its claim on the abandonment of surgery in America, this effort gave the viceroy occasion to call for a report from Serrano—and one about as devastating as he could make it. Now, three months later, Serrano was grasping the opportunity to destroy the jurisdiction of the protomedicato. With a keen perception of what was important to colonial officials, he fastened upon the fees absorbed by the personnel of the protomedicato that, since the government was already financing the chairs in the School of Surgery, might well be saved or diverted to useful purposes.

Serrano's effort in 1804 could be carried, in part at least, upon the tide of growing state power. The Alemán case in 1798 had already stripped the protomedicato of jurisdiction in purely civil and criminal matters—those that were neither a *caso* nor *cosa* of medicine. But the agitation culminating in the cédula of March 2, 1804, did not turn out as Serrano wished. Whereas the Junta Gubernativa de Cirujía in Spain had sought to assume control through subdelegations until the establishment of schools of surgery in America, the king only authorized the creation of a new commission composed of the regent, oidor, civil fiscal, senior alderman, city attorney, and a member of the ecclesiastical chapter. Serrano argued in vain that, since the anticipated school of surgery had already been established in Mexico, it was clearly the royal intention that it should assume jurisdiction in place of the royal protomedicato.[103] His argument, however, filed away with related papers called for by the crown attorney, came to permanent rest in the archives.

The internal evidence on the miserable state of pharmacy, despite some show of progress in the area of botany, is even more convincing than in the case of surgery. The chair of botany had been held since its founding in 1787 by Vicente Cervantes, a man who gave evidence of competence and displayed a yen and capacity to keep up with European developments. It was no coincidence that Cervantes and the surgeon Serrano, after waiting nearly two months to answer the viceroy's call for a report on the state of their subjects in New Spain, informed him on the same day and made almost exactly the same points. The impression is overwhelming that the protomedicato had grown so inured to custom that it regarded routine as nature itself. As ancient practice allowed the protomedicato to collect lush fees in every profession related to medicine, the protomedicato remained quietly but passionately devoted to the status quo. In fact, economic advantage was so important to the protomédicos that they could not make a decisive and honest effort to weed out the unqualified surgeons, druggists, and phlebotomists. In short, the protomedicato could no longer protect the public health in the only way that had ever been fully open to it—by maintaining the integrity of the medical professions.

Vicente Cervantes, therefore, the director of the botanical garden and professor of botany, made a report that was both a plea for the reform of pharmacy and a condemnation of the general state of medicine. As in the case of surgery, pharmacy was "in the deepest state" of neglect and decay, and separation from the supervision of the royal protomedicato was the first step in its revival and modernization. Surgery, at least, had a chair of anatomy and another of "operations," but pharmacy had no school to educate the youth electing to practice it. As a result, pharmacists, even when they had the shame to care, could not be properly qualified.

What caused this shocking condition? The first was that those who practiced pharmacy enjoyed neither honor nor prestige.[104] More than anything else, the protomedicato perpetuated this state of things by confounding the few who had some "industry and merit" with the many who had no precise knowledge of their calling nor the competence to understand what had been published in recent years in "all cultivated Europe." Direly needed were professors of pharmacy who would keep up with publications in the field and give youth decent instruction, and exclude— in their own tribunal—those with no mastery of the subject. "Honorable recognition" would inevitably follow.

As it was, candidates were examined, passed, and given licenses to practice who did not have the beginnings of Latin master works. Even those licensed sometimes shamefacedly admitted that their examination by the "expert" serving with the protomédicos was a shallow farce. In fact, this examiner might himself well be the last examined and most ignorant of all. The result was adulterated drugs and prescriptions incorrectly and badly filled. Cervantes, who "accompanied" the protomédicos for three years when they examined prospective pharmacists, had firsthand evidence. Others in Mexico also knew the reason for this doleful situation: the dependence of pharmacy. In fact, said Cervantes, all ardently favored the same separation of pharmacy from medicine in Mexico that obtained in Spain, "except for two or three" in the capital who had some personal connection with the protomedicato or whose "apathetic souls" were possessed by "torpor" and "indolence."

The remedies Cervantes proposed were similar to those put forward by Serrano for the reform of surgical education and practice. An independent new faculty would be set up directly under the Junta Superior Gubernativa de Farmacia in Spain. Though the new decrees governing the "reunited" faculty in Spain had changed the situation, Cervantes held to his view that a school of pharmacy was still vital. Such an institution would need, altogether, five chairs in Mexico City. Two of these, albeit on the periphery, were already there. Cervantes himself had held the chair of botany since 1787 and, through his regular duties, had given lectures and staged demonstrations for pharmacists. In the Real Tribunal de Minería Professor Luis Linder held a chair of chemistry and, in addition to those compelled to attend, allowed auditors. By adding a substitute professor of natural history and another in pharmacy at five hundred pesos a year each, the reformers felt they would have the necessary complement of instructors. As an astute petitioner of the crown, Cervantes undertook to show how this school could be financed without cost to the royal treasury. As it was, for example, the crown got only a little over five pesos[105] of the ninety deposited by the applicant for his examination and license. By collecting 3,750 pesos from inspections of some 150 drugstores, 750 or 1,000 pesos from examinations, and by adding the income from degrees, the total figure should come to 5,500 or 6,000 pesos. After paying the 3,500 pesos in expenses of the school already established, the government could still pay the 1,000 pesos for the two substitutes called for and still have a surplus to go as emoluments for inspections and examination.[106] This was an ingenious plan for a day when it was not only hard to raise money, but, after the crown had looked at every possibility with a microscope, to think of a plausible scheme for doing so. Though he hedged enough, Cervantes was still too sanguine.

Now came the turn of the royal protomedicato. Fortunately, it rendered its report without knowledge of what Serrano and Cervantes had said concerning the issues. The charges of the governing juntas overseas on the sad state of surgery and pharmacy "in these dominions," it said, were based upon information that, if it was not sinister, was certainly mistaken. And if it had known what Serrano and Cervantes, upon the same occasion, were reporting concerning the protomedicato itself, mere language would have had to give way to more adequate, volcanic form of expression. The first point was suave, though perhaps not applicable. New Spain, it ran, had had surgeons of such outstanding merit that their memory still lived. One of these, Antonio Velázquez de León, for instance, not only was outstanding in his art but was also the actual founder of the surgical amphitheater, which had two endowed posts, one the professor and director and the other the dissector. Likewise, before accepting an applicant for theoretical and practical examination in surgery, the protomedicato required him to present proof that he had four courses in his subject and that he had served the legal term of internship before accepting him for "theoretical and practical" examination of five or six hours' duration on two afternoons "with the greatest rigor." Many failed and, when they felt ready, were allowed to return for reexamination. With the help of the Royal School of Surgery, "this Tribunal" boasted that it had turned out many surgeons, comparable to the best and highly esteemed by the public, who satisfactorily met their professional obligations in hospitals and military posts. Moreover, with the appearance of any sign of carelessness or neglect, the protomedicato had the power to call the offenders for reexamination—something that could be documented with countless archive files.

Then came the admission of a slight flaw, so well calculated to support the truth of the main contention to the contrary. Some years ago, the confession went, many practitioners of surgery, armed only with the certificate of the professor of anatomy, presented themselves in towns and cities where municipal officials without further ado gave them licenses to practice. When this practice became known, the protomedicato prosecuted many as false practitioners and ignorant (*ignorantes*) and forbade the professor of anatomy to certify any until, on the eve of an examination, the protomedicato requested him in writing to do so.

The protomedicato was particularly unhappy with the implication that the creation of subdelegates of surgery in New Spain would remedy the flood of curanderos. If subdelegates would serve this purpose, it would have been done, for the protomedicato itself had subdelegates, duly paying their media anata, in such cities as Puebla, Veracruz, Guanajuato, Valladolid, San Luis Potosí, Zacatecas, Querétaro, and Campeche to inspect drugstores, validate titles, watch out for curanderos, and see to it that practitioners qualified in one branch of medicine did not practice in another.

The protomedicato laid most of the blame for the curanderos—who existed here "as well as everywhere else in the world"—at the feet of the local magistrates and the people themselves. The magistrates, they said, received these curers without examining their papers, or even without asking for them, and not only allowed them to practice but warned and protected them upon the appearance of the subdelegates and inspectors of the protomedicato. The papers of the cases they had instituted were "resting in the archives" of many places. Their pleas to intendants, corregidores, and justices attested to their efforts to weed out the charlatans. And, because many of these were in towns with no licensed doctor, the people always set up such a loud clamor for tolerance, it had to be heeded. In such a case a curandero might be allowed to continue, but without a license and not in competition with a trained practitioner. The protomedicato was quite right in saying that the legitimate practitioners, whether physician, surgeon, or druggist, would have been the first to remind the tribunal of any laxness on its part.

This contention accorded with the universal practice, but the contention that only the highest motives led them to force all foreign physicians, the moment they began to practice, to "justify themselves" or, if they could not properly do so, to submit to an examination is open to question. In fact, the protomedicato now made the point that the Inquisition would not have had its troubles with Dr. "Esteban Morell," the Frenchman imprisoned along with Murgier, if the protomedicato had been allowed to refuse him a license on the perfectly legal ground that the prisoner had no naturalization papers. Instead, the Superior Government, meaning, no doubt, the viceroy, overruled the tribunal. Thus, the civil jurisdiction and supervision over medical certification, especially by the magistrates in municipalities, led the protomedicato to make a host of appeals to the Superior Government that proved the zeal of the protomedicato rather than any neglect on its part.

The reform of medical organization proposed in Spain, under consideration by the viceregal government, now became another object of a detailed rebuttal by Dr. García Jove and his colleagues on the royal protomedicato. They answered first that the complete separation of surgery and medicine would harm the public health. The laws already forbade romance surgeons, who were in a majority, to practice internal medicine without being accompanied by a physician, though of course they often did so and only gave way "at the last moment" to a physician to avoid getting caught by the protomedicato. The subdelegates, they argued, would only be accomplices in this criminal practice. Who besides the protomedicato would be able to limit or apprehend violators of the law?

Though the protomedicato was willing to concede that the subdelegates, if they were willing to spend the five or six hours in the examination like the protomedicato, might be able to pass on the qualifications of the candidates in surgery, it would not agree to anything else. They scorned the idea that a candidate in surgery, after two years' practice, be given the privilege of examination on the basis of the "good character" references he might get from the justices and town councils.[107] Since the new laws required "literary exercises" before examination, this proposal was directly opposed to the royal position on the matter anyhow. And, from the higher ground of experience, the protomedicato was able to make the financial proposals of the junta in Spain look pretty brash. How could even a subdelegate collect a fifty-peso fine from a quack who was insolvent in the first place? Moreover, they were able to show that the estimates made by Serrano as well as Cervantes on the amount of money that could be raised to support special schools were grossly out of line with realistic expectations. With a statement from the royal treasury they proved that to reach such high figures, they exaggerated the fees collected, besides raising the charges for degrees that young men regarded as hardly worth the expense anyway. The protomedicato had opposed such levies to support the botanical expeditions for the same reason. Besides, though the crown had authorized a chair of physiology upon the founding of the Royal School of Surgery and Anatomy in the Indian Hospital, the decision, supposedly for want of funds, had never gone into effect.

This defense of the protomedicato ended on the same note that it began: that the reports it was in effect answering—those of Serrano and Cervantes—were mistaken when they were not vicious.[108] Early in 1805 the viceroy finally ordered the junta convened to review the information assembled.[109] Considering the choleric temper of Dr. García Jove and his willingness to argue with and foil a judge of the royal audiencia, this was a mild effort.

The antagonism between Protomédico García Jove and Surgeon Serrano that boiled up in 1805 boiled over in 1815. A year earlier the financial situation of the Indian Hospital was so desperate, the number of patients so reduced, and the half-real paid by the Indians so hard to collect, the hospital's executive board proposed that two surgeons assume the work of the two physicians, thus reducing the staff from four to two. Thereupon, Dr. García Jove, in alliance with Dr. Luis Montaña, addressed a "paper" to the viceroy[110] to show that none of the surgeons was qualified to treat medical cases. In the first place, they said, Licentiate Antonio Gutiérrez, the other surgeon, had come over with the Balmis vaccinating expedition and should return to Spain, not hold the post assigned him by the Superior Government. As for the Director of the Hospital, Antonio Serrano, he had rushed the protomedicato precipitately before it could get the proper ordinances in hand for his incorporation as a licentiate in medicine and in medico-surgery and before he could have completed the "prerequisite literary acts." Moreover, he had applied for incorporation of the degree five years after its date, which, therefore, was "clandestine, illegal and null"; in fact, such scattering of honors was a disgrace to the royal colleges and to Spain. They had said enough. All the pedantic citations of the world's distinguished physicians to prove that only physicians were qualified to treat certain cases went pale beside this accusation.

The reply from Serrano was as bitter as it was prolix.[111] Disregarding Montaña as a private practitioner, Serrano launched an attack upon

García Jove's calumnies and insults as a dishonor not only to him but also to the surgical colleges of Spain. And—a grave charge in the midst of rebellion—García Jove's scornful statement challenged the viceroy and the "august" and "royal authority" itself. In fact, he said, the surgeons had royal appointments, which the other two lacked, and when challenged to produce their titles in "both" fields, they not only had done it but also produced copies of their incorporation by the royal protomedicato. Then—the first thing that would be said today—Serrano indicated he could justify his appeal to Viceroy Calleja by showing that fifteen years before a royal cédula[112] had authorized professors to appeal directly to the viceroy when the protomedicato proceeded contrary to the laws of the Indies.[113]

García Jove's assertion that naval or military doctors reaching America could not practice but must return to Spain did not go down easily with Serrano, who replied sarcastically that "this *decano*" takes upon himself functions of a judge reviewing an official's tenure in office. Then he cited a royal order[114] requiring captains general and commanders to allow no one to disturb military doctors when they practiced among the people in the neighborhood of their stations. Besides, if any doubt arose in these cases, it was the function of the military chief and not the protomedicato to resolve it. Another order given at Aranjuez on April 10, 1799, expressly permitted the graduates of the Cádiz School of Surgery who were naval doctors to practice in the towns to which they were sent. In royal establishments under the protection of the captains general, doctors who were neither naval nor military could validate their diplomas before the ayuntamiento.

What bothered Serrano even more, perhaps, was García Jove's "diffuse writing" that came down to this: though a surgeon may have "united in him" both medicine and surgery, he might not practice medicine unless accompanied by a physician. To this he could only exclaim: "Poor fellow! To what lengths will he not go to save his post in the Hospital!" Even though a licentiate in medical surgery, not revalidated in medicine, in either the army or the navy, Serrano might practice medicine alone in the neighborhood where he was stationed. This slant enjoyed the debater's license, for García Jove had really put the most effort into an attempt to show that a degree in medical surgery was not the same thing as one in medicine alone.

José Ignacio García Jove was a proud man, touchy about his prerogatives, but his rivals sometimes saw him also as a grasping man, interested in holding onto anything that had a little income attached to it. His whole object in attacking the validity of his licenses, said Serrano, was "his pocketbook." And, indeed, the evidence indicates that García

Jove, though busy, was highly wrought up at the prospect of losing his position and salary as physician on the women's ward of the Indian Hospital.[115] Besides, he was the chief protomédico where the fees were considerable, professor of prima of medicine in the university—even getting two-thirds salary there after retirement—and a private practitioner as well. Serrano did not understand how García Jove could have done justice to his chair while active in it.

For his part the protomédico took the position that no graduate of the colleges of Cádiz, Barcelona, and Madrid might practice medicine without having studied in the university and the clinic as demanded in a royal cédula of December 10, 1803. In the end, to bolster his position, he undertook to ruin the reputation of the Spanish surgical colleges. On his side Serrano, who had never heard of this cédula, which may well not have existed, had to ruin the reputation of the university. Both angry men were successful, though Serrano as an observer on the spot was more concrete in his disdainful attacks. Probably, though, the issue was never resolved. The growing turbulence in Spain and New Spain and the lengthy time normally taken to resolve such disputes probably meant that Mexico became independent before either García Jove or Serrano could be justified—or put down.

The Protomedicato: Ships

"Origins" of institutions, particularly of institutions that had no origins, are especially hard to trace. As late as 1679 the royal government in Madrid did not know whether or not the fleets sailing for America (Armada de las Indias) had a protomédico. When in that year Dr. Pablo de Santa Cruz applied for the position of *"protomédico de galeones,"* the king had to ask the House of Trade whether there was any such post and who filled it.[116] The House reported that the fleet did indeed have a protomédico and had had one since time out of memory—always appointed by the general of the fleet. The doctor was, accordingly, allowed to present his "merits and experiences" to this general.[117] Of course, during the first century of American history, the fleets always sailed with a complement of surgeons with their assortment of medicines and food—particularly food—"for the regalement of the said sick people" aboard.[118]

The inevitable sailing between islands and between ports not served by the fleets as well as the outfitting and movement of small ships in time of war forced irregular—even illegal—practices. In Cuba where as late as the eighteenth century whole cities could not claim a single doctor, those ships, the chances are, either sailed without a doctor or sailed with an unlicensed one. The crown was so hard put to get anyone to put to sea on this onerous duty that its officers invariably winked at the custom of taking aboard mulatto surgeons who were legally ineligible not only because they lacked academic training and the required internship but also because they lacked "blood purity." So far were such surgeons from concealing their illegal status that they actually boasted of such service and, in seeking a regular license, argued—politely, of course—that if they were good enough to attend His Majesty's soldiers and sailors on dangerous voyages, they were good enough to practice ashore in time of peace. Then, as vessels began to be built in New Spain to sail from mainland ports, the viceroy assumed responsibility for seeing to it that all these ships had surgeons. So hard were qualified laymen to come by that in 1771 Viceroy Antonio María de Bucareli (1771–79) appointed Santiago de Dios, a religious of the Order of San Juan de Dios, as surgeon of the packet boat *Principe* at the port of San Blas. As a strange inducement, Bucareli exempted the friar from the duty of going to sea; he would merely "cure" the crew whenever it put into port.[119] The salary for sailing as surgeon from San Blas was 840 pesos a year, a salary far better than that of the prima professor of medicine in the Royal and Pontifical University in Mexico City.

In American ports of entry like Veracruz or Santo Domingo, naturally, the need for combining medicine with governmental authority was so great that no fleet surgeon could suffice. The tribunals of the protomedicato in the viceregal capitals, at least in Mexico, came to appoint deputy protomédicos in the ports to exercise their functions in ordinary matters. Yet to the very end of the colonial period there was no fixed hierarchy of unquestionable authority. The result was that doing anything trivial required the cooperation of the city, and doing anything of more importance required the intervention of the governor if not the viceroy himself. This haziness sometimes forced cooperation between the subdelegate of the protomedicato and the cabildo. Subdelegate Miguel Sauch, for example, one of the seven men practicing medicine in Veracruz in 1806, solicited and obtained an order of the town council instructing José Almayer to present his license "to go on treating the sick of this public or else abstain. . . ." Though such illicit practice was a universal problem, the medical inspection of incoming ships and passengers was of intense concern, especially when epidemics threatened. The physicians, however, looked upon such inspections (*visitas de sanidad*) as onerous assignments.[120] In fact, a suspiciously large number of them developed severe indispositions or an oppressive vulnerability to seasickness. Because the work was dangerous, burdensome, and not a well-paid professional plum, drastic steps sometimes had to be taken. When the subdelegate of the protomedicato decided that all practicing physicians in the city, except those who were suffering from some habitual disability, should take their turns, the first man to qualify not to serve was Sauch, subdelegate of the protomedicato: his attacks, he hoped, were "notorious."[121] Others had the same idea, for, within a week, the subdelegate inquired of the city council to learn whether Dr. Cristóbal Tamariz and Dr. Francisco Hernández were exempted from the duty; in reply he got a repetition of the previous reprimand for not taking part in the inspection. The list of practicing physicians now drawn up by the subdelegate did not contain the names of these two men. The subdelegate then undertook to have a porter notify the men on the list, and the city council voted to tell Hernández that he must take his turn.[122] The stubborn doctor refused to comply. Two years later the cabildo of Veracruz notified Governor-Intendant García Dávila that all the doctors had the previous day, on the ground that Hernández had the prime practice, signed a document refusing to take their turns unless Hernández did likewise.[123] The adamant physician, in turn, presented a series of medical opinions over twenty years old[124] (1782–84) showing that he then suffered from haemoptysis (spitting of blood) complicated by a large hernia brought on by chronic seasickness during five or six years at sea. He flatly attributed his troubles to "the unjust clamors springing from the rivalry of some of my companions."[125] As it lacked the power of the royal protomedicato, the cabildo asked the governor to call a conference of doctors, including Hernández, and have them decide. In the meantime, inspections should go on with Hernández doing his part.[126] When the governor turned to the subdelegate for an opinion on whether illnesses suffered so long before were enough to justify exempting Hernández from taking his turn, he got the opinion that long voyages might revive the haemoptysis but that a short trip from mole to ship would certainly not do so.[127] Hernández's rebuttal accused the subdelegate of "fluctuating between his knowledge and undue influence. . . ." He took it as transparent that anyone with "half-discernment" would know that "the turbulence of the harbor," where "the sea never changes," would be disastrous to an *"hemotoyas habitual."* Hernández argued, for obvious reasons, that opinions should be taken from doctors in other towns.[128] At last, growing weary, the governor exempted Hernández and ordered Miguel Sauch, the subdelegate of the protomedicato, who had formulated the list of those eligible to make the ship inspections, to strike out the name of Dr. Francisco Hernández.[129] The doctor "with the prime practice" had worsted his "envious rivals." He had not taken a turn for three years since 1806.

The governor's decision merely set the conspirators to work anew,[130] although the indignant note they sounded was altogether too self-righteous to fit the true character of the colonial physician. Their first step was to empower Dr. Florencio Pérez Comoto, retired surgeon of the royal navy and one of their number, to proceed against Hernández.[131] They forthwith appealed to the governor for a reversal of his decision. There were some doctors, however, who either thought of the case as a personal feud or who, because a general scrutiny might expose their own questionable legal qualifications, refused to give Pérez Comoto power to act in their names.[132]

When the litigants got through with each other, practically everybody was left with something to be ashamed of. In his appeal to Viceroy Pedro Garibay,[133] Pérez Comoto rehashed the whole case from 1806. When Hernández was not too sick, Pérez Comoto shrewdly insisted, he held one post as surgeon of the garrison battalion (*batallón fijo*), another in the Hospital of Loreto, another in the military Hospital of San Carlos, and still another as "doctor and surgeon" of the city itself—work that required him to see 450–500 hospitalized patients a day—all in addition to a profitable private practice. With the cabildo joining in the hue and cry, Governor García Dávila did only what was inevitable: he passed the problem up to the viceroy.[134] There in Mexico City, Dr. Hernández answered through his attorney that there were only 274 hospitalized patients—not 450–500—under his care and that he had taken Luna's post only at the urgent behest of the man's family because, otherwise, it would have fallen vacant. His crowning point was that his enemies and envious rivals were behind his persecution. The proper solution: to sustain the decision of the governor of Veracruz.

The lawyer for the dissident doctors in Veracruz directly challenged the very integrity of Dr. Hernández. He claimed that Pérez Comoto and his companions never took Hernández's exemption from the duty of health and sanitary inspection at Veracruz for granted, and Hernández had proved by the very documents he presented himself that it was false that the cabildo made an exception in his favor in 1806 on the insinuated ground that he was suffering from haemoptysis. Besides, there was no proof that he was still suffering from this affliction, though he claimed it had gotten worse and worse. He also responded to the charge that Pérez Comoto did not wish his father-in-law to be caught in the same trap with Hernández and "had his lips sealed." Far from being the truth, said Pérez Comoto, he had an "authentic" exemption from the ayuntamiento of Veracruz. "And in the other particulars of Hernández's writing there are found one thousand (other) falsehoods." Would the viceroy, in reaching his judgment, be pleased not to take into account Governor García Dávila's decision—a decision reached without hearing the interested parties.[135] As was natural, the fiscal advised consulting the experts on the royal protomedicato, and as was even more inevitable, the viceroy agreed.[136] The protomédicos García Jove, Vicuña, and Gracida thought that haemoptysis going back twenty-seven years, especially when there was no legal evidence in the file to establish the continuance of the disease, should not interfere with Hernández's taking his turn when this could be done on "a short, tranquil voyage," but not in stormy weather. The tribunal's considered judgment was that, within the bounds of the common sense and moderation suggested, there was no harm in Hernández's taking his turn.[137] The defending lawyer, Ignacio de la Campa Coz, however, insisted that there were plenty of proofs in the file to justify the exemption made by the governor-intendant. He asserted that the haemoptysis was not only there as before, but three years later was complicated by a hernia and "advanced age"—Hernández was fifty-seven years old. Even a short trip on tranquil water was now enough to aggravate his infirmity. After all, one might "leave the mole in a serene moment" only to have "hard winds sweep up," as they frequently did in Veracruz. The brilliant fiscal Ambrosio Zagarzurieta insisted that Dr. Hernández take his turn on the conditions set up by the protomedicato: that he should make his inspection only when it was "serene and calm," never when it was stormy—a compromise the viceroy quickly endorsed.[138] While this decision was being pondered, however, both a Dr. Rodríguez and Miguel Pages, "dedicated to surgery," offered to take Hernández's turn as medical inspector whenever it came up. The fiscal in Mexico City, "the eyes and ears of the king," however, learned that Rodríguez had no license to practice medicine and that Pages was only a romance surgeon—if that. Hence, upon his advice, the archbishop-viceroy ruled that Rodríguez could not substitute without certified papers. Also, as a romance surgeon had never been so honored, Pages could not serve under any circumstances.[139] The only man not taking his turn was Dr. Ignacio Ametller, a navy doctor, and as naval and military doctors were under the direct orders of their commanding officers and did not take turns, nobody was left who might substitute for Hernández.[140]

As was often the case with litigation in New Spain, Hernández refused to accept defeat; he turned again to the archbishop-viceroy, charging that whether a man was a surgeon or a physician made little difference in Veracruz. He must have gotten pleasure from reporting that Dr. Pérez Comoto, though only a surgeon, practiced medicine without qualifying as a physician.[141] Likewise, Joaquín de Ablanedo and Juan Crivelli were surgeons and therefore forbidden to practice medicine by the royal dispatch of 1797[142]—all an indirect reflection upon the efficiency, if not honesty, of the subdelegate of the protomedicato in Veracruz. The viceroy's ruling—that Rodríguez and Pages be allowed to substitute as soon as they were "habilitated"—did not change the status quo.[143]

In fact, it was not until well into 1810 that the viceroy cleared up the situation with a set of instructions that dealt not only with Hernández but also with the whole problem of medical inspections in Veracruz. First of all, all physicians, doctors, and licentiates of surgery, as well as regimental surgeons, should go on the list of those to be called for the inspection of incoming ships. Moreover, every physician and surgeon, "embarked" and practicing on land, whether from a warship or merely one stationed in the harbor, should likewise take their turns.[144] Though Rodríguez was "enabled" to serve for the time allowed him to get the diploma and license "that he had left in Spain," Hernández nevertheless found himself "by verbal order" compelled to make the inspections after April 1. He was irate, though, at the "studied malice of my envious rivals and enemies," who, he protested, withheld the order of February 23 from him and then accused him of deliberately disobeying it. That he had permission to use Rodríguez as a substitute did not please him; he wanted the ruling revoked utterly. The governor-intendant, however, merely sent the petition to Mexico once again and told Hernández that while waiting he remained liable for his turns.[145] In Mexico City the legal advisers of the viceroy thought that no unbearable burden had been imposed upon Hernández, and though they did not rebuke him for his insolent persistence, they did let the matter drop and ordered him to participate in the inspections.[146]

Offhand, one might not think that the effort of one Spanish navy doctor to avoid taking his turn as health inspector of incoming ships was a matter of earthshaking import. Yet in the case of Dr. Francisco Hernández, litigation went on under five separate governments in Mexico City and took over four hundred pages to record. It dealt with a trivial matter that neither party to the suit recognized as such—as they never did in cases of personal dignity. And, as in similar cases for three hundred years, the government, though a revolution was patently getting under way, never once rebuked the contestants for troubling it with picayune matters; its genius had always been to encourage these coming to the top. Moreover, any issue that probed medical personnel, especially at Veracruz, was like opening a party *piñata*. A port was the logical place for army and navy doctors, whether waiting for or jumping ships, to "disembark" and begin civilian practice. Then, the unlicensed practitioner's explanation that he had left his papers behind would work longer in Veracruz than in Cádiz. There, too, surgeons went over with impunity into the practice of medicine in disregard of clear statutes. Even foreign physicians could and did begin illicit practice. Yet Miguel Sauch, the delegate of the royal protomedicato, either did not detect or did not take note of any of these violations. In fact, after the king's fiscals and assessors in Mexico City had noticed how casually the illicit practitioner became a regular one, it was the town council, at the suggestion of the viceroy, that forced a registration of medical certificates in its secretariat in the old and customary way.[147] Without financing for his office, the proto-médico was no doubt too busy practicing himself to round up "intruders" by himself.

T HEY PRACTICE MEDICINE without fear of God our Lord and
without the bachelor's degree." The juxtaposition of the Lord and
the degree academic in this colonial complaint was not sacrilegious.
The Spaniards at home had required a university degree for the practice
of medicine—at least the bachelor's—since the fifteenth century, and
within the next three centuries they bolstered this law at home and
transferred it to the Indies. Here, despite this and many other carefully
drawn, rigorous statutes, practitioners ranging from the pathetically un-
lettered in the towns to the rank charlatan in the cities increased almost
geometrically. In the eighteenth century "ministers of death" and "enemies of nature" were typical of the phrases invented to depict this evil
to the royal protomedicato or to the viceroy himself. Time after time
the ever-plaintive critics touched "the direful consequences" that followed
these "funereal battalions" of "intruders."[1] They condemned first the
degradation of medicine and then the resulting disasters to the people.
They never lingered on anything so puny as a specific case that they
could carry before a judge. A miscarriage of treatment short of the demise of the patient was too slight for comment—and most of the time
even then was ignored.

Yet two types of critics raised their urgent and ineffectual voices as
medicine was "inundated" by empirics practicing so openly that they
regarded themselves as the only legitimate physicians in every town and
village. In the Spanish town the "Latin" doctor—the one behooded by
the university—regarded the intruder first as a competitor cutting down
on his fees and, second, as accessory to murder before the fact. The
modern reformer of the late eighteenth century threw his weight to the
side of the university man, but he regarded a radical change in medical
education as a prerequisite to any plausible effort to get rid of the
"plagues" of curanderos. Yet these two classes of critics saw the nineteenth century in full swing with the quack and the curandero more
rampant than ever before, if that is possible. Why should such universally
recognized need for improvement suffer such continuous and discouraging defeat?

The Spaniards, of course, never entertained any real hope that they could carry European academic medicine to the native population outside the main cities. The people in rural areas were too isolated, too credulous, and too poor to make such an attempt reasonable. To them, a man who invoked charms had a command over life and death that the traditional university doctor did not have. The pompous mouthing of unintelligible medical terms by an uneasy Latin physician, moreover, was as mysterious to them as any enchantment ever conjured up by a curandero. Even the religious who saw at first hand the dumb suffering of people without medical help often had no choice but to practice themselves. When the alternative was to allow a whole province to go without physicians, both the Spanish and the viceregal authorities chose to interpret the law mildly, prudently, and realistically. For example, in 1652 the king, informed that "many people practice medicine without the requisite examination and approval," made a clear distinction between unlicensed practice in Indian towns and those in which Spaniards lived. In the same breath that he ordered Viceroy Enríquez de Guzmán to ferret out the quacks in Spanish towns, Philip IV explicitly recognized a fait accompli that it was not illegal to practice medicine in the Indian towns without a license.[2] Hence, the ever-recurring struggle to enforce the laws requiring examination and licenses occurred only in places where there were whites.

Even in Spanish towns, when the outcries and petitions against quackery came, the solutions were not dogmatic and precipitate. There the empiric, when taking "refuge in the rule of Providence that all must die," went on as long as there was no one else legally qualified. Until they could attract university graduates, town councils either licensed curanderos or neglected to demand their papers. So did the royal protomedicato[3] itself, except in the capital cities where its members felt there were enough licensed doctors to go around. Even in these more favorable circumstances, however, the practitioners, trained in universities and duly examined, only served well-to-do white families.

A Chronic Shortage of Physicians in the Indies

Above everything else, the unremitting scarcity of physicians explains the distressing history of medicine in the Spanish colonies. The early conquerors waded through morasses, slept in deserts, mingled with primitive populations, and endured venereal disease—all without the help of doctors. Just as in the villages of Spain, common report soon singled out somebody in the ranks reputed to be in the secret of physic. Who knows under what ministrations the companions of "stout" old

Bernal Díaz del Castillo dressed their wounds from the grease they "took from a fat Indian left on the field" of Tlascala! In Peru a Greek artillery-man left the ranks of Pizarro's men to treat their wounds. When Val-divia undertook the conquest of Chile, his mistress took the role of medi-caster as she might have done in a Spanish hamlet.

Long after the conquerors passed on, leaving submissive towns and provinces behind them, doctors and medicines had yet to come. Thirty-four years after the discovery of Española, for example, the crown finally assigned 30,000 maravedís to pay for the medical services of Licentiate Barreda in that island.[4] The appearance of Licentiate Hernando Sepúl-veda provided a second physician, but he complained that "the things of medicine and the apothecary shop" were very dear and the people sick and without drugs, even though physicians were there to prescribe them. Sepúlveda, however, bared the plight of the people when he asked the town council of Santo Domingo to lend him four hundred pesos for seven or eight years to put a stock of drugs in the city, supply the poor with medicines, and charge the well-to-do "less than they paid in the convents." The alderman turned a cold shoulder, and the king, instead of acting on the request, resorted to the dodge of asking the audiencia for a report.[5]

The shortage of doctors in the Antilles was chronic from that day when Ferdinand sent "a doctor and a musician" to Española to assuage the ills of the body and soul of Columbus's struggling settlers until the last shot had sounded in the wars of independence. At the crossroads of empire, Havana was all but without medical care nearly a century after the occupation of Cuba, and in 1604 Governor Pedro Valdés (1602–8) drew up a memorial lamenting that for want of "a salaried physician" many citizens, traders, and other people "from the fleets" and in hospitals had died. The king parried this overture by asking "if there had been a physician in the city" and, if not, "whether it would be a good idea to send one from these kingdoms. . . ?" Indeed! Neither the king's secre-tariat nor the Council of the Indies knew whether there was a physician in Cuba.[6]

How long and how desperate was this plight? Soon after the French and Indian War in 1765, the Conde de Ricla, governor of Cuba (1763–65), learned that "many cities, towns, and places" in the island did not have a single practitioner and challenged the royal protomedicato for a solution.[7] It is a fair index to the next century that in 1820 the captain general of Cuba and the intendant of the army there were trying to get six students from the College of Medicine and Surgery at Cádiz to come to the island "to take care of the white population." The mulatto empirics might take care of all the rest.

Shortage of legal medical care was endemic in Puerto Rico. In 1707 the cabildo of San Juan petitioned the king to send a physician from "those kingdoms" and, anticipating a call for a report on how he could be financed, argued that the income from the hospital, convents, and private citizens would provide enough. So, His Majesty graciously allowed the city to find for themselves, if they could, this solitary disciple of Aesculapius.[8] In 1773 the same council represented to the governor "the need of having a practitioner of medicine and surgery." The governor turned to the king and he, in his turn, as monotonous as the call of the whippoorwill, inquired whether there was any income to pay a doctor. As San Juan was already hopelessly in debt, the king thought the city might try to induce a physician to settle there by allowing him "to charge his patients fees in proportion to their means and the success of the treatments."[9] How modern that first part! Thus, four or five years after making its overture, and at a time when the town council thought the city ought to have two hospitals, it did not even have a physician. The governor of Puerto Rico reported in 1812 that there was no protomedicato there and "hardly a single practitioner of surgery or medicine throughout the length and breadth of the island."[10]

Caracas—even the whole province of Venezuela—was long on the very brink of having only curanderos and an occasional "intruder." Dr. Lorenzo Campins complained in 1775 of the scarcity of men "in his faculty" and the complete "neglect"—*abandono* was the telling word— of the medical profession.[11] In 1800 Dr. Felipe Tamariz went before the royal audiencia to get action. That body considered the half dozen duly licensed practitioners in Caracas as hardly adequate to take care of the whites in a city of thirty thousand souls, two-thirds of them of "brownish color [*color quebrado*]." As two of the four surgeons of Caracas were in Havana, how could the remaining two serve the military hospitals and religious communities and treat all whites, Negroes, zambos, and mulattoes? The audiencia accepted the plain fact: for the "lowest classes" it was the empiric or nobody.[12]

If such is the record of the Caribbean provinces, that of Mexico leaves no room for boasting. Twenty-four years after the fall of Tenochtitlán, the audiencia in Mexico City under Viceroy Antonio de Mendoza fined the "said-to-be" Doctor Pedro de la Torre[13] half of his property and sentenced him to perpetual exile, on pain of "natural death," should he tarry in the country when released from jail.[14] Taken as proof that the Spanish colonial courts made short shrift of quacks, this case is misleading. The review of the "definitive sentence" some seven weeks later reflected a growing alarm; Dr. de la Torre, instead of paying the death penalty for delaying his exile, would merely pay five hundred pesos.[15]

Even after the review sentence, the campaign to retain this man, though he was patently practicing with forged papers, rose in crescendo. Between July 3 and August 5, 1545, the town council, the Bishop Juan de Zumárraga, the cathedral chapter, an imposing list of founders and important citizens—"the whole university of this land"—rushed petitions into the audiencia. The quick and resolute participation of the most distinguished surviving conquerors gave the sanction of dignity to the agitation. All these distinguished people shuddered now that a catastrophic smallpox epidemic—a "great sickness and pestilence that the Lord has seen fit to send to this land"—was raging. They trembled yet more to realize that, even before "Dr." de la Torre's sentence, Mexico had only four medical men. Now, one of these was no longer there, and another was in jail. Of the remaining two—both "rich and prosperous" and thus unresponsive—one was old and threatening to leave for Castile.

With the aid of an elaborate interrogatory, to which Bishop Zumárraga courteously responded, de la Torre's advocates established some impressive personal points. De la Torre had "come into fame as a good physician of experience and presence." A man of affable bearing, he was open to approach by Spaniards, Indians, Negroes, "masters, and servants." He attended the poor gratis—something roundly commendable in that society—and his successful cures among them made him "notorious." The ecclesiastical cabildo hit upon the idea that the audiencia should stay the sentence of exile while Bishop Zumárraga appealed directly to the king on de la Torre's behalf. The municipal council improved upon the idea with the suggestion that the doctors already in Mexico subject de la Torre to a rigorous examination and permit him to practice pending an answer to Zumárraga's proposed intercession with the king. On this note the record ends, but as every corporation in the city and prominent citizens as well seemed to think that the audiencia was acting in a hard and rigid manner,[16] one may guess whether the sensitive Dr. de la Torre, now at large on bond, returned to the practice of physic.

Over two hundred years later, every city and town of importance in New Spain—not to mention the miserable villages—was still in the medical doldrums. Between 1607 and 1738 the University of Mexico conferred 438 bachelors' degrees in medicine, an average of 3.35 a year.[17] So few degrees fell well below the demands of the country. In fact, in 1791 there were not enough physicians in the cloister to draw lots in the selection of councillors. Because of the unchanging salaries, professors of medicine slighted their medical classes in favor of their practice,[18] and there is good ground to estimate that all the other universities in the empire put together conferred fewer medical degrees than did the University of Mexico. Though academic degrees did tend to increase in the second half of the eighteenth century, the records of medical licenses, scattered though these be, show no substantial acceleration in rate. In 1800, the last year that might be considered normal in New Spain, the protomedicato examined six candidates in medicine and six in surgery.[19] The University of San Carlos de Guatemala, with thirty bachelors' degrees in medicine between 1700 and 1821, averaged just under one every four years.[20] Fed by this system, Guatemala was in such straits that in 1820 Dr. Pedro de Molina threw up his hands at the spectacle of perhaps eighteen practitioners for the whole kingdom of a million people. He was ashamed that the University of San Carlos de Guatemala had only one hundred pesos to pay the substitute professor of medicine who did the work.[21] One university in the country, that in León, was so far away that the candidates it graduated in medicine could not make the trip to the protomedicato in Guatemala for examination and, in consequence, suffered the stigma of being curanderos for the rest of their lives.[22]

In some places, according to the protestations of the time, the pressure of the curandero had driven all the white men from the faculty in the university and therefore out of the medical profession. In the middle of the eighteenth century, when the University of San Marcos de Lima had only four graduates in medicine,[23] one viceroy after the other attributed the collapse to the failure of the rector of the university to require certificates of blood purity for matriculation. The mulattoes, forty years later, wanted to know what 60,000 inhabitants of the City of Kings would do without the "forty-odd swarthies" who trod the streets, cured the sick, and comforted the infirm.[24] Even in romance surgery, where academic degrees were not required, those of "broken color" could not qualify for examination by the royal protomedicato. Hence, the mulattoes everywhere joined the endless queue of those illicitly practicing.

In Venezuela, as well as in Peru, the evidence of this drift is clean and strong. A Mallorcan physician in Caracas, Dr. Lorenzo Campins, complained in 1775 that owing to the scarcity of "legitimate practitioners," the curanderos, tolerated out of sheer necessity, had greatly swollen in number. When he had himself "incorporated" in the cloister of the University of Caracas in order to enter the oposición for the chair of medicine, which so far had neither professor nor student, he stated he was determined to "extirpate" the quacks "who had done such notable harm to human health." Nine years later, this bitter lament went on, those who had wished to enroll for medical careers had not done so because the toleration of mulatto and Negro empirics "had caused medicine to fall from its state of splendor."[25] The cloister of the university supported him with the claim that mulatto curanderos had toppled the prestige of medicine and kept youths of "good family" out of medicine.[26] In fact, the rector of the university declared that Campins was still the only medical doctor in the cloister.[27]

Despite the surfeit of evidence of this dearth of trained medical care, it is still hard to grasp that 162 years after Jiménez de Quesada had lined up his men to face Belalcázar and Federmann on the Plains of Cinnamon, there was only one properly trained physician in the whole kingdom of New Granada: Isidro Gómez de Molina, doctor in medicine from the University of Alcalá de Henares.[28] Though protomédico in Cartagena, Dr. Gómez de Molina fled that town in 1697 on account of the French attack upon it and retired to Tamalameque, where the oidor of the Audiencia of Santa Fe de Bogotá began a campaign to induce him to go up to Bogotá. Here there was neither a single professional physician nor a chair of medicine, which had gone unfilled for forty-nine years. Meanwhile, Panama, which had lost its two physicians—presumably the only two—started a hopeless agitation to raise funds to bring Gómez Molina there. When the money fell through and this physician fell ill, "Captain Durán" begged the audiencia to accept Manuel de Miranda, "a practical doctor," on the ground that, though he had no license, he had had some "good hits." The archbishop-governor appointed Oidor Licentiate Juan Gutiérrez de Arce as agent to find a doctor. The four "reported" to be in the kingdom, inexorably and one by one, declined to come to Bogotá.[29]

This discouraging failure lingered on in the second half of the eighteenth century. Not satisfied with the treatment accorded the licensed physician with the baccalaureate, the swaggering curanderos arrogantly demanded the obeisance done the doctor of medicine.[30] Little wonder that the enlightened protector of the Indians, Antonio Moreno y Escandón, despaired of establishing medical studies in Bogotá, a city of more than twenty thousand and the capital of the viceroyalty! In the Colegio del Rosario, he said, Juan Bautista Vargas held the chair of medicine with no evidence of his fitness, save a degree "conferred by the Dominicans." Though he believed that a properly filled chair of medicine would go far to curb the curanderos and open a career to youth, he felt that it would be better to drop the chair than to fill it in this unscientific way.[31] Years later, Viceroy José de Espeleta (1789–96) reported that the efforts to engage a physician and pay him through municipal revenues had invariably failed. The only resort left open, then, was to rely upon subscriptions from powerful families and to leave the poor and the victims of accidents to the curers. His plan was to bring physicians from Europe and to pay the first one a thousand pesos a year, five hundred of this from the secular cabildo.[32] Even so, Bogotá, now "a city of twenty-five thousand souls," had only two doctors and some "tolerated" curanderos in 1800. Even these two doctors lacked formal education, for when the viceroy tried to start the chair of medicine, he had to turn to a man who had not gone through the formalities of a medical education and examination himself. The viceroy thereupon proposed that Dr. José Celestino Mutis, head of the botanical expedition, supervise the examination of Miguel de Isla, who, if he passed, would then "read" the chair. The royal audiencia insisted that the chair should be filled by oposición—something patently impossible. The king, however, administered a sharp rebuke, "exempted" Isla from the required medical courses, and allowed him the doctor's degree—steps normally too touchy even for the king to take. Moreover, he ordered the use of the city's surplus lands if necessary to finance the chair and set up an interim board composed of Dr. Mutis, Dr. Isla, and another qualified physician to examine those thought fit "to preserve the public health."[33]

It is just as striking that in 1800 the presidency of Quito should have had only one or two physicians in its main cities and sometimes only that many in all. Guayaquil, for example, had three licensed physicians. One of these soon died, another fell into prison for debt, leaving only one to care for a city of nine thousand inhabitants, "unhealthy anyway because of its climate." This solitary soul, unfortunately, preferred "the society of his friends" and the cash "of the most powerful." The rest would have to die with only the solace of a curandero.[34] When, the next year, the city proposed to bring two boys from each town to study the arts and then medicine in Quito,[35] the king's skeptical ministers suggested that without the great number of physicians and surgeons Francisco Calderón had proposed, the people of Quito and its province had kept themselves "healthy and alive for many years without noticing any difference from the other provinces where there is an abundance of such practitioners." Thus, tacitly asserting the uselessness of medicine, the Council of the Indies put the cold hand of interminable delay upon the project by calling upon the president and audiencia of Quito for a full report.[36] Before this exchange could take place, however, Governor José de Aguirre Isisarri wrote the viceroy in Bogotá that the people of Guayaquil paid with their lives for turning to curanderos in their desperation. The drug trade was out of control and prices soaring—all with no sign of a protomedicato to inspect them or even examine and license bleeders and dentists.[37] President (Baron) Carondolet (1798–1806) tried to get financing for the chair of medicine that had been authorized in the University of San Fernando, but as one Pedro Aguayo had never produced the eight hundred pesos he promised, and as the available property in haciendas yielded only thirty-three pesos, he had to give up.[38] Thirty-three pesos to start a chair of medicine?

From the provincial towns without a single physician, or with one or two, Lima and Mexico City, the seats of royal and pontifical universities, often appeared to have doctors "in abundance." The petitions from these remote places were, therefore, mournful in the seventeenth century and despairing in the eighteenth. Querétaro, for example, had only two legally qualified doctors in 1787 to take care of a hospital, nine religious establishments, two schools, the jail, factories, "all private houses," and the rest of the population of 35,000. One apologist said that "it would be stupid to say" that this could be done.[39]

"Ministers of Death and Enemies of Nature"

The whole history of colonial medicine, as it really was, is the story of the all-too-natural filling of this awesome gap in doctors. The man who filled it in the cities sometimes, though rarely, began as an attendant of a licensed physician, holding his horse perhaps. More likely, though, he worked as a servant or a male nurse in a hospital—say San Juan de Dios. Quick of wit, and with little to lose, he began doing favors for the sick and injured. Presently, with a reputation for many cures and fame for his charity to the poor, he attracted the favorable attention of the prior of a convent or an abbess in a nunnery. If in surgery, he might then actually apply for examination and a license. Other intruders were of more exotic cast. "Bold foreigners," coming into the empire illegally, slipped quietly into medicine. It was marvelous how many of these poor physicians coming out to the Indies had had their ships overhauled by English men-of-war and been stripped of their baggage and, of course, their medical diplomas and certificates. If they could hold out ten or twenty years, acquire "root" property, produce progeny from a native mother, and establish their Catholicism, they even had a good chance of securing naturalization and "toleration."

Though these curanderos were "generally such idiots and so gross that many of them could not even read," every provincial city had its half-dozen "more or less." Of the half-dozen practicing in Querétaro in 1787, two were friars, one a Frenchman, perhaps, and one an Italian. All of these "practiced tranquilly" and "even with applause" alongside examined physicians. When they could not have a Latin physician, literate inhabitants preferred the foreign intruder. The benighted populace then turned to the friar, for they knew he could read medical works, and because he often was obliged to try his hand at prescriptions and cures, he gained both a knowledge and a reputation he could not escape. Not even the Frenchman, who had the "best assortment of drugs imaginable," allowed the poor "to turn away comfortless and empty-handed."[40]

The cold fact is that in north central Mexico the sick were treated by empirics or not at all. In 1795, for example, the surgeon, Dr. José Sánchez Camaño, after two months of practice in the valley of Santiago in the intendancy of Guanajuato, complained bitterly that territorial justice "tolerated" the horde of curanderos, barbers, and old women. He besought the viceroy to see that these did not practice.[41] When the viceroy inquired into the case, the civil and religious authorities answered his inquiry in a refrain. There were, they said, some misfortunes, but in places where there were no examined physicians, the inhabitants could only appeal to those who, because of their experience or reading, could prescribe or apply some simple remedies to common ailments.[42] But lo! Dr. Sánchez himself was a fraud. When the case came to the attention of the royal protomedicato, it discovered that it had never heard of or admitted any Dr. Sánchez Camaño to the "medical cloister" and intimated that this particular medicaster was deliberately trying to confuse himself with a "professor of ability and judgment" by the name of Camaño in San Luis Potosí. The case ended in the arrest of Sánchez Camaño but not in the ruin of the local curanderos.[43] Some years before, in the mining area of Real de los Catorce, there was extended litigation to drive out charlatans—all of the dispute between men who were themselves illegally practicing![44] Of these, one was an unlicensed foreigner and the other two Mexican intrusos. Such tragic facts, in the self-righteous view of the royal protomedicato, left the health of the public in the hands of "ignoramuses" who were nothing more than "ministers of death" and the "enemies of nature."[45]

Inspection of Physicians and Surgeons

Yet the Spaniards never abandoned the idea that any evil in America, however hoary and deep-seated, could be arrested by the firm use of authority. Two obvious and traditional means of applying it were open to them: punctual inspection (visita) and rigorous prosecution. They never approximated either. Inspections had certain disadvantages: they were delegated and unfortunately combined with the far more remunerative business of collecting fees for inspecting drugstores. In fact, the protomedicato's instructions to its agents to demand the licenses of physicians and surgeons as well as of druggists came as an afterthought. When the inspector lived in the town visited, especially when he was an aggressive and overbearing man, his rivals—whether practicing legally or illegally—resorted to every obstructive artifice and stratagem to foil his efforts and mar his record. To begin with, he had to have a commission from the royal protomedicato, an order of compliance (*auxiliatoria*) from the viceroy, and a written permit (*pase*) from the cabildo or local magistrates.

Two inspections at Querétaro, one in 1768 and one in 1787, show a division between success and failure that is instructive if not typical. In 1768 the protomedicato chose Dr. Miguel Díaz Chacón as its lieutenant to conduct these inspections of the medical life of his native town, which the viceroy and the cabildo of Querétaro promptly approved.[46] Tacit in the instructions[47] of the protomedicato to the visitor was the feeling that Querétaro exemplified every characteristic shortcoming of medicine in the Spanish empire. Going beyond a mere inspection of apothecary shops, the protomedicato required Díaz Chacón to call upon all physicians, surgeons, apothecaries, and bleeders and to demand their diplomas and licenses to practice. That there were no fees or scale of fees for inspecting physicians and surgeons shows that this procedure was irregular, if not rare. Thus those whose papers were in order went their way without paying anything. Those without papers, however, would stop practice and stand by while the visitor reported them to the royal protomedicato for further action. Against the recalcitrant, the visitor himself had orders to institute proceedings in the local courts and remit the records to the protomedicato in Mexico City. In other civil or criminal charges involving medicine, surgery, pharmacy, or phlebotomy, the inspector would consult a lawyer and take the proper steps. Because those away from Mexico City were not expected to have licenses in any event, phlebotomists got two or three months' grace to give them time to submit to an examination by the royal protomedicato, after which they might expect fines the same as any other intruder. Pending the arrival of a "licensed master," however, the protomedicato authorized the existence of two or three bleeders—depending upon the population of the town. As the mundane purpose of such *visitas* was ordinarily the inspection of drugstores, however, the rest of Díaz Chacón's instructions reflected fear of the traditional abuses in the drug trade.[48]

In 1768 Dr. Díaz Chacón met these terms and conducted an uneventful inspection in Querétaro, but when he undertook to do the same thing in 1787 with a private letter from Dr. José Ignacio García Jove, president of the tribunal of the protomedicato, the city attorney of Querétaro challenged the whole procedure as irregular in the hope, apparently, that it would bog down.[49] To the protomédicos, this hostility meant that "the quacks were patronized by those who should be their exterminators." All the charges made by the accusers, they insisted, were true. Dr. Domingo Melica, an Italian, was openly practicing medicine in defiance of the law; and Dr. José Guillén, though "not vicious," in disregard of a warning given him in 1780 went on violating two laws: that apothecary shops should be operated only by licensed pharmacists and that no man could write prescriptions to be filled by relatives, much less write and fill his own. Besides, did not the city attorney admit that the religious, Nava and Zagarraga, both practiced medicine? As a climax to its statement, the protomedicato asked whether the city attorney would be responsible if Dr. Melica made some disastrous blunder.[50] The cabildo denied that its order was merely to allow the unlicensed to go on practicing while drawing out the litigation.[51] Díaz Chacón himself, after three years had already elapsed, complained in 1790 that though he had the viceroy's license to carry on the commission, his enemies had found ways to defeat the inspection. Meanwhile, with drugs illegally handled and curanderos rampant, "nobody knows to this day how the matter got lost." Now exceedingly wroth, Díaz Chacón let the viceroy know that the empirics and the cabildo had held up the inspection of the medical professions for eleven long years. In fact, just at the beginning of January, a curandero administered herbage to a young lady who died nine hours afterward without the sacraments and without a confessor, though begging for both. The curandero, he concluded, went free.[52]

Called upon a second time to state its view and making use of such bitter testimony as that of Díaz Chacón, the protomedicato tried to din it into the ears of the viceroy that, in defiance of his authorization, the cabildo of Querétaro had postponed a reckoning of eleven years. The result: the drugstores were in a state of "abandon," the curanderos despotic, and the legitimate doctors "oppressed."[53] The opponents of Díaz Chacón, however, had a case, and his inspection, whether it took place or not, had its consequences. The subdelegate inspected the drugstores and declared them all in fine condition. The cabildo of Querétaro made a convincing apology for the state of medicine there. Suffering from some kind of mental inertia, Guillén was now too sick to practice if he wanted to. Of the two religious practitioners, one had gone to Mexico City to become secretary of that province, and the other had retired on account of "this hullabaloo." Of those originally charged, only Dr. Melica, the Italian, remained. Still, because of his "accredited instruction" and "honorific titles," the municipality felt he should go on practicing during the two years the crown had allowed him to get his naturalization. Innumerable Europeans were "living here" in spite of the laws, and Dr. Melica's profession was "useful to the republic"—a legal ground for tolerating a foreigner in the Indies. With the death of Dr. León, "only two doctors, one of them Díaz Chacón, remained to take care of a city from 45,000 to 50,000 souls."[54] This visita, then, beginning with so much firmness, just died with no accomplishment beyond that of producing alarm. The government in Mexico City took the position of Querétaro and suspended Díaz Chacón's commission.[55]

Thus, only the case of Melica remained suspended, but by 1794, of course, his time had run out, forcing the Superior Government to rule that he must either present his documents to the protomedicato and get a license or cease practicing. Drs. Díaz Chacón and Ramón del Guante, two of the original enemies of quackery in Querétaro, examined Melica and found him afflicted with symptoms of "nervous hypochondria" that rendered him "profoundly irritable and immobile." A better diagnosis is that the sight of Díaz Chacón and Guante rendered him profoundly irritable and speechless as well. The remedy: a more humid climate! The dry one of Querétaro "would only exacerbate Melica's symptoms" and render them incurable.[56] Then, at the last moment, it turned out that Melica was telling the truth when he claimed that his brother had dispatched his letter of naturalization. By this document, reaching Mexico before the end of April 1794, the Council of the Indies decided that, since he had established his blood purity and produced proof that he was a doctor from the University of Turin, he should be given the protection of the crown.[57] He then carried his case to the viceroy against the "tricks" of the other doctors to get him out of town and won there, too.[58]

Repeatedly baffled in its efforts to "put limits" on the illicit practice of medicine, pharmacy, and surgery in Querétaro, the protomedicato, nothing daunted, returned to the hopeless fray in 1794. As Díaz Chacón was now a marked man in his own town, the tribunal assigned Joaquín Muro to this task only "to have obstacles put in his way as happened before." Not very well advised by his fiscal, Viceroy Revilla Gigedo refused his permission on the grounds that the laws of the Indies[59] assigned the handling of drug inspection to viceroys, presidents, and governors. Moreover, other laws authorized the ordinary justices, and not the protomedicato, to prosecute persons without the required degrees and licenses. Accordingly, partly because it was expensive to have an inspector coming and going from Mexico City, the senior alcalde of Querétaro, accompanied by a Spanish druggist, José Francisco Aranda, undertook to inspect all the pharmacies in town.[60] Who the "expert" was when the "visitors" came to the shop of Aranda himself the record does not say. As invariably happened when the civil and not the medical officials conducted the inspections, "all was in good order." Appointed yet again in 1796, Dr. Miguel Díaz Chacón sprang a sudden inspection in Querétaro and, deliberately concealing his commission, entrapped and fined Aranda and another Spanish pharmacist, Francisco García, who had previously spurned an order of the protomedicato to submit their papers and licenses. Viceroy Branciforte, however, annoyed with the ineptitude of the protomedicato in the smallpox epidemic then raging, denied it authority to stage drug inspections and ordered the fines returned.[61]

These rebuffs and frustrations in Querétaro meant that the authority of the protomedicato had been foiled and its prestige sullied. So dimmed was the luster of the protomedicato that late in 1797 some anonymous carper addressed a letter to the viceroy complaining that during the recent smallpox epidemic the druggists proved so ignorant and incompetent that it was astounding how they ever won their licenses in the first place. He thought that if the viceroy would ask the druggists themselves, "he would learn much to censure in this indolent and condescending protomedicato."[62] His view was that the ignorance of the protomédicos was great and the damage to the public greater. The viceroy went so far as to call attention to reports of incompetence during the epidemic and repeated that examinations might not be rigorous enough. When the royal protomedicato answered, however, it voluntarily acknowledged that a similar "denunciation" made in Revilla Gigedo's time was found to be false. Perhaps, the protomédicos mused, their critic was machinating "the bastard satisfaction of revenge" for failing an examination. They rested their case in the hope that truth would triumph over calumny.[63] No longer particularly concerned, the viceroy urbanely and tritely hoped that the right thing was being done,[64] ending exactly twenty years of complete and utter futility.

Prosecution of Illicit Practitioners

"Curanderism" was so universal that evidence of it is left behind only when some competitor with a license, and sometimes without, appeared and, professing to be overcome with horror at the damage being done to the health of his majesty's subjects, by some dose of mercury or *"píldoras de opis,"* cried out to heaven and, less often, to the authorities. These intermittent and ineffectual outbursts usually followed some grievous outrage. A typical petition to the royal protomedicato was that of Miguel de Lemus y Tapia, calling for the required letter of authorization to prosecute all types of intrusos in San Andrés de Chalchicomula in New Spain. To support this strong request, Lemus charged that Diego Rusi, from "overseas," had treated a patient for a fistula, "which not only did not relieve him" but "left him dying in awful pain." To a woman, shortly after childbirth, he gave a "remedy" that "left her dead in three days."[65] The protomedicato gave the petitioner the proper writ, but required him to work through the king's magistrates instead of constituting itself a court. Six years later the licensed physician Manuel Villegas

Clavijo of Taxco got a similar warrant to proceed against "the many" who practiced without a license or elaborated and sold drugs in the same illegal way.[66] If these prosecutions, or any others like them, amounted to anything, the records of the protomedicato do not show it.

In 1723 Dr. Marcos José Salgado, a protomédico of New Spain, entreated the king to act against "intruders" who, protected by "powerful personages," practiced medicine without reference to the protomedicato.[67] This, he reasoned, was a gross infringement of his rights as protomédico and in prejudice of the other physicians who "spent their patrimony on their degrees and examinations." Salgado was not so slow as to neglect mentioning the harm the intruders' blunders caused the public. The crown responded by giving verbal support to the protomedicato in enforcing the laws against curanderos, even against those who had practiced for a long time.[68] The records of the protomedicato indicate that this typical ambition ended in a characteristically empty paper victory.

Complaints against members of religious orders were few, yet the vitality Dr. García Jove gave to the royal protomedicato at the end of the eighteenth century did upon occasion involve them. In 1795, for example, the protomedicato got word that the lay brother Antonio Bera of Monterrey "claimed to cure without distinction all types of ailments" without establishing his ability for "such extensive accomplishments." Since Bera had taken up medicine at the request of the town and diocesan council, his guardian wrote the protomedicato that it would "not have the slightest cause to return to this complaint."[69] The prior of the Carmelite convent in Mexico City was not, however, so urbane and placating. An "erroneous" charge from the protomedicato that the agent (*procurador*) of the convent had given medicines improperly stuck under the skin of the reverend father. The procurador had merely administered a prescription of an established doctor but only on the advice of Dr. Gracida, a protomédico, and with the understanding that the patient would call that physician if the fever did not subside. The prior's succinct conclusion went to the heart of the problem: "Poor unhappy ones who have no means to pay for a doctor and medicine!"[70]

The curanderas, the female medicasters, had a baffling defense even when they were transparent quacks. When arrested, they had the adroitness to swear that they undertook treatment only when there was no time to go for a doctor for fear the patient might die. They were, they said, merely nurses giving prescriptions written by licensed doctors, which they arranged beforehand to certify. To deny them this right would have made it necessary, on the basis of strict logic, not to allow mothers, sisters, daughters, or "other charitable persons" to give medicines to their relatives in their own houses. And, since there were many patients without these family connections, those with means hired experienced women to come into their homes to render this service. Others, lacking "root property" such as houses or other substantial means, made shift to rent a bed in the house of some curandera, which, at best, was a nursing home and, at worst, a clandestine hospital. If she had become famous, the operator enjoyed special terms of endearment and sometimes of awe.

One of these was Doña María Antonia López, La Beata,[71] brought to the bar of medical justice in 1791. Reared as the ward of a physician and married to a surgeon, she had a better chance to learn medicine than any country curandero. Affecting religious dress, she often laid hold upon the soul as well as the body of her patients. In fact, La Beata herself collected more than fees; a man no less highly placed than a colonel, Francisco Rivero, left her a legacy in 1790.[72] Owing to the dyspepsia of Dr. García Jove, the presiding protomédico in 1791, however, the tribunal was especially active against its "enemies," like La Beata. Word had gone abroad that this woman "went about publicly treating all kinds of illnesses," and that she kept patients in her house as a kind of hospital "in serious detriment of the public health," enough to get the order out for her arrest.[73] The depositions in this preparatory process (*sumaria*) reveal, in unconscious asides, how slippery medical prosecution really was. They show that the defendant claimed that she took persons into her own house because she could not go hither and yon nursing.[74] They also reveal that she had many resident patients with others coming in from the streets.[75]

In the midst of this case a scandal involving the protomedicato itself broke. Dionisio Castellanos, a copyist drawn in by the clerk of that tribunal to assist him, went to La Beata's house and offered to sell her information "greatly to her advantage" for twenty-five pesos. A woman left the house, however, while the bribe—"half in advance"—was being solicited, and police officers (*comisarios de la Acordada*) soon appeared and made inquiries. Castellanos was then arrested—"seized by the throat," he put it—and thrown into jail at the instance of the protomedicato. After the evidence was gathered, the tribunal, making dire threats, barred the greedy amanuensis from serving it, or anybody having business with it, as a clerk.[76] This defection of the tribunal's copyist interrupted the preparation of this case for a whole fortnight. Then, when a solitary woman deponent testified that La Beata had applied an unction to her for clogged lungs, the protomedicato had proof at last of a fact long known.

The testimony of La Beata herself[77] is a classic demonstration of the curandera's agile defense. True, she said, she had treated various people for syphilis, including the Carmelite friar Juan San Angelo. She claimed, however, that she treated other individuals only when allowed no time to look for doctors. Her other treatments were under the direction of a doctor, something that often required her to go out at "inconvenient" times—presumably when the doctor would not. What she had received had been neither fees nor charges but gratification made by the patients themselves. Except in the doctor's prescriptions, she did not claim to have anything more than some sarsaparilla, guaiacum, and a few syrups compounded of these simples. Nor did the clerk and bailiff (*ministro executor*) of the protomedicato, Francisco Carabantes, when they went to the defendant's house, find any patients or any medicine beyond a little sarsaparilla. But, since La Beata had four weeks' warning, what did they expect?[78]

Carrying out a sentence that involved corporal or even capital punishment was easier in Mexico than collecting a stiff fine from a poor defendant. Nevertheless, in view of La Beata's confession, the fiscal of the protomedicato advised the tribunal to fine her according to Spanish law.[79] When the fine amounted to fifty-five pesos four reales, she claimed that, as a sister of a Franciscan missionary, it would be unseemly for her to go to jail. She tried to settle for thirty pesos, but finally in 1792, when someone else agreed to make up the difference in monthly installments, the case came to rest.

Conclusion

Spanish colonials fully understood the plight of their medicine. Had it not been for their jeremiads on the scarcity of doctors, no one today could well establish the case that there was a shortage. They were not tempted, as are the facetious in these times, to say that even if the natives had enough academic physicians to go around, they would have been no better off. In fact, in all the records turned up, only one contemporary official made this argument.[80] The Spaniard in the cities actually winced when he heard how the poor natives went on bathing, or even stepped up the pace of it, when stricken with measles or smallpox. The colonial physician, of course, knew next to nothing about the etiology of disease, but he was drilled in diagnosis and therapeutics. Moreover, difficult as it was, he kept in touch with the new medical literature from Great Britain, France, Italy, and Spain.

The inveterate curanderismo in the Spanish colonies was owing, in good measure, to the failure of the crown to find or earmark sufficient funds for medical education. More particularly, though, this evil was a consequence of the scarcity of legally qualified physicians, the isolation of the populace from the legitimate physicians who did practice, and an oppressive poverty that left the majority of the people dependent upon the charity of doctors they could not have reached even if they had had the money. The alternative was the curandero, and, though he was called an intruder, he was more the result of demand than of aggressive intrusion. For this reason, prosecution of "curers," even in the less superstitious "Spanish" cities and capitals, was half-hearted, infrequent, and ineffective. Viceregal officials, but not established doctors, preferred a prudent and humane interpretation that bent the law to the circumstances.

The cardinal error of medicine in Spanish America—as true of the republics as of the colonies—lay in retaining standards so rigid and high they could not be reached, or if reached, by far too few. What was indicated was something like the British method in the South Pacific in modern times—the selection of some healthy, bright young natives for instruction in the elements of bonesetting and in coping with common diseases and accidents. Prominent citizens sometimes advocated bringing youths from the towns and villages, but they could never bring themselves to suggest limited training for a second class of practitioners. Because surgery was so low in the scale of prestige, the Spaniards did approximate this solution for this art; they allowed men to practice once they had assisted and observed a surgeon for five years. The majority of these, unhappily, had to be examined with the prerequisite certificate of blood purity or else not at all. So deep-seated was curanderismo, that these licensed romance surgeons eased inexorably over into the practice of internal medicine until, as the legitimate physicians bewailed, they "reached the execrable extreme of holding consultations."[81] Even they found quackery more profitable and prestigious than legitimate practice.

IN THE SPANISH EMPIRE the more persistent the violations, the more often the law was repeated. The crown itself recognized this when, all but in despair, it prefaced a law with the plaintive introduction that "there is no prohibition more often repeated than that forbidding foreigners to go to the Indies without our express license."[1] Why should this be so?

For one thing, the very factors that encouraged the curanderos across the country, through the villages, towns, to the very walls of the viceregal capitals, invited not only the legitimate foreign physician but also the foreign fraud. A full quarter of a century after the conquest of Mexico City, for example, the 150,000 inhabitants of the city and the millions in the countryside faced the inevitable sweep of epidemic diseases over the unimmunized population with one solitary doctor—and he was under sentence for forging his license. Little wonder that both the town council and the cathedral chapter, headed by the bishop, begged the crown to be merciful!

Yet the mere lack of physicians was not the only thing that favored the foreign intruder; the foreigner also had all the allure that makes the word "imported" so magical in colonies and new countries. Even in Spain, Benito Jerónimo Feijóo, a realistic, sensible reformer, recognized that though French medical treatises were full of "obscurity, uncertainty, and falsehoods," Spaniards took them for little less than revelation. The French, he remarked, said that their medicine was the worst of all. Few Spaniards accepted this view, however, and if a French physician of no more than "median reputation" crossed the Pyrenees, the Spaniards "thought that they had gained a man capable of restoring souls from the other world."[2] In America, where the subject population could regard a bulbous nose as a sign of occult curative power, even their white conquerors could not be blamed for investing the foreigner with power over life and death.

Spanish Law and Foreign Practitioners in the Indies

To begin, who was a foreigner to the Spaniards?[3] Everybody except a native of "these kingdoms" was a foreigner.[4] As Portugal was not one of "these," a Portuguese was a foreigner. Citizens of countries in "friendship and alliance" with Spain, as potential emigrants, were also aliens.

In such a jealous regime the prerequisites of naturalization were hardly less complex than being born again—and in the right place this time. Though these laws specifically forbade any foreigner or "prohibited person" from going to the Indies, foreigners might go when naturalized and, like Spaniards, secure a license. The first requisite of naturalization was that the applicant be Catholic, but this was so taken for granted that ten times more laws dealt with the foreigner in trade than with the foreigner's religion. Even so a man had to be in the Indies for twenty years continuously, even if he had entered legally, before he could become a citizen. For ten of these years he had to hold real estate or "root property," not just movable goods, valued at four thousand ducats. This carefully inventoried property could be acquired by inheritance, by deed (*escritura*) supposedly through his wife, by purchase, or by other title, all to be determined through legal documents—not just the testimony of witnesses. Something else as much calculated to tie a man down as real estate—marriage to a native—was the third condition of naturalization. Even so, the Council of the Indies had to declare formally the conditions of naturalization fulfilled legally before the king's "letter of naturalization" could speed—at eight knots an hour—upon its way. And of course, legally speaking, no man could stay for twenty years unless he had been legally recognized as a proper emigrant for a payment (*compuesto*) and duly licensed by the Casa de Contratación—or classified as in a useful "mechanical trade." Some ten laws forbade the foreigner's trading, especially in gold, silver, or cochineal, but it was their enforcement that proved so difficult. Not even foreigners entering the empire with a license might remain in a seaport. Instead, the duty of governors and viceroys was to retire them a safe distance from ports and to watch their occupations and activities closely. As for the "foreign bachelors," the injunction was not to "retire" them from the ports but "to throw them out" and, if they were without proper papers, to "throw" them out of the Indies. When the English Lords Proprietors were taking their first slices of the Spanish empire, Spanish viceroys and governors in America got orders to round up all foreigners without entry permits and remit them to the House of Trade in Seville. But these required entry licenses, the crown admitted, were the most futile prohibition in all the laws of the Indies.

The laws against entry made up only a part of the barrier against foreign physicians and surgeons. The protomédicos were under a special charge to protect all the royal laws in the handling of medical problems. The law that no one might practice either medicine or surgery without a proper academic degree and a license, by implication, applied to foreigners. In fact, the Castilian laws on medicine made applicable to America in 1535 carried a requirement that no one "prohibited by the laws" might lay claim to any medical title if he had not been examined, approved, and graduated in a recognized university. And in America by the time of Philip II, every man wishing to practice had to appear personally for examination. And, of course, a foreigner without a license to be in the country in the first place and without a diploma from any university was obviously suspect.

Philip II put it upon the statute books that any man graduated in surgery or medicine "outside these kingdoms" of Spain should be obliged to submit to an examination by the royal protomedicato before practicing in Spain.[5] "Natural law" dictated, though, that the university, as with those in Spain, should be an approved one.[6] It also stands to reason that, if a man were allowed to come before a tribunal to test his scientific fitness, he would have the royal permission to stay in the country for that purpose—either by "tolerance" or by naturalization.

The laws probably had some deterring effect upon those who might have wished to lead their lives in the Indies aboveboard, but those who had to sneak into an empire were not abashed about sneaking into a profession. Consequently, long periods passed when not one bit of evidence appeared in the documents, either that foreigners were entering or that they were present. Then, some headstrong foreigner, perhaps even deranged, would force attention upon himself by scoffing at the monarchy or even at religion. To handle the individual case that had so uncomfortably emerged was not enough; to protect themselves against the charge that they had allowed seditious elements to infiltrate, harried viceroys and governors called for a census of all foreigners, especially those "known to be in this state." The internal evidence is plain that they knew there were many.

When the crown ran into cases where the colonial officials had "suspended the law" and tolerated foreign doctors, it showed its impatience by ordering those relaxing to "round up" these foreigners and to "remit forthwith," or by the next ship, all those illegal residents. As these infractions were treated as separate cases, the Council of the Indies avoided coming face to face with the problem of composition (*composición*)—making exactions on foreigners living illegally in the Indies. Thus, when the English physician Juan de Binde Banque went from

Jamaica to the Bay of Campeche with five companions, they were all arrested and carried to Havana, where they "remained in great misery." An envoy extraordinary of England reported this incident and begged the Spanish king to order these men released. The king responded, however, by commanding that the men be sent to Spain at the first opportunity so that the proper resolution could be made of the case.[7]

In the sixteenth and seventeenth centuries the issue of the foreign practitioner was really like a jet from a punctured hose, but new pressure built up after the arrival of the Bourbons in Spain, though the law that citizens of friendly and allied countries were to be considered foreigners and excluded from the Indies remained on the statute books. Then especially after the Family Pact of 1733, officials in America lost their fear of foreigners in general and Frenchmen in particular. In fact, only in the viceregal documents, the very highest category in America, is any distinction made between the British and the French. Sometimes, there seemed an almost perverse custom that made local officials refer to a Frenchman as English and to an Englishman as French. And, when we run through the garbled spelling to which every name was subjected when each new factotum took up pen, it is a surprise that the poor devils were not labeled Chinese.

There were two stages to the disenchantment with foreigners in medicine under the Bourbons. The first came after 1700, when the duly licensed creole physicians, especially those on the tribunal of the protomedicato, began to feel "inundated" by the foreigners among the native-born medicasters. (The ignorant local empirics did not endanger the profitable practice in the mining towns and metropolitan centers.) The second stage came when the eighteenth-century revolutions left the Spanish regalists with a growing state of dread. Either the Frenchmen who had long been present were tempted to vaunt their superiority by assuming a "revolutionary" tone or the creoles and peninsulars for the first time began to attach importance to what they said. And nearly all these appeared within striking distance of the Caribbean and Gulf ports.

In the first half of the eighteenth century the government was lax in admitting foreigners and casual in handling those who had entered covertly. Not everyone accepted this drift with equanimity, however, for the Latin physicians—both Spanish and creole—felt the competition. Upon occasion, too, the large number of foreigners practicing without licenses, when added to the legitimate concern about curanderos, began to worry the members of the royal protomedicato. In keeping with the eighteenth-century disdain for the American as an intellectual being, viceroys sometimes appeared with Frenchmen in their retinue. In 1723 the chief protomédico of New Spain, Dr. Marcos José Salgado, did not mince words: Mexico was being "buried" by "various subjects, many of them foreigners, who under the protection of powerful persons" had taken up the practice of medicine without being examined, approved, or licensed. For him it was galling indeed to have to sit by while these foreign fellows were summoned to the salons of the great houses. Dr. Salgado thought this practice was injurious to those men who had spent their patrimony, not to mention their youth, in preparing for the examinations required by law, but he also hit the refrain that the practice caused grave damage to the health of the king's vassals, who risked their lives and spent their money in vain. He then petitioned the king to issue the necessary orders and cédulas to force the viceroy and audiencia to give the support necessary to the protomedicato to arrest, try, and punish these bold empirics.[8]

The crown attorney, a lawyer first of all, opined that the memorial did not come with supporting documents, that no action could be taken upon the simple assertion of a single party. He thought that all remedies necessary were already in the laws of the Indies. Upon his recommendation, though, the council approved a royal cédula enjoining the viceroy and audiencia to give the royal protomedicato all the aid necessary to prevent the slightest injury in this most serious matter.[9]

Though foreign doctors filtered into all the viceroyalties, these foreigners, "especially Portuguese New Christians not very certain in the faith" had poured into the ports, mostly on the slave ships, ready to trade and, perchance, to subvert the Indians.[10] Most numerous in the Caribbean and in Mexico, they steadily increased in numbers during the eighteenth century. Of the nine foreigners involved in litigation, or otherwise getting their names into the official papers of Mexico during the first half of the eighteenth century, four were French, two Scottish, one English, one Portuguese, and one Italian. In the second half, among a total of eleven so involved, seven were French, one English, and three Italian. The natural deduction is that those for whom records are lacking appeared from the various countries in about the same proportion. There is no way, however, to be sure what the total was, for much of their practice was clandestine. In fact, so much was stealthily concealed that Latin physicians, in Mexico City at least, complained that foreigners and curanderos had inundated them.

Foreign Physicians in Mexico

By the end of the first quarter of the eighteenth century Mexican physicians had begun to feel the competition of foreign practitioners. In 1723 Protomédico Marcos José Salgado had made a bitter complaint about the "inundation" by quacks, many of them foreigners, but the best he could get was a condescending response from viceregal officials. Five years later the whole tribunal of the protomedicato begged the king to expel the foreigners who were practicing without license and without permission to be in the country in the first place. Of course, the first concern of all established physicians in Mexico City was with the incurable problem of the curanderos, who, though tolerated in the remote, purely Indian villages, also made their way into the cities. Though these might menace public health, they created no economic jeopardy, for the Indians could not pay fees to attract the Latin physician. So, it was when foreigners, without license, joined these native medicasters that both the professional and economic hackles of established physicians began to rise. It was fashionable to look to foreigners, especially Frenchmen, for everything superior in medicine. In consequence, these exotic types were welcome "in the greatest houses" and hence much desired by all others in the society.

The protomedicato, now as always, made out the case that these men—unexamined and unlicensed either by the protomedicato in Mexico or Madrid—were not only dangerous to the public health but that they also undermined the privileges conceded to the protomedicato by the king. Specifically, the protomedicato petitioned the king to order the proper authorities in New Spain to ship out all those practicing without being examined and to punish those resisting with "fines and prisons" to discourage such actions in the future. Giving advice accepted by the Council of the Indies, the fiscal cited the law that required any man practicing surgery or medicine in New Spain since the early seventeenth century to have "the degrees and licenses of the protomedicato required by law,"[11] that the fiscals be asked to take this into account, and that in their residencias lack of enforcement be taken into account.[12]

Still, despite these timid efforts at restriction, elbowing from foreign practitioners had begun to push aside even the most secure physicians in Mexico. In 1741, for example, the administrator of the Royal Indian Hospital directed a complaint to the king: Dr. Juan de Baeza, he said, was a person of such good conduct and reputation that he was elected to treat the Indians. Moreover—that crowning glory of a successful practice—he had been called "to the principal houses of that city, even to that of the archbishop." Despite all this, though, someone too fearsome to mention had violently stripped him of his post and put in his place a "foreign doctor" just arrived in the kingdom—also with a name too powerful to bruit about. Worse than that, the foreign doctor lacked that prerequisite which creole physicians stressed so much—a knowledge of the predilections and characteristic sicknesses of the inhabitants. The burden of this plea was that Baeza had been removed without cause and should be restored to his post.[13] The Council of the Indies obligingly agreed and, what is more, gave instructions that the name of the person making the complaint be omitted from the cédula ordering the restoration of Baeza.[14]

Physicians of British origin also appeared in New Spain in surprisingly large numbers at the very time Oglethorpe was pushing Florida for its existence and English interlopers were having incessant encounters with Spanish coastal patrols that eventually erupted in the War of Jenkins' Ear. Despite its "repeated laws" against foreigners residing in America, the Spanish government had also authorized a Frenchman, presumably one with the proper degree and license, to go to Peru to practice medicine.[15] Immediately, Santiago Estevanzos—James Stevenson—sent a memorial to the king of Spain, appealing on this precedent for permission to live in New Spain and practice medicine. The king turned to the Council of the Indies.[16] Estevanzos, on his own words, was a Scot, Roman Catholic, a "supposed-to-be" doctor, who had been in Mexico practicing medicine "for some years" with approval for teaching natives ("expertizing" them was the phrase) the medicines of Europe and holding solemn anatomical demonstrations that, since he petitioned to continue these, he must have thought overawed his auditors. But the practiced eye of the crown attorney ferreted out the unmentioned ingredients. Estevanzos had come to New Spain and had maintained himself there without a royal license, despite the repeated laws and cédulas forbidding foreigners to enter or reside there. Moreover, there were strict laws stipulating the years of study in approved universities[17] required to practice in the Spanish world: for the bachelor's degree in medicine, the examination, and the two years' practice with an approved physician. Either in surgery or in medicine, no one could practice in the Indies without examination by the protomedicato and a license from it.[18] The Council of the Indies also had other sources of information, a "certain report" that Estevanzos was not qualified. Moreover, his penchant for parading as an anatomist, most likely getting under the skin of the professor of anatomy in the university, had led to his banishment from Mexico City.[19] The king then ordered Estevanzos put under arrest and returned to Spain at the first opportunity.[20]

Like most of these medical knights of the road, Stevenson—for it now begins to be certain that that was his name—began a flexible campaign to return to New Spain that enabled him to push the crown for something, not one rung under but one above, what the government was disposed to grant. Within a year Stevenson had somehow established that he was a physician "with a doctor's degree from the University of Leyden in the Low Countries." On this ground, seemingly, the royal protomedicato in Madrid agreed to examine him and, more to the point, passed him. With this firm ground under his shaky career, Stevenson went straight for a license to return to the Indies to practice medicine undisturbed anywhere, especially in New Spain. The right to return to New Spain and practice there the king graciously conceded.[21] He might even take one servant—a Spaniard—his personal clothes, and equipment necessary for the practice of his profession, provided he was not married in "these kingdoms," was not one "of those forbidden to go over to the Indies," and was able to produce evidence of his identity. His request for naturalization was ignored; he might go despite the fact that he was a foreigner.[22]

This critical point past, seventeen years after beginning practice in 1711 and fifteen after starting in New Spain, Stevenson was brazen enough to present a vita (*relación de méritos*) as if he might be some proud conqueror instead of an adventurer on the brink of being exposed as a fraud. This bold step was designed to induce the king to give him the honorary title of protomédico general of New Spain without any salary whatsoever so that he could "continue his services with more honor." When the council permitted him to return to New Spain in 1727, it authorized him to hold anatomical demonstrations in Mexico and to "dispute the materials" involved, but it left it up to the viceroy whether to accord him precedence in public acts. The privilege and title he sought demanded learning and advancement, and in Mexico and Lima the two professors of prima of medicine by law[23] were the protomédicos given the honor of presiding over meetings and functions in order to give dignity to medicine and encourage its study. That Stevenson had "neither the learning nor the experience comparable to that which he solicits, nor even to much less . . ." was cause for rejection of the request. That such a man should "wish to precede all the physicians of New Spain and enjoy all the other privileges attached to the post was despicable," a patent and flagrant abuse of the professors of medicine in the university. The crown took only two words to agree with the recommendation: "as stated [*como parece*]."[24]

A foreign doctor never petitioned to enter the Spanish dominions; he merely appeared, either in the Indies or in Spain. The circumstances, even those supported by the most convincing and pathetic stories, were always suspect. How could a magistrate differentiate between a harried and a furtive soul if the aspiring physician had lost his diploma and license, as he invariably claimed? And if he presented diplomas and licenses might these not be forged? Hence, any English said-to-be doctor in the first half of the eighteenth century, or any Frenchman of the same stamp in the second half, was likely to attract patients for the same reason that he aroused distrust.

When he had a shred of plausibility, the expatriate English physician always appealed to the Spanish crown on the grounds that he was a harried and persecuted Catholic. In 1739, for example, Dr. Juan de Ynglevi (Engleby?), an Englishman professing to be a graduate of Montpellier, appeared in Madrid with a strange medical odyssey. Living in Jamaica with his wife and two daughters, he found himself on the eve of the War of Jenkins' Ear required to abjure the "Catholic religion he professed." When he refused to comply, he was thrown into jail, where he remained until he "precipitately absented himself, with notable penalties and loss of property, and retired to the Island of Cuba." From there he went to Mexico City in the hope that Viceroy Juan Antonio de Vizarrón y Eguiarreta (1734–40) would take him under his protection. There, however, the royal protomedicato opposed his practicing with the claim that he needed the "examination and license" of the royal protomedicato in Madrid. Thus, with still more "penalties and loss of property," one can be sure, he had turned up in Madrid, submitted to the examination, passed, and received a title on March 21, 1739. Now he could approach the throne with a petition for a passport and naturalization for himself and family in the Indies, especially in New Spain, and practice medicine freely there.

Such an unwarranted concession required some persuasive arguments. Ynglevi had the classic ones. He "had always professed the holy Catholic faith," and he would treat the poor absolutely free of charge. The crown sympathized with his zeal for the faith and the losses he had sustained in his prolonged flight from Jamaica and acceded to his supplications.[25] And so, in a few weeks he found himself with a license authorizing him to return to his wife and daughters in Mexico City, taking with him "the brown" servant he had brought into the country. Though treated with respect, Ynglevi had to swear not to aid or abet any person entering the Indies by stealth (*polizón*).[26]

George Abercromby, a Scottish resident in New Spain, lacked several of Ynglevi's requisites. He was a doctor by profession, but his credentials were far from being of "general acceptance and usefulness to the public," something a trifle short of an M.D. from Montpellier. He was, though, "Catholic, Roman apostolic," married to a vassal of the king from Veracruz. He had also lived for more than twelve years in Yucatán, having come there as a factor of the South Sea Company in San Francisco de Campeche. For twelve years he practiced medicine there, winning the respect of his neighbors—neighbors who stood often in mortal fear of certain if not swift death in their families.

Then Abercromby returned to Spain, and Alejandro Gutiérrez de Rubalcaba, president of the House of Trade, allowed him to go to England to settle his accounts with the company. That done, he went back to Spain by way of Holland and made an application for naturalization in New Spain. In support of his application he offered strong recommendations from the governor of the province, the provisor, the vicar general, the bishop, the ecclesiastical and secular cabildos of Mérida de Yucatán, the rector of the University of Mérida, and the city council of San Francisco de Campeche. These revealed "not the slightest note of scandal" in all of Abercromby's twelve years in that country. In the Spanish bureaucratic system, however, he had the misfortune not to approach the throne armed with a letter from the viceroy in Mexico City. Moreover, since he had not resided in Mexico in twenty years or "held root property" for twelve consecutive years, the crown rejected the petition.[27] Nevertheless, the crown was still inclined to encourage even those physicians who had no better title than "general acceptance."

What pretext could be scraped up for tolerance in this case? In the first place, if a legally qualified practitioner even came to such a remote place, he came by accident. Besides, physicians were not included in the repeated orders requiring the expulsion of foreigners from the king's American dominions; their profession was "useful to the commonwealth." Abercromby had "abjured" his Protestantism, accepted baptism, and been "born spiritually" in San Francisco de Campeche. Thus in 1745, when England and Spain were at least technically at war, the king of Spain gave Abercromby the right to return to New Spain and practice medicine and later in the year supplied him with a letter of naturalization.

At the same time the king invoked all the precautions the laws specified in such cases. When he came to embark, Abercromby had to swear that his servant was not leaving a wife behind or practicing any other deception that would make him one of those *polizónes*—idlers without license to emigrate to the colonies.[28] Neither might this versatile Scot engage in trade and overseas commerce, nor live within twenty leagues of any seaport or coast. This last condition he protested as "morally impossible," because "the interior towns of those provinces" were reduced to such poverty by want of commerce that not one of them could support a doctor.

Because he lacked the legal qualifications for naturalization and because some doctor—trained or not trained—was needed, what was more natural than to fill the gap and at the same time exact the price of a royal *gracias al sacar?* This little balm was to be "200 pesos at fifteen reales de vellón each." This smoothed the way for the Scot "to live and reside in my kingdoms of the Indies . . ." and, as a citizen, to enjoy all the honors, favors, and benefits enjoyed by those born in "those king-doms." Now, he could not only practice his profession of medicine but also hold all political and military offices and engage in trade except with "other foreigners."[29]

Yucatán was also the door through which William Joseph Bates, a native of London resident in Mérida, came to enter Mexico and, in the same convenient and informal way, to take up the medical profession. His entrance into Mexico was more precipitate, however, than the arrival of his practice; he was cast up in a storm at Ascension Bay. Allowed out of considerations of mercy to go into the interior of New Spain, Bates soon came to Valladolid, where by October he was already "instructed in the dogmas of our holy religion" and baptized and launched into the practice of medicine. There the next year he married Doña Josefa Es-cobedo and sired a son who did so well in the Royal and Pontifical Triden-tine College that the proud father began to have hopes that he would "follow a literary career," take academic degrees, and go into a profes-sion. This in turn necessitated a letter of naturalization.

In 1785, therefore, Bates went to the crown with his petition for citizenship. Beyond being Catholic and married in the country, he now proved that he had "root property" surpassing "by many degrees" the minimum of four thousand ducats required by the law; he had also been in the country for twenty-one years practicing medicine "with the great-est applause, application, zeal, disinterestedness, and charity." Besides, during the American Revolution, he had made a "donation" to the crown for use against his fatherland, had served as interpreter for some prisoners of war, and at last, in view of "the voluntary payment of one hundred pesos," the king condescended to grant his petition for citizen-ship.[30] Moreover, the price of naturalization in the next fifteen years went up to 8,200 reales.[31] That Bates was certain to practice medicine without a proper license was passed over in silence.

Though one would expect Portuguese and Italian physicians, speak-ing romance languages and professing Catholicism, to be the most numerous in the Spanish empire, they appeared much less frequently than did the British and French. One of them, Dr. Domingo Melica, a citizen of the Piedmont, claiming to be a doctor in medicine from the University of Turin, reached Mexico in the mid-1780s. He apparently presented himself to the tribunal of the protomedicato in Mexico City for examination and license to practice, but since Viceroy Matías de Gálvez (1783–84) had sent the protomedicato a royal cédula forbid-ding any foreigner to practice medicine without express license from the king, the tribunal simply declined to examine him.[32]

Still, the protomedicato could move in devious ways. It had issued a commission to Dr. Miguel Díaz Chacón, a physician in competition with Melica, to conduct an inspection of the medical profession in Querétaro. The design, according to those not in Díaz Chacón's coterie, was to lessen competition by disqualifying all those about whose right to practice there was any irregularity. And there were irregularities in the papers, if indeed they had any papers, of nearly all those practicing medicine in New Spain.[33] In the spring of 1790, then, Melica asked Viceroy Revilla Gigedo to concede him naturalization rights.[34] Melica got fifteen days to produce the documents entitling him to practice as well as the "license whereby he has come to these dominions."[35] Reporting on Melica's "career and conduct," the corregidor of Querétaro judged him to be successful "but envied." Perfectly reflecting this envy, the protomedicato in Mexico City stated officially[36] that Melica's being a foreigner worked against him. In the first place a royal cédula transmitted to the tribunal by Viceroy Matías de Gálvez made it patently illegal for him to practice medicine without the express license of the king. Indeed, it was on this ground that the protomedicato had refused to examine him "more than five years ago." Melica had not even paid the necessary fees. He clearly could not legally "treat the public."

This case, however, got mixed up with the quarrel over the control of medical practice in Querétaro. As a result, a visitor of the royal protomedicato in that city, who had obtained his appointment in a "sinister" way, forbade Melica to practice on the ground that the protomedicato had not examined him and that he was a foreigner. The viceroy decided, however, to grant Melica two years in which to get his naturalization papers, provided he presented himself within thirty days with papers to obtain his license.[37] Melica passed his examination before the protomedicato with honors on October 24, 1791.[38]

He had now legally demonstrated his blood purity and his qualifications to practice, but two years was too short time to get the zealously guarded naturalization papers from distant Spain. The Council of the Indies, to which he promptly appealed, rejected his application on the legalistic grounds that he had been in Mexico only four of the twenty years necessary for naturalization. Nevertheless, the council advised that, since Querétaro had only two doctors, Melica should receive a "letter of tolerance" allowing him to remain in practice in that city. All this argument, though, turned on the "100 pesos *fuertes*" Melica had submitted.[39]

French Physicians in Mexico

French physicians and surgeons began appearing in New Spain at the time of the Family Compact in 1733. Like the English, the French first made their appearance in Yucatán and Campeche where there were no Mexican physicians to denounce them as "unlicensed" when they got in ahead to treat the denizens of the "great houses." The natives were more than friendly; in fact, they were pathetically eager. They were subject not only to all the tropical ills but also to the epidemics that always hit the coast before they made their inexorable way across the rest of the kingdom. And on the coast, for some reason, the regions of Yucatán and Campeche were favorite starting points for plagues that ran west and north into New Spain and south into Guatemala.

One Frenchman from Bordeaux, Juan Lucás Toniero (Turneaux?), won naturalization in 1739 in circumstances that appear deceptively easy. Favoring him in that year was the alliance with France in the approaching war with England. Then, too, when he tried for his papers, he was qualified on every count. He had been living in San Francisco de Campeche for twenty-two years, had been married to a woman there for seventeen years, had four children by her, had acquired houses and other root property through her and by other means, had practiced medicine with charity, had answered the bell in the case of alarms, had appeared for all musters, and had paid 150 pesos into the treasury. For all this, he was allowed all the privileges of citizenship in the Indies, including the right to engage in trade and commerce—something foreign physicians found hard to manage in the zealously guarded mining region of central Mexico.[40]

A license issued in 1738 to Joseph Dumont, a Frenchman and "honorary physician of the king's bedchamber," indicated a growing liberalism in the treatment of foreigners wanting to practice medicine in the Indies. He might go to New Spain for that purpose, but he could only take his personal belongings. He might not embark in case he was married without his wife's consent and in "conformity with the law" on that subject. Once there, he might not engage in trade and commerce.[41]

Even more unorthodox was the application of the surgeon D. Baltasar Rous (Rons?) for naturalization in 1758.[42] Rous had appeared thirteen years before in Mérida de Yucatán where he got authorization to practice surgery. According to the leading lights of the cabildo in Mérida, he did this with the "greatest approbation." After two years he continued practice in Campeche, where he had a wife and children. Among his merits was the punctuality with which he responded when called, the "Christian zeal" with which he attended the poor, supplying not only his services free but also the medicine and food needed by his patients. And what was especially marked, he had shown his dedication for preserving the health of the Spaniards.[43] The fiscal of the Council of the Indies suggested Rous served a useful purpose and was therefore not legally liable[44] to expulsion as an ordinary foreign intruder, especially since the law aimed, most of all, to exclude foreigners from trade.[45] The Council of the Indies then confirmed the fiscal's recommendation that Rous not be expelled and that he be given naturalization to allow him to remain in Yucatán to practice, provided he did not engage in trade and commerce.[46] In all this Rous never once alluded to a formal education in surgery. Neither did he mention submitting to any kind of examination. "General acceptance" and the "applause" of the public were his titles. Even the fiscal and the Council of the Indies itself preferred to ignore this troublesome question. What was wanted was a competitor with a legitimate title, legitimately arrived at.

The surgeon Germán Ducruette of the Duchy of Savoy ran a group of hurdles in getting a license to practice in Mexico that might have kept another man waiting and litigating for a quarter of a century. He first went to Jamaica, whence, claiming he was not able to practice his "holy Catholic religion," he went to Guatemala in a Spanish brigantine that had been forced into a Jamaican port by a storm. In Guatemala surgeons were all but nonexistent, and the captain general, who did not generally arrogate this function, issued him a license. Thereupon, he practiced, as the petition always put it, "with general credit and applause" until he took it into his head to go to Mexico City to set up there. He submitted to examination by the royal protomedicato and received his license in September 1757, but then found himself threatened with expulsion as a foreigner under the terms of a new cédula issued on March 6, 1750. The Marquis of Amarillas, the viceroy, however, exempted Ducruette from this law, and the Council of the Indies upheld him.[47]

Before the French Revolution, especially in those times when the French were the allies of Spain, as they were during the American Revolution, French physicians and surgeons got into the Spanish empire with relative ease—even if they did enter illegally. José Laporta, a surgeon approved in the College of Montpellier and therefore assumed to be a Frenchman, was in such good graces with the Spanish government that he practiced surgery with skill and success in "different hospitals" before he obtained the post of chief surgeon in the Hospital de San Miguel in Guadalajara in June 1766. The very next year the Marqués de Croix ordered him, along with Guillermo Cis, to march as surgeon with the military expedition into Sonora. After this, in October 1771 the government made him surgeon of the Regiment of Spanish Dragoons, which he forsook in 1777 to return to Europe for reasons of health, but in 1781 he was petitioning for a post in a ship sailing from Cádiz to Havana in order to return to New Spain.[48]

Because the opportunities were fewer, French physicians rarely appeared on the Pacific Coast of the Spanish empire. Juan Bautista le Blond, however, was first received as a physician in the protomedicatos of Santa Fe and Peru. Then, from Paris, petitioning the Count of Floridablanca to go to New Spain to practice medicine, he was turned down in January 1786. Thereupon he sought out the Count of Aranda at Versailles and convinced him to present his case for naturalization to the Spanish government with the aim of going to the Indies; he "had an affection for those dominions and they agreed with his constitution." Besides, he was "a man of accomplishment, well disposed toward our nation, of which he speaks well on every occasion," and he came with a recommendation from the Count of Osuna. Aranda wanted Floridablanca to agree to "protect" le Blond in Madrid—to encourage his hope of naturalization—so that he could come to Madrid with that end in view. The minister, however, simply turned over the petition, as was perfectly orthodox, to the Council of the Indies.[49]

One of the most famous foreign residents of New Spain in the eighteenth century was the French physician, Esteban Morell. As in nearly all cases of foreigners practicing medicine in the Spanish empire, Morell simply showed up in America. He went from Guarico in Venezuela to Havana where, under the protection of the captain general, the Marqués de la Torre (1771–77), who issued him a license, he practiced medicine for some time. Then, betaking himself to Mexico, he had the royal protomedicato "revalidate" him. On the grounds that foreigners "holding mechanical jobs and employment useful to the Republic" might not be liable to expulsion under the law of 1750, with a decree of February 20, 1791, Viceroy Revilla Gigedo gave him permission to go on practicing until the king decided the matter. In November the Council of the Indies approved this resolution of the case but advised the viceregal government to keep Morell's conduct under a sharp eye.

Encouraged by this seeming tolerance, Morell then went to the mining guild and got a declaration that royal approval meant that his rights now extended to the working and claiming of mines. Another miner, however, in litigation with Morell contradicted this interpretation and asked the Superior Government for a clarification. The fiscal found that the legal advice and proceedings of the mining tribunal had been defective and that Morell had merely received permission to remain in the country to practice medicine. The assessor, though, thought that the royal order in question did not state precisely whether the permission was to allow Morell simply to remain to practice medicine or to continue some experiments on machinery for draining the mines. Taking all the facts together, he thought it was intended that Morell work mines if he chose, though he advised that the case remain open until the king had been consulted.

Meanwhile, in Madrid, the *Gazeta de México* of August 21, 1795, arrived carrying a news item that on August 9 the Tribunal of the Holy Office had condemned the French physician Esteban Morell "for formal heresy, deism, materialism, with the purposes of committing voluntary suicide. . . ." If this was true, of course, there was no need to consider further the doubts raised by the viceroy. Nevertheless, the Council of the Indies advised a rebuke for the mining guild. Besides, Morell was not in Mexico with royal approval or with a letter of naturalization—express requisites for the operation of mines by foreigners. And the council remarked on the "ease and abuse" with which the royal protomedicato incorporated and gave degrees to foreigners who were not naturalized as required by law. Besides, the council's report opined that in the future no one could be licensed under pretext of his capability or special talent. Neither should anyone be allowed to practice medicine or surgery who had not gone out to the Indies with a royal license or, being a foreigner, had not obtained a letter of naturalization according to the laws of the Indies.[50] And for this purpose a cédula was ordered sent to the royal protomedicato.[51]

Foreign Doctors in the Spanish Caribbean: Cuba, Española, Puerto Rico

Though by 1582 the laws explicitly required a man to have a license to practice medicine and surgery, local officials lightly gave medical posts to unqualified persons, even sometimes when it was unnecessary. One licentiate, Fulano Peláez, was the victim of this whimsy. He was very talented in medicine and surgery with a title to practice both. Besides, he had served for four years as physician and surgeon in the armada sent to relieve the people of Florida, and upon his return to Havana he went on as naval surgeon, treating whites, soldiers, and slaves. In treating the poor he had gone so far as to forgo fees and even to take patients to his house to give them beds, meals, and free medicines, "making admirable cures." Despite all this "without any cause or reason whatsoever," Governor Francisco Carreño (1577–79) stripped him of his post and gave it to the Portuguese, Antonio Rumbo, a "mere barber," upon the request of certain people "with no interest in the public welfare" who were annoyed with Peláez for certain reports he had sent to the Council of the Indies. Taking the case as routine, the king asked the governor to take up the case and do what was necessary without doing any injury.[52] In these first years of the Babylonian Captivity, there was no special reason to be alarmed about the Portuguese in Cuba. Also, there seemed no apparent disposition to enforce the laws on preparation for a medical career.

Two centuries later Edward Hamlin of London, long a "physician and surgeon by profession in Havana," is but another indication that foreigners in the Indies, until they ran afoul of a rival or became ambitious for naturalization as an aid to their business, could remain as long as they chose. Surely these latter must have been the most numerous, but successful anonymity then means a gap in documentation now. Hamlin had the boldness to make an appeal for naturalization eleven years after he married Josefa María de Santiago in Havana "with 23,000 pesos," and, silent though he is on the subject, he was surely there some time before that.[53] Yet this is only one instance of foreign doctors assuming that they could disregard such elementary matters as the time and legality of their entry into the kingdom in the first place. If they knew anything about the Indies, they must have known that the fiscal, "that spy upon those that defraud the king," would discover this convenient oversight the minute the application came under his eyes. Though Hamlin might have entered Cuba as a factor of the South Sea Company in Santiago, his remaining in the island to practice medicine and surgery in Havana was bound to be irregular. Since marriage with a woman of the country, especially one from a prominent family, was one ground upon which these doctors sought naturalization, it is strange that no document gives any indication that marriage with a man who had no right to be in the country was the least bit difficult.

Hamlin not only practiced medicine illegally in Havana but he also appealed for "citizenship papers" in 1765—just two years after a war with England had seen Havana captured by an English army. His muster of arguments, however, as they always were, was strong. He had four children by his Cuban wife, a plantation with four adobe outbuildings, a single house in another place, slaves, and personal property. In October 1756 he "was named doctor for whites of that plaza with the right of military *fuero* [special privilege]." In 1761 he became physician to the infirmary of the Royal Tobacco Factory, with a salary of two hundred ducats, and to the Second Battalion of Infantry of Aragon, then in Havana.

Despite all this, Hamlin "voluntarily" left Havana and from Cádiz put in his application for naturalization and the continued enjoyment of his military fuero. The council immediately asked the Casa de Contratación in Cádiz to report secretly on Hamlin, how he came there, and how he behaved during the siege of Havana by his fellow countrymen.

The secret report must have been unfavorable. The king informed the Audiencia of Cádiz and the governor of Havana that he had not only decided to deny Hamlin citizenship in the Indies but also the right to reside anywhere in the king's dominions—in Spain or overseas.[54] Secret reports to the king were not the only ones. Presently the fiscal of the audiencia in Cádiz was making a shamefaced inquiry concerning the "whereabouts" of Hamlin, "who had furtively absented himself from this city."[55]

Just as the high remuneration for American-born physicians in the United States has often forced insane asylums and other public medical services to turn to foreign physicians, it became necessary for the Spanish colonial to turn to the foreigner or to leave the isolated or humble people in the hands of curanderos. This recourse was irregular and therefore silent. In 1792, however, when the captain general of Cuba attempted to execute a royal order calling for the summary eviction of all the foreigners in the island, Miguel Peñalver y Calvo, a sugar mill owner, revealed that he had two English physicians drawing salaries on his property to treat "nearly 300 sick Negroes." He argued that to eject these practitioners would mean a return to the miserable conditions that prevailed "for want of Spanish physicians" before the Englishmen came. Some haciendas and sugar factories, whose owners had slaves by the hundreds, he added, were in the mountains far removed from any town or any help. It was thus absolutely essential to have such physicians, even if they could be obtained only by paying excessively high salaries. "The hospitals as well as the university did not turn out a sufficient number, nor of the training required, to take care of this island." Thus, some sugar mill owners "had to take bleeders with the name of surgeons, who probably do more harm than good to humanity."

The people in the whole district of the Quivocán Sugar Factory, in fact, had made one of these English physicians their "titular angel" on account of his skill and charity in treating all sick workers around that factory. In effect, Peñalver argued that physicians in these circumstances as "useful to the republic" as these two be allowed to remain and thus encourage others to come. The king acceded to this request "for the time being," but with the inevitable injunction that the conduct of these two Englishmen be kept under observation.[56]

Despite the intensification of Spanish xenophobic activity during the French Revolution, there is no precise moment when foreigners were not theoretically and officially suspect around the Caribbean. The very establishment and activity of the Inquisition at Cartagena in the seventeenth century are proof enough of this perennial concern. Yet this concern waned more often than it waxed. Any time there was a world crisis, a poor foreign physician, illegally resident, could get into some minor trouble and fan the problem up again.

So it was in 1748 when the Frenchman, Miguel Huc, "received by the cabildo" of Santo Domingo as a physician, fell afoul of the alcalde ordinario. When that circumspect doctor was asked to examine a leper, he ignored the call. When the alderman twice served legal notice on him, Huc not only refused to treat the leper but also broke into a tirade in which he made light of the alcalde's authority. The police officer promptly threw the intemperate disciple of Aesculapius into the calaboose. Thereupon, the vicar general of the archbishop claimed the "ecclesiastical privilege" for Huc on the pretext that he was the archbishop's physician and, in a summary fashion, declared the alderman excommunicated. The alcalde responded by appealing the case. Huc countered by asking the audiencia to release him to treat some sick people, which it allowed. Not only did the audiencia show leniency toward Huc but it also required the alcalde to present his case before the audiencia, thus depriving the alcalde of jurisdiction in the first instance, which the laws conceded him. The cabildo, whose officer was thus depreciated, took exception and appealed to the Council of the Indies. It asserted that this French doctor, aided and abetted by the provisor and the archbishop, was one cause for the "quarrels and public disturbances which the French physicians in all times had caused in that city, that their policy was to acquire wealth and move back to their country." Then, instead of suspending Huc's license, the audiencia apparently supported his pretentions. In the view of the cabildo, the audiencia's sustaining of the contumacious doctor greatly damaged the authority of the cabildo.

In drawing up its suit for the Council of the Indies, the town council advised that, "for the preservation of these dominions," all foreigners be ejected, as commanded by the royal laws. In this document the town council singled out the French as more prejudicial than other foreigners in America, because they were intimately acquainted with the government forces and properties as well as because they were so free in matters of religion. These could result, at the opportune time, in great injury. On the basis of such arguments, the cabildo called for expulsion of foreigners from the island, especially Frenchmen, even though they claimed to be taking asylum there. The city modified the rigor of its request enough to say that, in some cases, these men might be taken from Santo Domingo to places where they could do no harm.

In an especially sharp rebuke to the royal audiencia, the Council of the Indies criticized the legality of its proceedings and demanded that the documents taken from the alcalde when he was stripped of "jurisdiction in the first instance" be returned to him. More important, the council ordered the audiencia and other officials to expel the foreigners not only from Santo Domingo but also from the other towns of the island, with the exception of those who were legally established there.[57]

The scarcity of doctors that led to the tolerance of curanderos in Mexico and Peru and to the tacit acceptance of black and mulatto empirics in Cuba also led to the encouragement of unlicensed French physicians in Española. So eager were the people of Santo Domingo to have a chance to make a choice of a doctor when members of their families fell ill, it took over eighteen years to clear up the status of Dr. Agustín Marco and Francisco Oller, French practitioners in the city. Not content merely to practice medicine and surgery, these two had gone on to set up drugstores, a combination of professional activity prohibited by Spanish law everywhere. When asked to report on the matter, the governor of Santo Domingo said frankly that authorities before him approved or condoned physicians in proportion to their scarcity, and there was need for these two in the interior towns of the island, where "the consummate misery of the people" made it impossible for the best-qualified doctors to sustain themselves. For the same reason his predecessors had not considered certain experienced and skillful foreigners as subject to the royal orders calling for expulsion of those not licensed by a qualified tribunal.

Such a course might even have been unjust and inhumane, not to say detrimental to the population. For example, Dr. D. Pedro Tevenard came from Guarico in Venezuela to Santo Domingo to treat the people of the city. Would it not be a violation of good faith to evict him after he had dutifully practiced his profession so many years? Likewise, the surgeons Marco and Oller, though unlicensed, had practiced since their arrival without any problem whatsoever. In this case the crown followed the governor's counsel of humanity and expediency but required everybody practicing without a license from the protomedicato of New Spain to submit to an examination. Since there were not enough qualified medical doctors in the University of Santo Domingo to constitute an examining committee, the governor had to appoint the three best-qualified ones in the city to conduct the tests.[58]

In cultural matters or in medicine, Puerto Rico was always on the rim of the Spanish colonies. It had no university and therefore a sorry medical history as well, especially in the regulation of the medical professions. Just as the island was not especially attractive to Spanish doctors, it had fewer foreign medical "intruders," although the peregrinations of Luis Rayfer, a French physician, embraced Puerto Rico.

The French Revolution had its quota of émigrés, of whom Rayfer was one. Claiming to be a physician and surgeon, "approved," so he claimed, in the University of Toulouse, he began practice with the idea of entering the Royal French Navy, but since he could not accept the new constitution following the overthrow of the monarchy, he preferred "to expose himself to the chances of a sad exile to preserve intact the principles of Religion and faith so inherent in him." Because of the proximity of Haiti and "the island of Santo Domingo," at the beginning of 1794 he managed to get into Santo Domingo, where he asked the captain general for permission to take up residence. Not only did the fiscals of the audiencia and the town council concur, but also an examining committee judged him "sufficient" in medicine. Thereupon he became a citizen and won his license to practice medicine and surgery. Then, taking all the proper, even classic steps to ingratiate himself, he presented himself to the captain general as a volunteer to treat "any soldiers that might arrive from the frontiers wounded or with medical problems of other kinds" while supplying any medicines needed from his own drugstore. The captain general accepted this offer and assigned him to Dajabón. In the same year he substituted him for Nicolás Nicolle as titular doctor and surgeon of the Cantabrian Regiment and the Veteran Battalion of Santo Domingo, where he served to the complete satisfaction of the commanders. With acceptance obtained in this way, in 1795 he bought a hacienda and got married in Española. Just when he was beginning to enjoy the fruits of his good work and conduct, he had to flee again, this time to Puerto Rico because of the cession of Santo Domingo to France. On the recommendation of the government and town council of Santo Domingo, Puerto Rican authorities allowed him to become a resident and practice his profession, which he did "indefatigably." During the siege of San Juan by the English in 1797, he treated the sick of the Castle of San Cristóbal and afterward those in the Royal Hospital under the orders of the chief surgeon there.

With this list of qualifications, Rayfer finally appealed for naturalization and the enjoyment of his rights and privileges. What he ignored, though, in seeking this reward for his prolonged and noble services, was that he had entered the Spanish empire illegally, resided and married there illegally, and practiced medicine and surgery there illegally. One even wonders whether, since he only stated he had a university education in medicine, he actually had a medical degree at all. This is the kind of thing a Spanish fiscal, especially of the Council of the Indies, would hardly overlook. True to his advice, the council this time denied the petition for naturalization and desired to know from the governor of Puerto Rico on what grounds "this foreigner" was tolerated in violation of the laws and asked for a report on his "expertness, marital status, age, conduct, and religion." Finally, should he be permitted to go on practicing in that city either because of the scarcity of doctors or for some other reason? This was an opening for another delay that, in view of the discouraging outlook for citizenship, seems to have lasted from then on.[59] Very rarely, it seems, did the council summarily order an intruder returned under arrest.

Conclusion

Except for the vicissitudes of war, the problem of the foreign physicians in the Spanish empire hardly changed at all in the course of the seventeenth and eighteenth centuries. If these intruders could not hope to escape detection without any formal title or papers, they falsified the documents. Those who were more venturesome or less chary or who could not get forged papers simply took their chances, hoping they could bluff Spanish authorities in the Indies or convince them of their expertise, particularly if a community was in crying need of medical care. Usually claiming that their documents had been lost, misplaced, or sunk to the bottom of the sea, these foreigners attempted to get recognition not only by falsely claiming that they had the requisite medical degree from Toulouse, Montpellier, Leyden, Turin, or some other place but also by achieving an excellent record of cures among the population they served. To make their case stronger, they also proclaimed their charity toward the poor who fell sick. In fact, in some areas these foreign doctors came to have such strong defenders among the Spanish residents that they attained more luster and prestige than their formally trained, legally licensed Spanish counterparts.

The tolerance and acceptance of foreign physicians by colonial and Spanish authorities and the place of these foreigners in colonial society testify to the sad state of medicine in the Spanish Indies. Doctors were scarce, terribly scarce, and foreigners served like the curanderos to fill a vacuum. That many had spurious degrees, suspicious backgrounds, and a marginal place was not important to people in desperate need of any sort of medical assistance. The real importance of the foreign physicians, unfortunately, will never be known. In cases where there was no jealousy or denunciation on the part of local Spanish doctors, no quest for a legitimate license, or no attempt at gaining citizenship, the foreign doctor practiced unlicensed and unchallenged, as vital to curing the sick as the curanderos and the licensed Spanish physicians.

❧ 7 Legitimacy and Blood Purity (Limpieza de Sangre): Birth, Race, and Caste, and the Practice of Medicine

AFTER THE MIDDLE AGES in Spain, when an established practice was finally set down in writing, it was often already a hoary, venerable law. The *Siete Partidas* of Alfonso the Learned, invoking the sanction of the "Holy Church," convicted and stamped a child born out of lawful wedlock as "Infamous"[1]—tainted and handicapped by a note of infamy. This is both definite and severe. Yet nearly everything bearing on the problem tended to ameliorate its rigor. Poor boys inclined to medicine rarely learned to read and speak Latin, the gateway to the universities and hence to the professions. Though not often concerned with medicine, the well-to-do could get letters of naturalization for their bastard sons. On the other hand, the poor were exempted by economics, and the rich more often by disdain, indifference, and influence. Besides, the relative silence of the documents before the eighteenth century, the disposition of the Spanish universities to graduate the able poor lad as a bachelor without fees, and the later tenderness of Spanish law for the abandoned child suggest that the Spaniards at home, as well as in America, disregarded a statute that required a man to possess what the "accursed" circumstances of his birth had already denied him. Could a man select his own father? one of the victims asked. In medicine, sure trouble came only when an empiric sought to cross over and set himself up as a "Latin" physician, a man obliged by law to have behind him both university degrees and a two-year internship.

The Status of the Illegitimate in Spain and the Indies

Since the laws of both Spain and the Indies required all "Latin" physicians to hold university degrees in medicine and to undergo an examination by the royal protomedicato, the first question that arises is: what were prerequisites for entering universities? The tendency in the sixteenth century was to overlook the prerequisite of legitimacy in colleges, seminaries, and universities. In 1594, for example, the Archbishop of Lima got express instructions "henceforth" to follow the canons of the

Council of Trent not to ordain any illegitimate.[2] In the next century the crown occasionally lifted the stigma of illegitimacy for a certain fee (*gracias al sacar*), because an illegitimate child might very well be challenged by other heirs and barred from inheriting property. But it was not very likely that a rival would challenge a man merely because he wanted to go to school and might eventually turn to the practice of medicine.

In the eighteenth century the economic nerve, touched at last, began to draw attention to the sensitive fact that illegitimates, when they had the means, position, and inclination to do so, had long been registering in universities and qualifying for professions without attracting attention. The agent of the University of Mexico, "Dr. and Master" Miguel Antonio del Castillo, revealed in a petition to the crown in 1728 the negligence of university rectors in admitting persons who "detract from the luster" of the university. Thereupon he wanted to require all "legitimate sons" to present birth certificates and the "natural sons" information concerning their parents. To enforce this resolution, the cloister proposed that the king appoint "four or six" doctors to examine the documents presented by the students matriculated the previous year and report back to the cloister. The fiscal of the Council of the Indies opposed this petition on the ground that it was contrary to the "liberty" granted everybody to attend the universities and against the established "practice of the universities of these kingdoms." He would agree, though, that "unknown persons" and others of "inferior quality" should be required to "legitimize their persons" before receiving higher degrees, even though a bachelor's degree was sufficient to practice medicine. The Council of the Indies accepted his opinion completely.[3]

Twelve years later the cloister of the University of Havana denied José Alemán Salgado, a bachelor of medicine practicing in the town of Puerto del Principe, admission to candidacy for the licentiate and the doctor's degree on the ground that he was illegitimate. To counteract the "great injury" and "shame" of this repulse, and incidentally to qualify for "degrees and posts of honor," the applicant appointed agents in Madrid to get him a "cédula of legitimacy." After calling for the statutes of the universities of Havana and Alcalá as well as the records of three cases of legitimation conceded "because of the sums the interested parties paid," the Council of the Indies accepted the fiscal's advice that a "rescript of legitimacy" might be granted, for which the applicant paid and got the proper certificate. As in every case of this kind, the authorities made it plain that, in addition to the "proper sum," aside from his illegitimacy, the candidate had to be preeminently qualified for all the honors he sought.[4]

A similar case arose in Mexico in 1779. Bachelor José Peredo wrote the king in February that "the accursed chance of his birth had deprived him of the considerable prerogative of legitimacy" and robbed him of the capacity to certify his purity of blood. Since both the statutes of the University of Mexico and the laws of the Indies forbade the institution to confer the doctorate upon an illegitimate, Peredo appealed to "the royal protection of his majesty" for the "grace of legitimacy" to enable him not only "to graduate as doctor but also to obtain chairs, the rectorship, the office of protomédico, and other posts of honor and privilege."

The applicant had a strong case. He had gained the reputation of being an outstanding student of mathematics and medicine and had won the plaudits of the rector and secretary of the University of Mexico. He had even gained the acclaim of the royal protomedicato and had great success in practice both in Mexico City and Oaxaca, where the bishop had named him "doctor of the bedchamber [*médico de cámara*]" and charged him with the care of the sick in the Hospital de San Cosme y San Damián. Above all, the royal university, eager to keep in everlasting memory a person who had "ennobled" the very halls where he "flourished," mentioned him in the prologue to the 1775 edition of its statutes as defending "many exquisite mathematical and medical conclusions," offering to "prove them with geometrical demonstrations." Above all, the editor of this celebrated publication mentioned Peredo along with the Mexican astronomer José Ignacio Bartolache, whose fame in this rare and strange composition rested upon his having concocted "martial pills" of iron shavings and defending their use in the halls of the Royal and Pontifical University.[5] When the fiscal of the Council of the Indies rendered his report, he particularly stressed that Secretary José Imaz y Ezquer had made no scruple over registering Peredo, who had both the bachelor of arts and the bachelor of medicine degrees,[6] and that the applicant was not included among the blacks, certain mixed bloods, and those of "infamy" debarred by a university statute. He accordingly recommended that the certificate of legitimacy should be issued. More cautious, the council asked that the Audiencia of Mexico report on whether Peredo was of the "prejudiced castes," a black, mulatto, slave or ex-slave, or *chino moreno*. If this information was ever provided, it apparently was never filed with the record of this case.[7]

The spirit shown in the fiscal's opinions in these cases was reflected in important legislation and legal opinion in the next twenty years. In 1784 a royal cédula at last recognized that to bar illegitimates from the professions merely threw people upon the charity of the state, individuals who had the capacity to be useful to it. Brotherhoods and other organizations set up under public authority were accordingly ordered to rescind all laws that made illegitimacy an impediment in these types of work.[8] In Lima two years later Dr. José de Iturrizarra complained that he had been appointed protomédico by Viceroy Agustín de Jáuregui and had held this post in technical disregard of a cédula of 1646, the law that required the protomédico to be professor of prima of medicine. Upon the death of Jáuregui, however, the University of San Marcos staged a trial lecture in which the chair as well as the protomedicato fell to Dr. Juan Aguirre. Claiming his personal enemies promoted this turn of events, Iturrizarra alleged that the post of first protomédico had been held by men who were not professors, because "it is rare that the professors have the preeminent qualities." The main point against Aguirre, though, was that he was illegitimate. The fiscal of the Council of the Indies then strongly urged the councilors *not* to forsake legitimacy and purity of blood as prerequisites for these posts. The council, however, upheld the selection of Dr. Aguirre and hewed to the legal line that the first professor of medicine should head the tribunal del protomedicato.[9]

The continued inhuman treatment of abandoned children also aroused the royal authorities, and the picture drawn of conditions in America is proof that many informed and humane people in America were aroused, too. "Not a few thousand," the reports had it, "died annually" because of the barbaric treatment they received on the roads as they were being carried to distant orphanages from the towns where they had been abandoned. Their nurses (*amas*) and wet nurses received so little money, especially when they were nursing their own infants, that committing a child to them was often equivalent to infanticide. All this, the king admitted, was a great horror against nature, injury to the Christian religion, and a detriment to the population as a whole.

Such notices as these moved the royal will to take "the most opportune and efficacious steps in favor of foundlings"—to care for their lives, provide decent rearing, and make honest occupations available to them at least as becoming the sons of Christians instead of taking them for bastards and illegitimate children begotten in incest and adultery. Having seen the oppression inflicted by visiting the sins of unknown fathers upon known children, houses for abandoned children strongly urged that these young orphans, "not generally declared legitimate" because this "quality is not proved," should be given "civil legitimacy" by royal intervention. Upon consultation with the Council of the Indies, the king in 1791 so ruled in favor of the foundlings in the orphanage of Cartagena. Then, in 1794 to apply the principle generally, the king issued a cédula to circulate in both Spain and America[10] commanding that orphans not be stigmatized and that all foundlings of both sexes be taken as legitimate for all civil purposes despite any laws to the contrary. Persons of this origin would become full citizens.

To the beneficiaries of so humane an outlook, the results were not slight. They would now be admitted to schools, Jesuit colleges (*convictorios*), and charitable establishments without distinction and share in dowries and gifts—provided that the statutes of such colleges and foundations did not literally state that their members should be "legitimate sons begotten in true matrimony."[11] Any person calling these abandoned children borderline, illegitimate, bastard, spurious, incestuous, or adulterous would have to retract their statement "judicially" and could expect a fine in accord "with the circumstances." These people would not be subject to "public shame, whipping, or the gallows," for it might just be that the victim was "from an illustrious family."

Though this famous cédula of 1794 legitimized "all royal dispositions to the contrary," American universities did not always heed it. In Caracas, at least, the university statute barring illegitimates from holding degrees remained troublesome to the very end of the colonial regime. In fact, only two months before the battle of Boyacá, José Joaquín González, orphan from Caracas, won his fight to graduate as a bachelor and doctor of medicine.[12]

Limpieza de Sangre in Spain

The Spaniards made a fetish of purity of blood—*limpieza de sangre*—but we should make doubly sure that we follow their practice as well as their codes before we understand their real concern with racial "taint." In the eighteenth century when Miguel Eugenio Muñoz reviewed and compiled Spanish medical law from the Middle Ages, he never once asked whether a man's skin was black, brown, or white.[13] In metropolitan Spain, purity of blood meant exclusively freedom from the taint of heresy, the Moslem religion, or Judaism.

A pragmatic of 1501[14] declared that those "reconciled" after the crime to the second generation of the masculine line and the first by the female could hold no office or practice any profession. And every such office that could be thought of was mentioned by name. Among these, though at the very end of the long list, were the professions of medicine, surgery, and pharmacy. Violation carried a penalty of confiscation of property.[15] The Catholic Kings reserved the right to declare what offices were included in the "prohibition."[16]

After toying briefly with the idea of using America as a dumping ground for all kinds of "infected" elements, the Spanish crown caught itself up short. America, at least, might be kept free of infection by imposing an immediate quarantine. Ten years after the pragmatic of 1501 the royal government declared that many of these "sons and grandsons of those burned at the stake" (*quemados*) were running to Española because they were now forbidden by law to hold "places" in Spain. Without a tremor, the crown excluded them from the Indies and applied rigorous penalties.[17] So it was most natural that when the medical laws of Castile were transferred to America, Antonio de Mendoza, the first viceroy to New Spain, got instructions to see to it that no person forbidden by Spanish laws and pragmatics to practice medicine, surgery, or pharmacy might practice in America or graduate as bachelor, licentiate, or doctor.[18]

The seventeenth century was well advanced, though, before the royal protomedicato in Madrid showed any extraordinary anxiety about "tainted" persons practicing medicine. The immediate occasion for this concern was a pragmatic of the "Prince" of Portugal, forbidding those without proper blood purity to practice medicine in that kingdom. The result was that disqualified Portuguese physicians, surgeons, and druggists left their own country, where they were known, and turned up in Spain "with false certificates of purity of blood." The royal protomedicato in Madrid, therefore, instructed all medical examiners to force all Portuguese aspiring to medical careers in Spain to present notarized certificates of blood purity. Physicians who claimed to be trained in Coimbra or other parts of Portugal needed certification from the Royal Council of Lisbon to "be clean and not one of those included in the pragmatic [of expulsion], if surgeons or druggists, to bring the proper certification."[19]

Bona fide compliance with this regulation, or any regulation implying disfavor of the Inquisition, could not be expected. Indeed, isolated cases, symptomatic of an epidemic, cropped up with fair regularity— often enough to imply rigorous administration of the law but infrequently enough to prove that the Spaniards knew that even these men must live. Occasionally, the Council of Castile in Madrid had to intervene to maintain the necessary vigilance. When Dr. Francisco de Medina, convicted by the Holy Office of Toledo, boldly continued to practice medicine in the town of Illescas, the council prodded the protomedicato to know what had been done in such cases.[20] In its report, the protomedicato claimed, if it did not boast, that it "had succeeded and was succeeding" in extirpating from the practice of medicine those found "impure and stained with so horrible a vice and infamy." The problem of Dr. Medina, a special and deliberate offender, they tossed back onto the council tables. Would the king take the proper steps to see that Dr. Medina did not practice medicine? The Royal Council thereupon ordered the corregidor of Illescas to notify Dr. Medina that he was to leave town and not come within ten leagues of it, neither was he to practice medicine either for pay or for nothing.[21] Five years later, though, the king found it necessary to order the Audiencia of Valladolid to ferret out all those persons sentenced by the Inquisition who were still practicing medicine, even though they had recanted, on pain of expulsion from "these kingdoms."[22]

Despite the vigorous language of the statutes and decrees—or perhaps because of it—the proceedings suggest that evasion was common. A well-placed empiric could allege that a trip to the protomedicato for examination was prohibitively expensive, and if he had to, he could play one jurisdiction off against another. In 1726 the protomedicato reported that Diego Zapata, sentenced by the Inquisition of Cuenca, had boldly come to court and boldly practiced medicine without even going before the medical examiners. The protomedicato pleaded that because Zapata was under the protection of powerful people, it could not proceed against him. In consequence, it sought royal approval for exercising its jurisdiction under law until Zapata was totally excluded from the practice of medicine.[23] Deciding to go to the heart of the matter, the crown ruled that papers supporting purity of blood should be cleared through the agents in the towns. Accordingly, all corregidores got orders to publish this decree in their districts. Universities received express written warnings.[24]

Over ten years later, though, the protomedicato still felt that the Council of Castile was intervening in its business. Isabel Coronel, acting for Manuel de Castro, forced the clerk of the protomedicato to produce the act of certification (*auto de aprobación*) of Castro, whose medical diploma had been lost by the Inquisition while it had him under arrest, though the clerk was careful to insert the royal ruling of September 12, 1699, that medical people of all kinds sentenced by the Inquisition could not practice medicine.[25] The council had peremptorily ordered the protomedicato to examine Manuel de Castro in complete disregard of the reasons that tribunal had offered for refusing to do so. To put an end to controversies, the royal government declared that admitting Castro to examination was the proper and exclusive right of the protomedicato. To carry out this resolution, the council found itself obliged to return the records of all such cases to the medical board. In this windfall the protomedicato got the exclusive right to pass on prerequisites to practice—such as degrees, internship, and certificates of baptism—without appeal to the council, though in case of rejection of proof supporting of purity of blood, the council might hear an appeal after asking the protomedicato for a secret report. At the same time the king roundly declared that the protomedicato had exclusive jurisdiction to deal with the crimes and excesses of licensed physicians, surgeons, and druggists as well as to handle the case of those who practiced without licenses. After devoting a whole chapter of three sections amounting to twenty pages to the problem of limpieza de sangre of physicians, surgeons, and druggists, Eugenio Muñoz in his *Recopilación*[26] suggests recourse to a work by Juan Escobar del Corro, an inquisitor as well as fiscal of the Council of the Inquisition, on how to establish nobility and purity of blood.[27]

Limpieza de Sangre in the Indies

The meaning of "note of infamy" gradually took on a new implication in America. In Peru the statutes of the University of San Marcos de Lima, in two editions of 1602 and 1735, reflected the Spanish experience—that no persons sentenced by the Holy Office should be admitted to degrees or be examined for them.[28] From the beginning, however, Mexican statutes went much further. These added blacks, mulattoes, chinos morenos, or any kind of slave or former slave to those who could not get degrees. The Mexicans attached the logical provision that these were not to be matriculated either.[29]

Given the outlook of the times, there was nothing irregular in the exclusion of blacks and mulattoes from higher education and medicine. The crown began the government of the Indies on a note of suspicion for the mulattoes and mixed breeds and forbade these "worst and most vicious" elements or any other of that race with more than a year in Spain to immigrate to America, "for there they ran away to the mountains, formed bands, and otherwise set a bad example."[30] Reports from Mexico that hats were being badly made "and not as they should be and are made" in Castile led to the exclusion of blacks from the hatmakers' guild in Mexico. In fact, no black could work at this trade save under a Spanish master.[31] No black slave or mulatto could even be examined for the trade of glove maker.[32] The cabildo of Lima was equally adamant that neither black, mulatto, *zambo*, or *berberisco* should even be examined for lace maker or embroiderer (*orillero*).[33] Mulattos and mestizos were also barred from the profession of notary.[34] Royal orders to this effect were reaffirmed in the middle of the eighteenth century when the whites in the professions began their vehement and effective agitation against blacks and castes.[35] Not even a beadle who kept dogs out of church, however able he might be, could be a black or mulatto.[36]

With the black and mulatto barred from such humble offices, forbidden to go on horseback, and denied the privilege of carrying weapons, could it be expected that the same society would permit the black, mulatto, or mixed blood to enter universities? In fact, it was in the role of menial ornament that the black first associated himself with Spanish universities. The question very early was not whether the black might enter a university, but whether the rector might "enjoy the preeminence" of going about with two black lackeys wearing sidearms.[37] Agustín Rascón, however, a mulatto son of a nobleman of Cholula, was not even allowed to "defend and adorn his person" with sword or dagger.[38]

Almost exactly at the middle of the eighteenth century a marked apprehension of the black in the universities and in the professions appeared in the Spanish empire, especially in Lima and the Caribbean. University statutes before 1700, if they did so at all, excluded persons of color in a casual, mechanical way. In the University of San Marcos de Lima, where the problem was destined to become bitter, the statutes had nothing to say on race, and it is unlikely that the phrase "note of infamy" meant anything more than it did in the Spanish legal language of 1501. Why then did not this historical tolerance of color, when combined with the vaunted Enlightenment of the second half of the eighteenth century, produce a contrary current?

Aside from pressure upon the professions by persons of color, there were other matters that stiffened the backbone of officials to discriminate. One was the lack of funds for paying professors in San Marcos de Lima, which forced that university to sell degrees (*grados de indulto*), increasing the already too numerous diplomas and dissipating their value from 2,500 to 800 pesos and threatening to fall as low as 500.[39] Thus "tainted" persons appeared among those with vaunted degrees, which were already losing their prestige for other reasons. In short, the university was falling into a decadence that disturbed every outgoing viceroy for a century. Besides, this was, after all, the half-century in which the Spaniards tried to regain all the efficiency of administration they had lost and, perhaps, some they never had. To talk of enforcing the laws against the inertia of the rest was no longer out of the question.

Several factors account for this sudden effort to reverse the easygoing practices of the viceroyalties. One explanation of this suddenly harsh course was the increase in the number of mulattoes among university graduates, or at least among practitioners of medicine, which began to give meaning to the phrase "a note of infamy" among white competitors. White doctors saw their fees in jeopardy, and the viceroys the prestige of white skin. White students now felt that this influx degraded medicine and lowered the social standing of its practitioners, and they refused to register in the faculty. Mulattoes, quadroons, and zambos now became "vile and despicable subjects." For the eighteenth-century white the pure-blooded black was too obviously "tainted" ever to have insinuated himself in great numbers into higher education and professional life.

José Pastor Larrinaga, himself a mulatto surgeon, in 1791 revealed, unconsciously perhaps, what had troubled the government forty years before.[40] He cried out to know what the 60,000 inhabitants of Lima would do if fifty-six surgeons did not daily tread the streets and plazas looking for the sick to cure, the infirm to comfort and preserve, and even the healthy to protect by precaution! The point of this outburst of rhetoric was a question: what would become of the City of Kings, "I repeat a thousand times," entrusted to "ten or twelve overseas surgeons, who are the only ones numbered in that beneficent locality"? Without forty-odd "swarthies or mulattoes," who would practice surgery? Spaniards from the colleges of Cádiz or Barcelona? No, not even the creoles would take up surgery, for they could become physicians! Even Larrinaga concluded that after two hundred years surgery was in such decadence that no one who could do so legally would cultivate the field.

Also it is not easy, indeed it is not possible, to tell which of the mulattoes in surgery and medicine in Lima in the second half of the eighteenth century were university men and which sheer intruders. Persons of color exploited the uncertainty of the law in Lima, where there was a greater black population than in highland Mexico. Viceroy Count of Castelar (1674–78) had responded to this problem by setting up a commission that decided mestizos, zambos, quadroons, and mulattoes should not be admitted to the university. This decision was incorporated into the laws of the Indies,[41] but unfortunately for Peruvian creoles, the law merely said that exclusions from the university should be based upon Statute 238, which made no mention of racial strains. Many mulattoes, therefore, pretended that exclusion decreed by Castelar's commission had not been specifically and concretely confirmed in the statutes. The Peruvian viceroy Count of Monclova ordered zambos, mulattoes, and quadroons excluded from the universities and their degrees rescinded as punishment for fraud. Indeed, Viceroy Marqués de Villagarcía (1736–45) in 1737 refused to allow one of these people to contest the chair of method on account of the "grave inconveniences" it would produce. Though Monclova, according to the cédula of 1752, had not included mestizos, this was probably a clerical oversight. At least when the Viceroy Count of Superunda (1745–61) pressed the crown, it responded with a cédula including mestizos with zambos, mulattoes, and quadroons, just as they had been in the time of Castelar.[42] The viceroys felt that the oppressive decadence of the university, which had complex causes, was due in an important measure to the negligence of the rectors of San Marcos in not requiring certificates of blood purity upon the student's matriculation to uphold these decrees. Bringing up the matter anew in

1767, Viceroy Manuel de Amat y Junient (1761–76), expressed his astonishment that, in the time of the Marqués de Villagarcía, "one of these" had been so bold as to try to enter the oposición in an effort to win the chair of method, the colonial chair of therapeutics, and the treatment of disease. Amat thought that this degradation explained the distressing fact that the renowned University of San Marcos of the City of Kings had only four graduates in medicine. He quoted a royal cédula in the time of Superunda dated 1752 authorizing the university authorities to ask matriculants whether they were mulattoes, zambos, quadroons, or mestizos, and, in case they enrolled through fraud, to "erase" their degrees from the records.[43] Such concern at the end of 1776 shows that these royal decrees had made little difference. Later, at the beginning of the next century the problem was to break out anew when some of Peru's most outstanding physicians turned out to be mulattoes.

Amat's stand did not eliminate the problem.[44] Strong and determined in this as in everything else, the viceroy complained bitterly of two lawyers of the "most obscure and sacrilegious birth" and of another one, a total bastard (*puro adulterino*) who had been able to register in colleges, graduate from the university, and "adorned" with these hoods, secure licenses from the audiencia to practice law. To reject them now would be taken as an injury. The seed of the trouble was the all but criminal negligence with which "the most vile types," by relaxation of the statutes, were allowed to register in the colleges and universities and thus set up the circle of deceit. Since "zambos, mulattoes, and other worse castes" sprang from an illegitimate class, the negligence of academic officials had thus failed to maintain not only their legitimacy but also their blood purity. He therefore called in almost strident terms for a royal order that would declare in general terms that no one be registered in a college or university before he had established in legal form both his legitimacy and purity of blood.

But a strident tone was the last one to assume with a crown lawyer such as the fiscal of the Council of the Indies. That exacting but self-confident functionary advised the council that there was no need for a general order if the statutes of the colleges and universities already covered the case. His suggestion was to have copies of these sent for examination from the three colleges of Lima and from the University of San Marcos and that this be followed by a royal decree enjoining college and university officials to enforce their own "constitutions." The viceregal government could produce only the statutes of the University of San Marcos, thus leaving in doubt Amat's assertion that these lost codes covered the case. At any rate, following the fiscal's original advice, the government dispatched an order concerning the admission of students, which was essentially the note on which the case settled slowly to rest in 1770.[45]

In 1767, just as these rigorous, almost venomous measures attained the force of law, a mulatto, José Manuel Valdés, was born in Lima of a Spanish father and a free black woman. Escaping the confinement of domestic labor, this mulatto youth went to school, where Augustinian friars noticed his ability and gentle eagerness. For José Manuel, in the knowledge that he had the ability to transcend his circumstances, the clearest outlet was a limited practice of surgery, for even the law permitted the protomedicato to examine a candidate without university training in surgery after five years' practice. For a young mulatto such as Valdés whose inclination and the clutch of circumstance indicated surgery and medicine, this was as near as a person of color could be to good fortune.

Without the possibility of enrolling in a university, save through irregular means, a man's chances of the best training available were very slim. In the case of Valdés, though, Dr. Juan de Roca recognized the keenness and charm of the lad when he was about fifteen and gave him instruction in surgical practice. In the limited professional circles of Lima it was natural also that Roca should recommend his promising charge to Dr. Hipólito Unánue in the days before this luminary became so engrossed in politics. So this suppliant enjoyed the tutelage of two eminent medical figures of Peru before he went before the royal protomedicato after five years' internship in the Hospital of San Andrés to be examined for certification to practice surgery. In 1788 he emerged from this trial with the title of "Latin surgeon," a singular thing in itself, for such men, unable to enroll in universities and "hear" courses in Latin, usually reached only the stature of "romance surgeons." The ability to understand Latin was the sole academic prerequisite for enrollment, though Valdés had mastered both French and English.

For nearly two decades, under temptation to extend his practice into the area of medicine forbidden to those not trained in universities, José Manuel Valdés remained in modest obscurity. Because of his skills, however, the public came to regard him as better qualified than most surgeons with more privileges, and he could and did build up an irresistible prestige. On this foundation his friends made their plea before the cabildo of Lima to award the doctor's degree to Valdés, who did not even have the bachelor's. According to a procedure now becoming common, the cabildo "elevated" the plea to the viceroy, who in turn elevated it to the crown. At last, in 1806, came a royal cédula erasing and silencing the "note of infamy"; Valdés might receive degrees as if he were a white man, provided, as was always stipulated in these cases, that he took and passed all the examinations imposed upon the orthodox candidate. In fifteen days Valdés won every academic degree—the bachelor's, licentiate, and the doctorate—plain indication of his impatience to be rid of artificial handicaps.

Of all the mulatto physicians licensed in America by the Spanish crown, Valdés justified this "grace" with the greatest contribution to medical literature.[46] In a surgical dissertation on cancer of the womb in 1800, he maintained that the disease was not contagious. Six years later he defended as his "doctor's thesis" the proposition that balsam of copaiba, applied to the severed umbilical cord, was "efficacious" in the prevention of infantile convulsions, the dread "disease of seven days." So critical was this discovery that Valdés's work also appeared in Spain. From the date of this rare thesis and for nearly forty years, however, the great bulk of Valdés's work concerned epidemics—no small wonder, for the City of Kings had been struck by an epidemic of some kind at least every four years during colonial days.[47]

The increasing pressure to deny blacks and mixed bloods the right to enroll in universities in Peru had its counterpart in other areas of the empire. The records of the University of Mexico show that, somehow, cases involving concern for blood purity arose with increasing frequency.[48] Undoubtedly, most persons of "humble quality" practicing pharmacy, medicine, or surgery kept quiet, hoping that nothing would occur to draw attention to their unlicensed status. Such a clandestine life could not, though, be very comfortable for a proud man. Occasionally, too hot to simmer any longer, a case boiled over. This occurred more often when disturbed times enabled an empiric to hope that with his record of public service he might break down the legal barrier; and war and foreign invasion offered the best opportunity for him to emerge, though practitioners who, for want of licensed doctors, had sailed as surgeons on the king's ships thought, particularly when they had not volunteered, that they should be allowed to practice on land what they practiced at sea. Failing either of these heroic props, a man who could get the prior of a convent to vouch for his charitable work often felt this alone entitled him to practice medicine, surgery, or pharmacy. Very often, though, men who had grown accustomed to practice without a license fought their cases all the way to the throne when they suddenly saw arbitrary color barriers raised before them.

Getting a license to practice any branch of medicine in Cuba under these circumstances took on the nature of a complicated confidence game. For support in this venture Juan Fernández Valiente of Havana, who suffered a "want of blood purity," turned to the royal protomedicato in

Madrid, which authorized the captain general of Cuba to select a "physician and druggist of his choice." In response to an appeal from Fernández, the king issued the proper confirmation for his post, ordering the captain general to carry out the dispatch of the Madrid protomedicato as soon as Fernández presented it.[49] When Fernández began to bruit about his concession in Havana, however, the local protomedicato, which had apparently rebuffed Fernández originally, let the king have proof that the concession was based upon fraud—"sinister" misinformation—in Spanish law the soundest grounds for reversing any ruling. The royal government then ruled that all such appeals should be made before the Havana protomédicos and not substitutes, and that the applicants should appear personally, supported by the doctor under whom they had interned.[50]

The war with England and the siege of the castle of Havana in 1763 were a boon to all mulattoes in the irregular practice of medicine there. José Francisco Báez y Llerena,[51] after having practiced surgery for more than thirteen years with the full knowledge of the first protomédico, Ambrosio Medrano, and expecting not the slightest obstruction, suddenly found himself forbidden to practice surgery at all on the ground that he was not a white man. His defense reflects many aspects of Spanish administrative standards. He promptly turned to the crown with a strong petition that he be exempted from the disqualification of blood purity. (1) During the war with the English he served as surgeon on the privateer *Nuestra Señora del Rosario,* and none died, though many of the crew were gravely wounded. (2) Though his father was the natural son of José Báez, his parents, despite their color, were by the paternal line white Spaniards and old Christians. Moreover, his pardo father had held distinguished posts under the crown in Cuba and the other Spanish Antilles. On the professional side, José Francisco had studied under Ambrosio de Medrano in the Hospital de San Juan de Dios and interned under the surgeon José Tomás Alvarez de Sena, who taught him what there was to teach of his art. In these circumstances Báez y Llerena was naturally shocked that the charges now brought against him were not mentioned when he first presented himself for examination. The crown attorney felt the same, for on his advice the king issued a cédula lifting the handicap of color and setting aside all laws and customs in this case.[52]

This was not to be the end of this case, however, for in 1772 Manuel Francisco, brother of José Francisco, reopened it, asking that his sons be declared qualified for any public office, to prepare for professions in the universities, to marry born whites, also to be entered in the books set aside for the registration of whites.[53] Manuel Francisco alleged that he had been of great service when the British invested Havana, procuring meat at the risk of his life. The fiscal of the Council of the Indies,[54] however, felt that certain tasks, such as providing meat, were not the same thing as spilling blood "in defense of the fatherland and of the crown," for they might have been for "lucre" and self-interest.

In Cuba the mulattoes seemed to feel that being white by the paternal line was a most persuasive argument. In this case, though, the fiscal stated strongly and clearly a "fixed principle" that with respect to his "quality" a person's status followed that of the mother, though in the matter of distinctions and honors it followed that of the father. The fiscal felt no repugnance, however, in the petitioner's plea that mulatto designation should not be allowed to stand in the way of his sons' holding public office or attending and graduating from universities, "for the study of the sciences should not fall by luck to certain types of subjects (principally in America)." The fiscal felt that in the future the applicant might record baptism of his children in the books used for whites. The Council of the Indies agreed.[55]

A good record in the war against England emboldened many physicians and surgeons to have the fact of their practice confirmed in a royal license, but no case emerging in these war years so clearly defined the position of blacks. In Havana, where blacks and mulattoes were more common, the English attack on Havana and the unprecedented call for medical assistance brought out numerous empirics who, after hostilities were over, sought to cash in on their services and pressed the protomedicato to license them forthwith to practice for life. By this time it was also conventional to prove that a man was "Spanish without any defect that should bar him from a learned career," and there were only occasional instances in which blood purity was strongly contested.[56]

Castes and the Practice of Medicine: Case Studies

More people—many more—practiced medicine in the Spanish colonies fraudulently than ever arrived legally. Of course, most of these were quacks or, in the softer Spanish term, curanderos. Many other practitioners, however, had gained licenses and set themselves up as trained physicians by fraudulent means. How many no one knows, for the chicanery was detected only when a practitioner made application for license or, more rarely, when he was discovered after establishing a reputation for the marvelous cures he had wrought. (In fact, the superstitious nature of the age was more likely to judge favorably of a fraud than of an honest man who was obliged to live and practice within the limits of his "science" as he knew it.)

It was natural that pardos should proceed on the assumption that they were white so long as there was a good chance no one would denounce them. Sometimes, though, a bold soul pretended in the most solemn way to have the education he had not. In 1761, for example, Juan de la Cruz y Mena, practitioner of medicine and surgery in Bayamo, Cuba, undertook such a deception on behalf of his sons.[57] Cruz y Mena built his case upon the exaggerated statement that the rector and cloister of the University of Havana had refused to confer the degree of bachelor in surgery upon his two sons "despite their having studied and practiced in that city the requisite time."[58] When the Council of the Indies referred this petition to the "king's mouthpiece," the fiscal, he called attention to the lack of any legal proof of the points made and advised the rector and cloister of the University of Havana to submit their version of the case.[59] The university's reply contended that although the two pardos "studied in these schools," that they had been denied degrees in surgery was a plain case of "obreption and subreption" because the petitioner had passed over in silence the fact that he was a mulatto. Besides, the cloister had never refused the degree. In reality, each lad had come before the secretary of the university to register. That officer, on the ground "of his inferior quality," had persuaded each son not to make the attempt to matriculate. In such a patent case of fraud the council wearily rejected the application but said nothing of punishment for the deception.[60]

In 1763 Miguel José de Avilés made an appeal to the crown closely paralleling that of José Francisco Báez y Llerena. Avilés had perfected the "art of surgery," he claimed, but was unable to obtain a license from the protomedicato of Havana because he was a "free pardo."[61] In his petition to have this disqualification lifted, Avilés presented his merits and services to the king—a procedure that, if the case was strong and no obvious fraud practiced, was nearly always crowned with success. He had practiced for more than a year among the poor patients in the Hospital of San Juan de Dios with such success and disinterest that he was able to present a certificate of proof from the prior, Fray Alejandro de Fleytas. Moreover, a pardo himself, he was keen enough to see that this had not kept the protomedicato from qualifying him to treat soldiers wounded during the English siege. Avilés could not openly boast of attending the wounded as a surgeon but only of actual combat as ensign in the Company of Pardos in the attacks and encounters with the English soldiers. He also hit upon the happy idea of asking that he be qualified just as was José Francisco Báez y Llerena in 1760.

The fiscal was impressed with the parallel between the two cases, but he felt that qualifying a man to practice surgery during a siege might be a matter of necessity and not sound practice in peacetime. He accordingly recommended that the king authorize the protomedicato of Havana to admit Avilés to examination. If he passed and there was no other impediment than his being a mulatto, the protomedicato should issue him a license to practice surgery.[62] The council did not demur, and the king dispatched the confirmatory cédula.[63] Avilés took the examination, passed it, and received a license to practice as a "romance surgeon" anywhere in the king's dominions.

Avilés most certainly would have gone on undisturbed had not the reaction against mulattoes in medicine in the mid-eighteenth century also struck Cuba. Governor and Captain General Conde de Ricla (1763–65) had proposed in February 1765 that physicians and surgeons be sent to the towns of Cuba and that pardo practitioners be eliminated. The crown then went so far as to ask Ricla's successor, Diego de Manrique (1765–66), and the bishop of the Havana diocese to report on this proposal. In the meantime Avilés was restricted to practice only in his own area. When informed that he would have to accept what the king ruled on the governor's proposals to eliminate mulatto practitioners, he petitioned the crown to allow him to practice anywhere in the empire, also taking advantage of this overture to propose that the disqualification of his sons to present themselves for examination in medicine be set aside. Having heard only from the bishop, the king rejected Ricla's scheme to get rid of pardos and renewed Avilés's unlimited license, but, as usual in such cases, he put off the request that the crown exempt his sons from their racial disability so they might enter medicine or surgery.[64]

Avilés had a point in insisting upon the extension of his license to include other places in the empire, for the mulatto empirics of Cuba sometimes tried to improve their lot by moving to New Spain, where even by 1788 no mulatto had ever been licensed to practice. One of these, José Vásquez de Sila, a native of Havana, had practiced surgery since 1762, "learned a lot" during the English siege, attended the sick in the Castillo de la Punta "in the War of '78," and served on the brigantine *Galveston* at sea. Just as in the cases of José Francisco Báez y Llerena and Miguel José de Avilés, his progress in surgery had been recognized when the protomedicato assigned him to the care of the sick and wounded during wartime. The implication was, though this is concealed, that he was not examined and licensed. Nevertheless, with this accreditation he went to Yucatán, where he heard there was a shortage of practitioners. Here, when on the verge of developing an outstanding reputation, he ran afoul of both his competitors and the authorities. His competitors—motivated by jealousy, according to him—denounced him for practicing without having been examined by a protomedicato and held him up as unworthy to practice medicine because he was a pardo. To the first object, he answered "Quite so." And to the charge that he was a pardo, he "confessed it in full voice," for what could he do about the quirks of nature that took place before he was born? He was, though, an industrious and honorable vassal. He held that the laws debarring those of his status from practicing did not apply to them when they practiced surgery "of the romance type." Moreover, he was willing to pay the stipulated sum for the king's grace.

Generally willing to give his advice without more to-do, the fiscal recommended that the protomedicato render its learned opinion. With more facts in hand than Vásquez had vouchsafed, the protomedicato reported plaintively that he had practiced without a license and that the ayuntamiento had resisted his overtures for lack of documentary support and doubt on the "quality of his blood." The applicant had, in fact, come in person "to insinuate his pretensions" but then turned to the viceroy when his wheedling failed.

One after another the protomedicato chalked up the score against Vásquez. Though the laws of Castile admitted romance surgeons to examination if they could produce proof of five years' internship—three in a hospital and two with a physician or surgeon[65]—Vásquez's documents were from the fathers of San Juan de Dios of Havana, who were neither physicians nor surgeons. Though once an orderly, Vásquez had lacked the discipline necessary for his certification as a surgeon. Neither could he present, as Viceroy Croix had decreed, a certificate from the professor of anatomy of the amphitheater or from the College of Barcelona or Cádiz. Though the king had made a certificate of baptism a prerequisite to examination by the protomedicato in 1737, Vásquez could not even present this. "Lastly," the protomedicato reported roundly, the candidate is a pardo, and "there is no indication in the archives that up to now the protomedicato has ever licensed one." Though willing to assume without positive proof to the contrary that Vásquez could produce a certificate of baptism and other missing documents, there was no possibility that the candidate could take black spots off the leopard. He had not presented, neither could he present, the required certificate of blood purity required by the royal decree of March 14, 1726. As a parting shot, the protomedicato advised that the "incorporation" of this person would be a scandal to other "professors" of medicine and might even occasion dissensions such as those in Campeche. So far as buying a certificate of royal grace was concerned, the fiscal must make that decision. This, they observed in an aside, would certainly drive many mulattoes to enter medicine through that loophole. The protomedicato felt, though, that Vásquez's honorable family and his services in war should be given consideration. It therefore recommended the "prudent" step of his going to some place bereft of practitioners. How much this tells! It is the injury he does to the legal practitioners' pocketbooks and prestige and not the injury he might do to the poor people operated on "in places bereft of practitioners" that moves the protomedicato. In any event, the viceregal government accepted the advice and turned Vásquez down in a case that took only about three short months to decide.[66]

Whom the gods wished to destroy in the Spanish empire they first involved in litigation. Such a man was Santiago Padilla, pardo and practitioner of medicine and surgery in Cartagena de Indias, who made an application to the viceroy for the post of fiscal of the protomedicato in 1806.[67] To support his claim, Padilla could prove that he had had a year of logic and physics in the Dominican college of Cartagena and had served with a licensed practitioner in a charitable hospital. He established that on March 20, 1782, he had been examined by the protomedicato and duly given a license to practice surgery and algebra, under the authorization given by the royal government to American protomédicos to examine those who had worked with a surgeon five years, even though they had no academic training. Surprisingly, though, authorities made no issue of the fact that Padilla was a pardo. As in Cuba there was a disposition to let mulattoes practice in time of war when surgeons for naval expeditions were needed; in accordance with this need, Padilla had actually served in 1781. On the other hand, a number of mulatto surgeons in Cuba had served with even more distinction during the English attack on Havana, and yet the question of their "quality" was raised, and no license was granted and no exemption given for their color handicap. It was not to practice surgery but to become fiscal of the protomedicato that Padilla sought in 1806. Playing down his color, he sought to win this post by emphasizing his acceptance as physician and surgeon by the distinguished Spanish families, his charitable work in convents and with the poor, and his work with the navy and the pardo militia—the classic justifications of the practitioner who had not "trod the flagstones of universities." In fact, he had never had any formal academic training in medicine, and according to the laws of the Indies, the fiscal was supposed to be a lawyer. The laws of expediency in the Caribbean, though, often prevailed over those of kings. Cartagena had no medical school, and even if there had been one, a mulatto was not qualified to enter it. Moreover, medical men had been chosen fiscals of the protomedicato in Cartagena before.

Padilla's case clearly shows how a mulatto practitioner in the Spanish empire without university training went about establishing his reputation and right to practice medicine and surgery. From remote times Spanish law held that an aspiring physician, after he had taken a degree in medicine, should intern with a man licensed to practice. But without formal training, the irregular method used by Padilla was the classic one for accrediting those who, at the top, were not Latin physicians and, at the bottom, were not willing to practice as a mere quack. Such a man would not only accept but also eagerly seek certificates from priors, guardians, and provincials of religious orders. Padilla, for example, produced testimonials from Fray José Mariano Saborido, vicar and "president guardian" of the Convent of San Diego, that he had tended the religious there without pay for sixteen years. Manuela de San José, an abbess, acknowledged both his "charitable" help and his taking the slight salary of fifty pesos so that the one hundred pesos saved could be invested in something else.[68]

Military officers and public officials were more than acceptable sponsors. Manuel de Aguiano Ruiz y Díaz, colonel of royal engineers, certified Padilla's skill and acknowledged that he was his household physician. Manuel Antonio de Irigoyen, captain in the royal navy, gave the same kind of testimony at the request of the applicant. Antonio de Narváez y Latorre, field marshal of the royal armies, testified that Padilla had cured him and his wife of *"terciana dobles fuertes."* Francisco Espejo, gentleman of the order of Charles III and a treasury official, certified the "eulogies" of Padilla, credited him with great charity, and mentioned him as his family's and domestics' physician.[69] To establish the point of his charitable work and of his prestige with important families, Padilla produced testimonies from two more friars and four more military and naval officers, one of these being head of the "Hydrographical Expedition to America."[70] Another went so far as to attest that Padilla had studied surgery under "masters with the best reputation."[71]

The obvious truth was that Padilla wanted to set up in medicine on the basis of certification by men who were not themselves physicians or surgeons. For the protomédico who reviewed the request, Juan de Arias, this was patently clear. He also believed pardos in the profession dissuaded many white youths who might enter medicine or surgery from making it an honorable and lucrative career. This, he said, kept many towns that lacked licensed physicians from having them.[72]

When in the course of the official procedure the report of Protomédico Arias came under the eyes of the applicant, Padilla's mounting wrath laid bare the true snarls in the case.[73] One of these was "the contempt" with which Arias "treats everybody in this country who dedicates himself to these faculties." Arias carried this distaste, Padilla argued, to the extreme of viciousness and malevolence. With heat as well as reason, he then proceeded to counteract the Arias report point by point. The first was the relatively innocuous one that the "municipal laws" required a lawyer and not a physician or surgeon for the post of fiscal of the proto-medicato. Though this was the "rigor" of the law, Padilla repeated what Arias had admitted—medical men had held the post. Besides, the man Arias presumed to appoint, Dr. Germán Gutiérrez de Piñeres, was the protomédico's personal friend. With an obvious effort at restraint, Padilla defended himself as best he could against the charge that he was unfit and of limited talent. The sole point, he said, that there "is not in this city any place to learn the first rudiments of surgery" is sufficient argument from which to gather the progress Padilla, who never left the country, could have made. Besides, all the education in the field that one was able to get through voluntary attendance at a hospital—"what learning in surgery is reduced to here"—could never be more than superficial.

Though Arias admitted that the fiscals in Cartagena had been medical men, he insisted that they had always been white because this pattern "corresponded to the honor owed the tribunal." With this object in view and no doubt at Arias's suggestion, in 1804 the viceroy ordered him not to admit in the future any man who does not have "blood purity and other requisites prescribed by law." Moreover, medicine, that beneficent and necessary science, "is found in this kingdom to be in the most abject state because of having admitted persons of inferior class to practice it, because, looking upon this vulgar preoccupation as ignoble, honorable men keep their sons from learning medicine."

When Arias's report reached him, the viceroy returned Padilla's application to Cartagena with the request that the governor report on the matter. The governor, in turn, went to the protomédico, Licenciado Juan de Arias. By sticking to the letter of the law, that official took positions hard to refute. In the first place, he said, the place was not vacant because the appointment of Dr. Germán Gutiérrez de Piñeres had already been announced, and though previous fiscals had come from medicine or surgery, undoubtedly this was owing to the difficulty of finding a lawyer without salary or perquisites of any kind who would be willing to take the post. Wanting the highest dignity for this post and following the example of the protomedicato of Madrid, Arias said he asked Dr. Gutiérrez de Piñeres to accept this portfolio and to appoint him promotor fiscal in accordance with Spanish law.[74] Arias showed that his predecessors had made appointments and now he had appointed Gutiérrez de Piñeres, a man of accredited abilities, a lawyer qualified, as the law required, to prosecute offenses brought before the protomedicato and to examine the reports on blood purity and other necessary requisites for admission to the protomedicato.

Padilla, Arias said bluntly, had neither the qualities of birth nor education. With respect to the first, he was born a pardo, and with respect to the second, "only necessity, the supreme law," could have provided the occasion to obtain this position on the basis of the Padilla affidavits. Here, however, he stressed Padilla's military record, pointing to the various expeditions in which he had held medical posts. Indeed, it was because of his service in one of these that the government approved him "in the class of physician."

Padilla admitted that he took Arias's statement on the matter of race as offensive, particularly concerning the penetration of men of color into medicine, which kept out those of a higher status. Unfortunate mortals who could only submit their ills to those born "under the sky of Europe"! After all, Cartagena had no medical courses that color could discourage the whites from entering. Padilla implied that the European physician, preferring to attend the rich and powerful, could hardly be expected to attend the poor in the daytime and at his regular hours, much less at bad times. Alluding to the "love and piety" with which "the king our lord" has looked upon his American vassals, Padilla took advantage of the increasing instances of persons "of his class who had been accorded honors" in the fields of theology, law, and medicine. Though one died before receiving his title, he had been appointed protomédico. Many others received rewards for participating in the conquest of Darién, in which he himself was involved. He added a damning postscript by saying again that the assessor was an intimate friend of Arias's.

At Padilla's request witnesses were called in Cartagena to testify on a number of points, but especially questions four and five: whether they had had information that Juan Manuel Castelbondo, a pardo of this city, deserved his title of maestro in the capital of the kingdom and his appointment as protomédico[75] and whether other pardos had received degrees of doctor or other honorific titles. The witnesses certified that Juan Manuel Castelbondo's intelligence, mastery of medicine, and faithful fulfillment of his obligations had led to his appointment as physician to the troops in "this plaza" of Bogotá and he was ultimately appointed protomédico by the king, though he died before this title arrived. Moreover, these witnesses produced names of pardos who had been "decorated" with the doctor's degree and other "honorific" titles. Pedro Carnacedo graduated as doctor in sacred theology and Alejandro Castelbondo got the doctor's degree in Bogotá after becoming a priest. This same Alejandro Castelbondo also got the post of physician to the Hospital de San Carlos de Cartagena. Other pardos had become surgeons of coast guard vessels based in Cartagena, and the viceroy had named Tomás Pérez y Castro as surgeon of the troops stationed at Portobelo. Of course, the witnesses did not neglect to mention the various honorable posts Padilla himself had held.[76]

Padilla made a strong case, but the official position was against him. The viceroy in Bogotá revealed his view when on November 10, 1807, he decreed that only those with certificates of limpieza de sangre could be admitted to examinations in surgery and medicine. The governor at Cartagena thought that perhaps the laws of the Indies might contradict those of Castile, but was reassured by his assessor—an enemy of Padilla's. After hearing his own legal advisers, the viceroy denied Padilla's application.[77]

In 1797 a royal policy that allowed a pardo to graduate from the University of Santo Tomás in Bogotá involved the crown in an inconsistency that, with pressure from some of its victims, it had seemingly corrected. In 1793 in Venezuela the celebrated protomédico, Felipe Tamariz, had kept the pardos José de Castro, Juan José de la Torre, and Diego de Obermexía from attending the "School of Anatomy" that Dr. Manuel de Carmona was holding in his house in Caracas. Since everybody practicing medicine with royal approval, as these men were, had to attend such a school, Tamariz's action was tantamount to debarring them from the profession.

As nearly always in these cases, the white doctors represented that there were enough of them, but the pardos were able to show that this assertion was false and self-interested. The royal cédula covering the case ruled that those practicing medicine with royal approval might not be kept out of classes in anatomy or any other subject they had to have. Protomédico Tamariz was invited to state his case, though, to see if he had any good reason for barring these pardo practitioners.[78]

Very often the arguments for allowing a mulatto to practice medicine were the same as those adduced for licensing foreigners who "found themselves" in the Indies. Francisco Colina, a mulatto who had come to Caracas from San Felipe, made typical arguments before the Audiencia of Caracas in 1798.[79] Having had an overwhelming desire to study and practice medicine from his "earliest childhood," Colina had followed his bent, assisted approved physicians, and then applied to the royal protomedicato for examination as a romance physician. Not only did he produce certificates from his doctor-teachers, but he also buttressed his case with the plea that, finding himself in Guanare, he remained for the space of two years because of the "absolute lack of medical practitioners there" and because of the town's entreaties that he remain to treat the residents.

Finding that the unfortunate rivalry between the governor and the protomedicato prevented him from getting the examination he sought, he could only try again before the royal audiencia. He argued that because the interior of the country totally lacked physicians there was no "express and determinative" legal prohibition that would bar those of his caste from practicing as romance physicians. Besides, he argued quite soundly, the many examples of approved pardo physicians should be persuasion enough.

At this stage the Superior Government, as was natural and routine, turned the case over to the fiscal. That officer advised that the case be postponed and handled with the file (*expediente*) that had been formed concerning the power of the protomedicato to regulate drugstores and examine physicians, and also the recent cédulas on termination of the pardo curanderos.[80] Colina's counsel contended that the audiencia should have him examined since the functions of the protomedicato were suspended for the time being, but the court, though returning the originals of some documents presented, turned the case over to a clerk of the court—tantamount to refusal to allow the examination.

In 1795 Protomédico Tamariz listed eleven white physicians and three white surgeons practicing in the city of Caracas. Two of the whites were romancistas and one a surgeon. When he came to the mulattoes, Tamariz called these mulatto practitioners "mulatto curanderos," not even dignifying them with the doubtful honor of romance physicians. The mulatto surgeons he called starkly "surgeons."[81] Of the eleven mulattoes, three practiced medicine and all the rest surgery, with no one practicing both. Clearly, the fact that the whites involved in this listing were overwhelmingly physicians and the mulattoes preponderantly surgeons shows that those with the best chance of getting an education chose medicine rather than surgery as the more dignified of the two professions.

Race and Caste: Dawn of a New Attitude

The middle decades of the eighteenth century, the time when one would begin to look for the full flower of the Enlightenment, was one of the low periods for persons of color in the Spanish empire who were struggling to pull themselves up. At the same time, to take a single case, medical faculties were nearly everywhere losing the slight prestige they once had. Young white men of good family simply did not enroll in medical courses. Alarmed officials explained that this was because pardos and others with this "stain" or inferior "sphere" squirmed around the regulations and into medicine in such numbers that it drove out the young white men, who could not bear to rub shoulders with riffraff. It seems just as likely, though, that the pardos, denied easy, bona fide access to the professions, simply filled the yawning chasm that lack of interest among whites had created. And then at the beginning of the nineteenth century, a new humane movement set in that began to favor a humanism that included men of other races. In 1803 a Franciscan provincial in

Guatemala initiated a policy of soul-searching in Spain reflective of this change.

Though it took place in 1803, the Franciscan José Antonio de Goicoechea proposed the first clear, unequivocal statement "on the need of honoring to a certain degree the mulattoes and zámbos in that kingdom and in all the Indies." The Council of the Indies, meanwhile, sent the request on to its fiscal, who proposed putting the papers in the same file being amassed from Caracas on conceding the address of *"Don"* and "other distinctions" to pardos. The main, unresolved case was one in which the authorities in Caracas had been resisting for some ten years a royal demand that Lorenzo, the son of Diego Mexías Bejarano, should be exempted from his pardo status and be enrolled in the university. Though he had been willing to supply the five hundred reales of vellón for this type of grace, the constant repetition of the cédula indicated that the royal will had been nullified.[82] Though the fiscal had made certain suggestions that were about to be carried out through royal cédulas, these steps, up to 1806, depended on the working out of some general formula on the status of pardos. The crown attorney favored the idea, but the constant application to the Contaduría General to find what effect the proposed concessions would have upon tribute payments and upon the fees collected for gracias al sacar indicates that the crown was touched deeply in that sensitive but inanimate region—the exchequer.[83] So far as the medical professions were concerned, the Americans were still opposed to the idea, not only because legal medical practitioners were touched in the same place, but also because the pardos were considered too far down socially to most of the well-to-do whites.

During the Napoleonic Wars, however, a government in desperate need of money and with a strong humanitarian, liberal bent changed all that—or at least attempted to do so. Caught in this change at the outbreak of the wars were two Guatemalan pharmacists, asking to be lifted out of their "sphere" of pardos. One of these, Mariano Fernández, informed the Council of the Indies that he had practiced pharmacy in various hospitals and drugstores. Further, when he had established his competence and fulfilled the other requirements, the captain general of Guatemala authorized him to open a public drugstore in October 1808. Fernández not only wanted this concession approved but he also wanted exemption from the handicap of pardo so that he could practice with complete freedom. Drawing special attention to Mariano's charitable work with the "poor Indians" and his scrupulous behavior, regency officials sanctioned the captain general's action and exempted him from any racial handicap in the practice of his profession.[84] Francisco Fernández, apparently the son of Mariano, petitioned the same year on December 2,

1810, saying that he "found himself practicing pharmacy" without being able to take an examination or to get a license from the protomedicato because he was a pardo. Moved in part by the example of his father, the government ordered the examination and, of course, exempted him from his pardo status upon payment of the seven hundred reales stipulated in the tariff of fees for gracias al sacar.[85]

The cases of the pardo pharmacists from Guatemala soon became important precedents. At the very time that the Council of Regency resolved neither to require nor admit reports on noble status, the cédula exempting Mariano Fernández from the "condition of pardo" was pulled out and reconsulted in various offices of the government, a government that had taken on a liberal stamp.[86]

Deliberations of the Cortes of Cádiz had already opened the way for a relaxation of the proscriptions against blacks, mixed bloods, and Indians existing in Spain and the empire. On August 17, 1811, the Cortes issued a decree intended to "open the career of honor and glory to the honorable families of the monarchy, thus handing out reward for the heroic effort which Spaniards of all classes have made and are making to maintain the independence and dignity of the nation." A short time later, legislation made those of African origin in Spain and the empire not in slave status full citizens of Spain. Then on March 9, 1813, the liberal Cortes went a step further by a decree to military bodies, colleges, and academies that certificates of purity of blood would neither be required nor permitted. Neither would the army and navy permit "expressions or distinctions which tend to foment trouble between individuals" and to promote legal inequality or the rivalry between classes. Eleven days later the Regency sent the decree to the Indies.[87] But it came too late to have any influence in America. Moreover, the return of the reactionary Ferdinand VII to Spain in 1814 and the continuing colonial wars of revolution subverted the new liberal legislation that had been intended to open the way for status and preferment to men of color not only in the medical professions but also in other fields.

Obligations and Fees

THE FEELING THAT MEDICINE was an obligation first and a profitable career second was already established in Spanish law at the time of the conquest of America. When the doctor took his oath, he swore to perform the duties of his calling and to attend and treat the poor as a form of alms without charging fees or expecting salary. This he asserted with all the solemnity that he swore to defend the Immaculate Conception "in public and in secret." But fulfilling his obligations did not rest solely upon the virtue and charity of the physician; there was legal compulsion when necessary.[1]

The Cortes of Valladolid of 1538, just three years after Spanish medical law had been extended to America, enjoined the doctor to keep in mind the cure of the soul, for even the cure of the body sometimes required it. The worst offense in the "cure of the soul," and one frequently enough committed, was the failure of the practitioner to advise his patient, especially the seriously sick one, to confess as required by canon law. The civil law on the point was drastic: the doctor or surgeon in such cases must advise the patient to confess, at least by the second visit, on pain of a fine of ten thousand maravedís for each failure.[2]

The mercy and charity implied in the idea of hospitals, as they were in Spain four hundred years ago, did not mean that the body should be spurned merely because the soul was more important. Spanish hospital records are full of evidence that much money went to feed the indigent patient.[3] Any modern man who has overheard the inquisitorial processes issuing from the nooks and booths that line the entrances to charity wards in modern hospitals will understand that it is still difficult to determine who a poor man is. Some Spanish physicians felt that a poor man was in such distress that he lived from charity alone. The view that prevailed, however, was that in common law he who lived by the work of his hands and had no property should be treated as truly poor. Every day, though, poor men sold their miserable furniture to avoid "going to the hospitals," a phrase that sounded then more like a death knell than a peal of hope.

In cases where funds were so desperately raised, custom required that the money should go first to feed the patient and second to pay the doctor. If anything remained, the druggist could collect, because he contributed not only "his bodily work" as the physicians and surgeons did but also his own means in the purchase of medicines. When a man died without sufficient property to pay the expenses of his illness, funeral, and "the intercession for his soul," these costs took precedence "by common and well-known rules."[4]

Some practitioners in Spain evidently attempted to evade their oath to visit and treat these poor people gratis. In the eighteenth century, nevertheless, the traditions of the medical profession went beyond the law. It was clearly understood that the salaried physician should not charge a fee, though an occasional commentator thought that a patient, once well, might make a voluntary payment.[5] In America a doctor able to prove that he treated the poor without charge and, especially, bought drugs for them at his own cost, in any struggle for preferment found himself ranked far above the doctor who did not. Even a midwife had to promise to take charity cases.[6] In 1800 such a policy left Dr. José García y Bernal so poor that after four months' illness he appealed to the rector of the university for money to sustain his family.[7] In 1800 the royal protomedicato of Caracas took time, after drawing up a solemn tariff of fees and charges, to exempt poor people from the obligation to pay a doctor's fees. Commenting that love of one's fellows and interest in the public health should be sufficient to induce the physician to attend the poor with even more love and care than they did the rich, the protomedicato threatened those doctors who demurred with "serious steps."[8]

Could a patient contract with a Spanish doctor to cure him in consideration of a certain sum? For a long time some authorities said yes, but they argued that the contractual pay was not due if the patient did not recover. Other authorities were worried over whether a patient was under obligation to pay when the cured disease supposedly returned. For a while some authorities thought that when the disease came back after a long time, the doctor had kept his bargain. The difficulties of this problem led legal authorities to the conclusion "that the transaction and other contracts between the physician and the patient are of no effect." This is the opinion Muñoz endorsed when he reviewed the subject in the middle of the eighteenth century. How, then, should a patient be charged? "In proportion to the work, the difficulty of the treatment, and to the property and possessions of the cured." This was "the soundest rule and the one most often followed in practice."[9] There was, however, no problem in the position that the physician should treat the penniless for nothing, for there was no other way he could treat them. The heart of the matter, though, was the likelihood that he would not treat the penniless at all.

On July 4, 1776, quite unbeknownst to those making themselves famous in Philadelphia, the town council in Mexico City set in motion a train of complaints against the medical profession that brought to a head a perennial problem of colonial medicine. Among the endless jeremiads against the deceptions of druggists and the techniques of barbers that left their patients "maimed," a councilman lodged a protest against the physicians who refused "to go out after nine o'clock at night except to powerful houses and then only when carriages are sent to bring them." The issue was serious enough to have the viceroy and council request a full report from the royal protomedicato. Though promising to continue prosecuting criminal druggists and crippling bleeders, the protomedicato, itself made up of practicing doctors, sounded a note of caution on night visitations. They referred with such awe to "what happened to Bachelor Ylario Regulado" that one can only infer that this physician had been killed in visiting a patient at night. Indeed, the protomédicos continued with emphasis, "for this reason the very confessors do not go out, even to take the holy oil, without an escort. . . ." In short, it was not reasonable to expect a doctor automatically to place his life in jeopardy to answer calls, even emergency calls, at night.[10]

Calls in the dead of night always have been the bane of the physician, and where these involved contusions, abrasions, and fractures of Saturday night revelry, they were likely to be an uncompensated bane as well. After three hundred years in Mexico, in consequence, the difficulty of getting doctors and surgeons to answer calls "at unseasonable hours of the night" had not been resolved. Yet sometime in the 1770s new attitudes occasioned by the Enlightenment also began to call for increased humanity in medicine and greater efficiency in policing. Sometimes the two went hand in hand; and they all went faster once the viceroy took up the gauntlet.

Such was the long train of actions set in motion by Viceroy Antonio María Bucareli in his ban of May 14, 1777. A report of the Mexico City town council the preceding February deplored the tragedies resulting from lack of medical attention to those wounded in frays and brawls. With no one to stay the blood, unnecessary deaths might and did occur. Besides, delay, especially long delay, often made the treatment of wounds futile. So much for humanity; neglect of the injured made less likely the apprehension of the "aggressor." A man often died in an obscure place, and after a long lapse witnesses could not be found, and the victim, needless to say, could not tell his story. All of this, the police declared, resulted from the "custom" of the surgeons in not attending these miserable fellows "without a prior order of a magistrate." To get a prior order from a magistrate might be as difficult as to get a surgeon out of bed at three o'clock in the morning with slight prospects of a fee. Hence, the police urged that the surgeon go immediately to the victim's side and report the visit immediately or at the "first comfortable moment." The royal judge could then take cognizance of the case and set up investigative procedures that would prevent the hiding of crime and avoid risking the life of the wounded man.

Always sensitive to the shifting of the Spanish winds, Mexican officials learned too that in the preceding summer the Madrid government had issued a decree in an effort to eliminate or lessen the same evils in Spain. Thus bolstered, Viceroy Bucareli decreed in 1777 that surgeons in Mexico City and throughout the whole kingdom should first answer calls to treat the wounded—whether wounded "by hand or by accident"—and then report to the judge within eight hours on pain of a fine of twenty-five pesos for failing to respond to the call or to report the case; for the second failure to report, the fine was fifty pesos and two years' exile twenty leagues from the city, and for the third, one hundred pesos and four years at hard labor.[11]

Since such orders came only at intervals—and always in the time of energetic viceroys—the inference is that the sad, often tragic conditions they were designed to correct actually persisted. A dozen years later Viceroy Revilla Gigedo had the same problem cluttering his desk. The first to feel his wrath were the guards charged with keeping the streetlights (*guardafaroleros*). By his new regulations a watchman found drunk at night might expect eight days in the public stocks before the jailhouse door. For covering up a robbery, the full vigor of the law would be brought to bear on him. The penalty for having the lights out or dirty was a warning, and for the second, summary dismissal. It also became his duty to see that the word was carried from mouth to mouth when a doctor or midwife had to be called from outside the district.[12]

A certain irritation with the presumption and continued lack of response among medical men also began to appear. In September 1790, for example, owing no doubt to the obstruction of the narrow streets, the viceroy issued a proclamation that forbade leaving mounts at the doors or entranceways to houses, and followed it with a statement of penalties for violation of the new decree. Presently the royal protomedicato got word that Bachelor Manuel Gómez, a properly licensed physician, had had his mount seized by the police and taken away. The harried bachelor could only redeem his horse by paying a large fine.

This indignity, the culmination of many suffered by other physicians and surgeons, occasioned a protest from the royal protomedicato.[13] These learned gentlemen told the viceroy firmly that it was absolutely essential that the mounts of physicians and surgeons be left at the street doors of courtyards of houses opening into the street. Practitioners— proud ones, the implication is—could not go afoot through dangerous neighborhoods and trudge the length of the streets to attend the sick. Such a requirement would mean that the sick often went without treatment and the doctors without the matching increment. Leaving the horse in the middle of some street with just anybody, even when just anybody could be found, or sending the animal to some public entrance hall to be left alone there, would have no result except to have the beast stripped of riding gear—"which takes place every day, and many times the thief [takes] the beasts themselves." What was there to do but leave the horse at the street door? So said the protomédicos "Dr. and Master José Giral, Dr. and Master José Francisco Rada, and Dr. and Master José Ignacio García Jove" on October 11, 1790.

The efficient and probably annoyed Revilla Gigedo answered the next day that the doctors could take a boy to care for the horse or else they could have someone come out of the courtyard to do it. Then, aroused by the failure of the protomédicos, nineteen doctors and surgeons prefaced a firm protest with the charge that the viceroy's suggestion would be costly for all, impossible for some, and at the very best difficult and vexatious. They felt that most medical men could not afford to have a servant stand by at all hours and that they would be obliged to abandon the profession, "or walk alone" against the order. A patient so poor as to be utterly alone, therefore, would not be visited at all. It would be better to have the sole attendant wait upon the doctor as he prescribes and gives his instructions for nursing than to guard the doctor's horse. The adverse effect of the drastic regulation would be felt most by the poor "to whom so many graces and exceptions have been extended." The protomedicato attached its solemn endorsement to this bold petition.[14] Nevertheless, in reviewing this petition, the crown attorney held that while the mendicant religious involved might be exempted from the law, in his view the medical man should be wealthy enough to pay someone to care for his mount. He advised the viceroy that if there were any doctors so needy that injury might result to the poor, the protomédicos should furnish a list of their names. In those days of exaggerated pride, no better twist could have been suggested to put the quietus on the medical protesters. The viceroy reiterated his original order and repeated the fiscal's stinging points.[15]

A viceroy grown testy through opposition from those practicing medicine was in no mood to hear of their other faults. At 12:30 a.m. on the night of July 14–15, 1792, Francisco María de Herrera, the senior alderman of Mexico City, reported that a wounded man in San Juan de

Tecpán was "bleeding with all violence," but no doctor could be found to go to him. Manuel de Otero, the ward magistrate who reported the incident, stated that at 12:30 "o'clock the night before last" someone knocked on his door and reported that in San Juan de Tecpán there was a man "bleeding violently and likely to die." Two night watchmen were then ordered to find and send a surgeon. Two-and-a-half hours later, at three in the morning, these men returned to say that they could get no doctor to go. They therefore decided to take the man to the Royal Hospital and report the incident to the city judge to institute proceedings. (Meanwhile, no doubt, the patient went to his mortal rest.)

Under oath, the notaries swore that the men had gone to the door of Dr. Francisco Prado where, after "having been at the door calling for something like an hour," a woman came to the balcony and said the doctor could not come out because "he had broken out in a sweat." A porter at the house of Dr. Ignacio Lucero excused his master with a polite phrase, saying "he was not in." In two weeks' time after the case was drawn up, the fiscal advised the viceroy to have the surgeons involved appear and make their defense. But nothing happened.

Eight months later, on March 14, 1793, the viceroy wanted to know why there was "so notable a delay." The notary, it appears, had misplaced the papers, but when these had been pried out of him by proper judicial orders, the surgeons at last appeared. Dr. Lucero claimed that he had performed an operation "on the liver of a man named Manuel" and that, as indicated in such serious operations, he was attending this patient until two in the morning. "Not precisely remembering," Prado thought that he was not called or "else he would have complied promptly." Annoyed at the lack of "correct administration of justice," the court fiscal said little could be done to find the truth after such a long delay. Upon his advice, though, the viceroy on May 26, 1793, instructed the protomedicato that all physicians, surgeons, druggists, and midwives should respond when called by the sick and by local magistrates. The viceroy also issued clear instructions to the ward magistrates to inform the patrolmen of the new regulations.[16]

Twenty-two years later the problem was as far as ever from solution. In 1815 Viceroy Félix de Calleja (1813–16), amid all the troubles of civil war, had to take time to issue an order on the subject. As a preface, he said he had been frequently informed that the physicians of the capital, forgetting the principles and institutes of their profession, refused to answer calls at "unseasonable" hours of the night. Much as he regretted it, such a "grave and important omission" required him to take steps to prevent a scandalous and inhuman proceeding in the future. Hence, any failure to go to the sick and wounded at whatever hour of the night would force him to reinvoke the penalties established by Viceroy Bucareli. This time, though, Viceroy Calleja took care that the illness was authentic and the call necessary. He required that the policeman or night watchman, when asked for help, should be approached not by some helter-skelter servant who might stir up three or four doctors but by the owner or some trustworthy person of the house. A policeman would accompany the doctor back to his house as well as away from it. This decision was, upon second thought, issued by ban not only in Mexico City but also in other places throughout the kingdom.[17]

If the Mexican officials failed in this aim, it was not because doctors had no clear understanding of their legal and moral obligations. In 1795, for example, a corregidor in Durango reported that the chief of police told him that four physicians summoned at midnight by the policeman on duty refused to visit a woman though she was very ill, receiving the "holy oil"—extreme unction—at 12:30 that night. The dutiful corregidor cited all four physicians who, "having bathed" for the night, refused to go to the sick woman.

How these four men excused themselves reflects the undependable state of medical assistance. Dr. Juan Losano claimed he had instructed the police on duty not to call him that night since his wife had been in childbirth the day before. Dr. Juan Bermúdez explained that his "habitual rheumatism" required frequent baths after which it became dangerous for him to venture out. Dr. José Jurado thought that, because he had syphilis, he could expect disastrous consequences from going out at night except in a coach. Dr. José Carmona was "constipated as the result of a catarrh" and feared a dangerous fever as the penalty of venturing into the night air.

The corregidor was not to be foiled by these random excuses. He took an affidavit from the policeman on duty, who could not sign the legal paper "because he did not know how." With this illiterate officer and an Indian woman servant, Josefa Cháves, the corregidor proved that all except Losano had been called to help the woman. The determined royal official now addressed the charge to the viceroy, who turned it over to his fiscal. Having just failed in his prosecution of Dr. José Francisco Rada, a member of the royal protomedicato, on the same grounds, the fiscal was in a choleric mood with the whole medical profession. Though he judged the Durango doctors' excuses "frivolous and specious," he came immediately to the abuses perpetrated by physicians in Mexico that needed "much reform." Had not Francisco de la Riva gone "unshriven to eternity" without "temporal help" on account of the same frivolous excuse by Dr. Francisco Rada? The fiscal thus recommended "severe correction" and a fine of twenty-five pesos each for Bermúdez,

Jurado, and Carmona. He also advised that the chief of police instruct his men not to call a doctor upon the mere statement of a servant but to confirm the information through the owner of the house or through some other responsible person. As a crowning stroke, the fiscal advised the viceroy to instruct the protomedicato to call a general meeting of physicians to rebuke the Durango doctors and "exhort those assembled to serve the public without giving rise to lawsuits." The assessor, however, only supported the recommendation that the medical men be assembled for the purpose recommended. The proper orders went out that the corregidor in Durango instruct his men not to call a physician, surgeon, or confessor until the need had been confirmed through a responsible person.

Responding in their consultative capacity, the protomédicos made a sharp set of their own recommendations. They wanted the night watchmen to call one doctor, the one in the patient's own district, and not end up by bringing three or four together at the same bedside. They objected also to the police practice of escorting the doctor to the patient but not back home again. Most of all, though, they could not understand why patients thought they ought not pay a doctor who had been brought by a policeman. They besought the Superior Government to drop the loose statements against Dr. Rada, who had been exonerated in court. Luckless Rada! Just the year before, while making a visit to the Inquisition jail, he had his dress sword or dagger jerked from him by the French revolutionary, Jean Marie Murgier, who presented the point of the blade to the doctor's Adam's apple as he took him hostage.[18] The Superior Government adopted every one of these recommendations, though it was careful to state that "when the patient can," he should pay the doctor escorted to him just as he would pay the unescorted one.[19] Though complicated, the case had taken only eight months to resolve, but, as nature remained the same, so did this problem.

Court Testimony and Legal Certification

Although Anglo-American courts tried medical cases by lawyers with expert medical testimony, in Spanish colonial courts they were tried by doctors with expert legal help. This reversal does not mean, however, that expert medical testimony could always be dispensed with. In a matter so critical as life and death, the most brilliant theologian, and certainly the ordinary parish priest, had need of medical testimony in a score of unexpected ways. To authorize a cesarean operation, not to mention a burial, the priest needed the certification of the physician whether one was to be found or not. A viceroy, for example, could not determine whether to replace a sick public official or to wait for the incumbent to recover and resume his work. In consequence, a mere licensed physician could supply the medical opinion required while matters of state called for the solemnity of a consultation by the royal protomedicato. Except in the cases involving canon law, however, these medical props sprang more from customary than from statutory law.

The evidence is abundant enough that the protomedicato often served in such a legal advisory capacity. As there was nothing that concerned the Spaniards more than the mode of handling the American revenues, the apparent illness of Luis Gutiérrez, the treasurer of New Spain, forced the viceroy to consult the Council of the Indies on the proper course to pursue. Fully aware of the danger to his position, the sick man then presented a document from the protomédicos that declared, apparently against the prevailing feeling, that his infirmity, "albeit venereal," was curable and that it would jointly undertake a variation of "mercurial unctions," supposedly to get the distressed official back to work in due course.[20]

Even a prisoner in need of mercurial unction was not beneath the attention of high political or medical officers. When in 1796 the criminal sala of the audiencia sentenced Jacinto Rodríguez to two years' labor at the fortifications of Veracruz, Dr. José Rada, the physician of the Holy Inquisition, and Licentiate Bernardo Cozar certified that he needed the mercury treatment for syphilis. Viceroy Branciforte thus instructed the Royal Indian Hospital to take the prisoner, treat him, and let him serve his time as a servant in the hospital. In this case the prisoner made his recovery before the end of November, continued his sentence by working with a hospital porter, and earned a good reputation.[21]

Attending physicians had curious legal responsibilities beyond mere medicine that involved the lives of those they treated. When patients were on the verge of death, doctors were often unable to perform all the acts for the good of their souls as required by canon law. In case the female partner in a common law marriage was pregnant, in imminent danger of death, and unable to reach the church and go through a ceremony there, the doctor had to so certify in order to enable the priest to perform the ceremony at some other place. To enable the cleric to marry the mestizo Sebastián Antonio González to the mestiza María Loreto Juárez, the doctor reported that the girl was on the point of dying of "catarrhal exanthematic fever," or, in the vernacular, "of *tabardillo*."[22] In another case Bachelor Mariano García, a physician treating María Antonia Vásquez, a Spanish woman, certified that she suffered from a malignant parturient fever, with "palpitation of the heart," and that she was "in obvious danger of losing her life." Thus, in keeping with his

duty, the doctor delicately suggested that she receive the sacraments.[23]
Yet, tragic and pathetic as these instances are, they seem trifling compared
to another type of certification that the medical man was obliged to
give—that, in effect, all the inhabitants of a village were dead, supposedly in an epidemic. If they were dead, the reasoning was, they
should not be expected to pay the tribute.

Obligations Filled and Unfulfilled

It would be very difficult to find a medical problem in America that had
not been anticipated in Spain, either in statutory or customary law. The
principle was firm in Spain when the conquest in America was at its
height that no physician might excuse himself from attending the sick—
not even if that person was down with a contagious disease, nor might
he run from a city suffering from an epidemic.[24] Yet three hundred years
later these faults were as pronounced and distressing as ever. The vehe-
mence with which the Spanish government as late as 1834 noticed and
tried to correct the evil of the physician flying both from his patient and
his town when these stood most in need of him give proof enough that
the whole span of the colonial period had not been enough to hold the
frightened physician to his post.[25]

At so late a date the Spanish government noticed the continued
failure of some doctors to meet the "most sacred duties" of their profession. The minister involved did not hesitate to label running away
from a town in its moment of affliction as "criminal conduct" and
"shameful cowardice." To set these miserable examples off from their
colleagues who so bravely held their ground, the crown made it a royal
order that all licenses of physicians and surgeons flying before an
epidemic, especially of cholera, should be immediately confiscated. The
Superior Governing Committee of Medicine and Surgery and other authorities, making use of laws in force, got specific orders to declare all
chairs in colleges and all posts in public establishments abandoned by
these refugees to be in fact vacant and to proceed to fill them with other
men. As a fitting humiliation, the junta would send the government the
names of these replaced practitioners to be punished in the "*Gaceta* of
this court," in the *Diario de la Administración,* and in provincial bulletins
alongside the names of those who had honorably done their duty. To
take these steps, it is evident, did not require new legislation—merely
revival of existing, even ancient laws.

In America not even a missionary, old and sick, might return home
to die without royal permission, nor could a doctor expect to move freely
from place to place. In 1760 it took a decree from the viceroy of New

Spain to allow Dr. Antonio Martínez to return to Spain, though Martínez was legal expert of the protomedicato and physician of the Royal Indian Hospital.[26] Dr. Luis Montaña, a highly respected figure, caused an uproar when he abandoned the woman's ward in this hospital for almost two months in 1804 in order to accompany a well-to-do figure to Veracruz and another sick man on the return, at least part of the way.[27]

In the Spanish empire it was very difficult to hold the official or salaried physician or surgeon to his obligations, particularly at ports of entry. As patron, the king had appointed a surgeon for the Hospital of the Order of Charity of San Hipólito in Veracruz to attend the sick "between 22 and 24 hours." The prior of the Convent and Hospital of San Juan de Montesclaros, however, revealed that something was wrong when he petitioned the king in 1704 to authorize Fray Rodrigo de la Fuente to substitute for the surgeon when "he fell ill or absented himself, as happened." Without its own expert, the convent might go without surgical care in an emergency. After all, the petitioner said, de la Fuente had substituted for the surgeon on such occasions, had been "examined and approved as a master of surgery by the protomedicato of this kingdom," as his certificate showed, and had served both as "religious surgeon" of his order and as head male nurse. Despite the plea that this precautionary appointment would be of vital use to the order, the king went straight to the question; he ordered the corregidor of Veracruz to submit a report showing whether the surgeon met his obligations, especially whether he made the visits called for under the terms of his appointment. For any failure, the corregidor should reprimand the surgeon and force him to comply. The viceroy should name a man to substitute in the case of sickness or "legitimate absence" without increasing the salary.[28]

Crimes, Brawls, and the Medical Practitioner

Wherever the official or salaried surgeon had the responsibility of mending heads broken on the weekends and on holidays—a good deal more than half of the time in the calendar—he found himself obliged to respond and sometimes to work single-handed. Though he would not have given up his "honorific title" for all the spices of Araby, it did irk him that while he staggered sleepily through the streets to the side of some bloody beggar, his colleagues lolled in bed or, when they sensed a fashionable call, woke themselves with a sniff of snuff, issued forth, and collected a good fee. The insistence of the licensed surgeons that all the unlicensed ones be prosecuted also reacted against them in cases like this one. In 1759 the Guatemalan surgeon, Pedro de Zúñiga, complained bitterly that he spent most of his time repairing wounds inflicted in fights and brawls. As the only licensed surgeon in Guatemala City, he could not call upon the city's unlicensed surgeons for help.[29] Forty-one years later, in 1800, Guatemalans did not feel that the situation had improved.[30]

Medicine in the Spanish empire was often a police matter. And this was not just a question of calling a doctor, which, if the call came during late hours of the night, often devolved upon the police. Brawls were as common then as they are now, and the brawlers served by the unlicensed surgeon in the Royal Indian Hospital in Mexico City became so bothersome in 1763 that the administrator, completely bypassing the royal protomedicato, made an appeal to the viceroy to stop their entrance. Since the wounded often came in drunk, and suits arose from these unfortunate incidents, it was uncommon in the extreme to have a doctor or surgeon present himself, examine the patient, and make a report to the police authorities. Since the assessor thought that it was not only good policy but also in accordance with the "urbanity" with which the hospital should be treated, the viceroy decreed that no person might enter the hospital to examine these patients or make reports concerning them without the permission of the administrator of the hospital.[31]

In this borderland between the purely medical and the purely judicial, however, there was never complete certainty on admissions procedures. The authorities were still so confused in 1815 that it was necessary for a notary to summarize all the previous regulations available and establish the proper procedures. From this digest it evolved that, when a wounded person was brought in, the hospital should enter in the books the name of the wounded man, that of the person bringing him, and the jurisdiction to which the man belonged. Thereupon, the doctor was instructed to make an examination and leave his certified report with the intern or some other known person to be turned over to the proper authorities. This practice required that the examining surgeon should say whether the wound was recent or appeared to have been inflicted some days previously—a precaution that could lead to the uncovering of the person having to hide the crime. To prevent alteration or fraud, receipts were entered in another book for these certifications. Likewise, in case of necessity, a certification on the gravity of a wound or state of health should be immediately available—presumably for prompt prosecutions. This care implied, of course, that when a wounded man died, the surgeon should quickly certify the fact and notaries, when such a contingency was expected, should come by the hospital often—daily if necessary—to pick them up so as not to delay the start of the case. Aside from such particulars in individual cases, the hospital sent to the proper court a list of those wounded and their judges, with notations of those who died and of those who recovered, and a statement of whether or not the certifications had been picked up.[32]

"*The Spiritual and Bodily Leech*" *and* Ad Curam Corporum

The failure of many licensed physicians to fulfill their obligations—to minister to the poor, to tend to the wounded and dying weekend brawlers and roustabouts, and to brave dangerous city streets or country byways in the middle of the night to go to the bedside of a critically ill patient—left critical needs to be met in the Spanish Indies. Curanderos and intrusos were two elements stepping into this breach attending those who could not afford the services of licensed physicians or who were ignored by them. Also, naturally and almost effortlessly, because of the close links between soul and body, the clergy became intimately involved in meeting those obligations that medical men forsook or shunted aside, and in many areas of the Indies the clergy filled the gap left open by licensed doctors.

The quality of mercy cannot strain long at distinctions between soul and body. From the earliest times of the Christian church there was a great temptation and an even greater need for priests and friars to enter the practice of medicine—"to unite the spiritual and the bodily leech," as Joseph Blanco White, an Irish observer, phrased it in the nineteenth century.[33] At first glance there is no union more natural. In fact, Miguel Eugenio Muñoz declared: "the practice of medicine has been the ministry of angels and archangels." Elisha, he said, purified the pestilential waters of Jericho, while Saint Paul, Saint Luke, and a formidable list of religious and saints practiced medicine. Muñoz emphasized also that four supreme pontiffs were among those learned in medicine.[34]

Unfortunately, the friars and monks embracing the "bodily leech" realized they could turn a penny at the same time they performed an act of mercy. With an afflicted and benighted population flocking to these friars, the most venal ones were soon holding "clinics" little better than those of the forbidden enchanters (*ensalmadores*). In medieval Europe the practice of medicine became so vulgar[35] that the church council of Rheims (1131) and the Lateran (1139) recognized this abuse and eventually at the Council of Tours (1163) forbade monks and friars, under the menace of drastic penalties, to leave their cloisters to take up the practice of medicine. Very late, though, when the religious houses themselves direly needed medical attention, the pope annulled the canon law that forbade priests from practicing physic.[36]

At the time of the opening of America, priests had as their primary duty "the cure of souls," but every stage of the Spanish conquest also brought them closer and closer to "the cure of bodies." At the first stage whoever professed to have more than ordinary medical lore, or accidentally revealed that he did, found himself in practice. From this kind of forced draft the religious could not escape, especially when there were no "Latin doctors" or when the ministrations of these learned men fell short of expectations. When suffering from a grave illness, for example, Viceroy Antonio de Mendoza dismissed his physicians and called in the Franciscan Lucás de Almodóvar.[37] From that day until the Franciscans were at the height of their achievement in faraway California, who can doubt that the religious accepted the responsibility of medicine when they needed to? In the early days of the post-conquest epoch the great number of people in the streets of Mexico City plainly and pathetically suffering from syphilitic sores, the outward and visible legacy of the conquest, profoundly moved both priest and laymen. In the sixteenth century Bishop Juan de Zumárraga even founded the long-lasting Hospital del Amor de Dios to treat these wretched victims and saw it endowed with an encomienda.[38]

The intervention of the church in many classes of medical problems remained normal, and sometimes priests rose to medical eminence. Men of the cloth became professors of medicine, and some actually became protomédicos, because as long as they held medical degrees they could qualify for membership on the protomedicato. In the University of San Marcos de Lima, for example, the presbyter, Dr. Pedro de Requena, became the second professor of prima of medicine, a chair founded in 1635,[39] and, with no serious challenge, protomédico general. Still, before the publication of the Constituciones of the University of San Marcos in 1735, there was sometimes squabbling in the cloister over whether priests might serve in university medical chairs. The man made professor of anatomy there in 1711 and of medical "method" in 1727 was Dr. José de Fontidueñas, an ordained priest,[40] but a curious medical career had forced the issue. Dr. Francisco Vargas Machuca, who brought the matter to a head, served every chair of medicine in the University of San Marcos except that of anatomy. Now as professor of prima of medicine he should normally and automatically become the general or chief protomédico. Because he was a priest, however, his inauguration was held up. In 1718, accordingly, Philip V ruled that, with papal dispensation, Vargas Machuca might legally qualify, as he actually did after the proper dispensation by Pope Clement XI.[41] Vargas Machuca's fate, however, was that his life overlapped with the master of wit and irony, the poet Juan del Valle Caviedes, a chronically sick man who mercilessly satirized the doctors at a moment when their pomposity robbed them of the flexibility they needed to reply with the same ammunition. Priests practicing medicine in Lima at the beginning of the eighteenth century, to judge by the number who came under the poet's strictures, was a common thing. In Mexico in 1753, Fray Juan Antonio de Avila, presbyter of the Order of San Juan de Dios, took the second seat on the royal protomedicato without a ripple. He simply asked the king, when he became senior member of his faculty, to confirm him as second protomédico.[42] Since the cédula of 1646 so provided,[43] the king routinely confirmed the title.[44]

Although there were never enough men to treat the sick, clashes between certified doctors and practicing friars did occur, especially in provincial towns. There the people, but particularly the very poor people, begged the religious to pay medical visits to them in their houses, while civil authorities asked them to attend prisoners in the local jail. In Aguascalientes, for example, where the Order of San Juan de Dios had a hospital, Fray Ignacio de Escobar rendered both these services on the outside. When these suddenly ceased, however, the magistrate, Pedro de Herrera Leyva, protested. Speaking for the hospital, Fray Pedro de Cardozo replied that the physician Anastacio Segura, the only doctor in this town, had been raging against "my religious" for practicing medicine in the neighborhood. An order from Cardozo's superior, reinforced by a ruling of the protomedicato in Mexico City, had forced Escobar to stop attending the sick in jail and visiting the poor in their houses. Herrera now made his second and most cogent argument. With Escobar pushed out of practice, he said, a city of eight thousand people could turn only to Segura, who was often out of town, and, the implication is, not available to the poor when he was.[45] It was usually more profitable to go off with some mineowner or some rich hacendado than to stay in town troubling himself with so many other types of people.

These are but a few examples of the ways in which the clergy filled the vacuum caused when medical practitioners did not meet their obligations to Spanish colonial society. But the religious were also active in other ways. The nursing orders of San Hipólito, San Juan de Dios, and Betelmitas were active in the establishment and administration of hospitals. In fact, the self-abnegating Hippolytes in Mexico invited members of other orders to serve in traditional administrative posts such as chaplains so that they might spend their time healing the sick.[46] In 1773, because their services were so badly needed in their own hospital endeavors, these same Hippolytes in Mexico were exempted from a viceregal order requiring a year's internship in the newly created school of surgery set up at the Royal Indian Hospital.[47] Often by default, clergy in convents throughout the Indies also set up apothecary shops to serve the needs of the surrounding community, although not always without charging large fees. Moreover, those religious demonstrating any natural talent for the practice of medicine and surgery, again by default, often established themselves as practitioners to serve the needs of those in areas where there were no licensed doctors. Like the curanderos and intrusos, the clergy responded both to the shortage of doctors and to their failure to meet their legal obligations when they were available. The religious found themselves forced to minister to the constituency's physical needs at the bottom of society's priorities as well as to their souls that ranked at the top.

⚒ 9 *Pride and Preferment:*
The Standing and Reputation of
Medical Men and Medical Practice

Social and Financial Privileges

THOSE WHO CAST their eyes back on the venerable history of medicine have been more puzzled than dismayed that around the staff of Aesculapius, the god of medicine, there should wind a poised serpent. Some suggest that the serpent bespeaks prudence, others help to the ailing. To a cynical modern like the Peruvian poet Juan del Valle Caviedes, the serpent might just as well represent poison. To every beholder, though, the serpent does more than suggest the dignity and awesomeness of the medical doctor; it hints at control over life and death. The doctors, who know better, can be forgiven if they do little to dissipate this notion.

In Spanish academic circles there was a distinct ladder of prestige, beginning with those who had the "cure of souls" at the top. Hence, to doctors who, with a little encouragement, could defy death itself, it was more than galling to find the lawyers on the rungs above them. Did not lawyers defend "things," while the physicians preserved and defended bodies[1]—just a little lower than the angels? As "counts of the palace circle," as "ministers of God" even, they should be praised and exalted "together with the Magnates."

What could be better, in the twilight of the peripatetic hold, than ancient authority for the elevation of the man of medicine? In Athens only the free-born might cultivate medicine. Under Roman law, did not the physician enjoy exemption from arrest for civil debt? Did not the very insignia invented by the ancients fit the case of the medical graduate? The bonnet or cap was an ancient symbol of "liberty, dignity, nobility, and victory." The ring, used by the Spaniards in the highly ceremonial investiture of the medical doctor, stood for "preferment" above others and "for science." The gown was the badge of honor, the staff the symbol of authority. And medicine should be taken as "more noble" than in ancient times, because it was not then "separated from the manual operation" belonging to surgery. Now, though, it enjoyed all the "greatest preeminences" such as "illustrious" and "excellent." The medical man preening himself could insist that the prerequisites for a medical career clearly indicated its nobility. Blood purity was necessary for the man who "professed" medicine, while the colleges preparing students for the legal career might or might not insist on such a requisite. No one in the militia, even to the rank of general, needed to establish his blood purity.[2]

That many such social tests were imposed upon the doctor, however, did not mean that he was the purest product of all. They could have been imposed because, as was more than patent in America, the dross of the population flocked into medicine. If those who were willing to practice could not qualify for a legal medical education, the intruder took command of every field.[3] From the honors of antiquity to a current claim was only one step. Because the protomedicato, in conception at least, was a medieval institution, it was born with sweeping jurisdiction and privileges. Thus, all members of the medical faculty, their subordinates as well as the colleges, their members, and all their "literary acts" were under the "governance" of the royal protomedicato. So high was the prestige of the protomedicato that up to the eighteenth century in Spain, surgeons, apothecaries, bleeders, oculists, dentists, or distillers were never selected for the king, royal family, armies, fleets, or hospitals without prior consultation with the protomedicato. Ferdinand VI even named a protector to preserve the extensive rights of the institution he had handled with "solicitous care."[4]

Both peninsular and colonial physicians knew how to make any honors bestowed upon them pay to the last maravedí. If, perchance, they had no honors, they knew all the sure arguments to make and the weak places to probe. Thus a coveted privilege was that of the military protomédico (*fuero de protomédico militar*). When in the eighteenth century the Spanish crown began to reclaim some of its governmental powers that had long been scattered among corporations, guilds, and towns, it empowered the royal judges to assume jurisdiction in military cases when the suits were royal or related to mortgages or properties connected with entailed estates (*mayorazgos*). Nevertheless, when the mayor of Barcelona sought to collect certain funds due the pious foundations of that city from mortgages held by a Dr. Thomás Claraso, a royal lawyer (*auditor de guerra*) stopped the collection on the pretext that Dr. Claraso was "protomédico of the army and of that principality, and physician of the royal bedchamber." The Royal Council in Madrid then rendered an opinion upholding the crown against the *"fuero militar"* of the protomédico.[5] That the point had been at issue for two decades did not mean that this or any other special privilege could now prevail against the crown; it merely meant that litigation was slow and often languid.

Short of winning in a conflict with royal jurisdiction, however, doctors and surgeons stood to gain much from the special rights, privileges, and exemptions of honored medical men. When these honors resulted from serving the crown, sailing on his majesty's ships, or attending military hospitals, there was no need to invoke the military fuero and thus run afoul of the royal prerogatives. In consequence, the post of physician or surgeon in an American military hospital was the best bridge to America. As an example, a Spanish military physician in Salamanca, serving "the Army of the Left" in 1812, begged because of his chronic asthma to go to the military hospital in Puerto Rico with the full "right to enjoy his uniform." He merited this distinction, he felt, for his services in the University of Salamanca, the Spanish army, and the city of Corio, where he had stopped a fever epidemic. Certainly this entitled him to the place in Puerto Rico where medical practitioners were so scarce.[6] This last phrase is the revealing one, for it shows the ultimate design of the applicant: to get into private practice in Puerto Rico while enjoying the power of his military post and the distinction of his uniform.

The medical profession was no exception to the Spanish rule that, when the need came, any man who could claim long public service might expect an extraordinary reward. Perhaps he might want a government post or, if aging, a pension, an outright financial gift, or some honorary distinction—something dearer than money, which was not spurned. That the government always handled these overtures as if they were natural and proper is an even better reflection of Spanish society.

Such supplications abound in every century. In 1685, for example, the physician of the royal bedchamber, Dr. Lucás Maestro Negrete, after thirty-four years of medical work in various places, petitioned the crown to assign him an adequate sum from the income of the vacant archbishopric of Charcas or from other Peruvian churches to provide a "dowry" for his twenty-four-year-old daughter who was "inclined" to a religious life. After all these years of medical work, he claimed, he had not even been able to provide for his four sons, much less this daughter. The government in Spain then assigned two thousand pesos to him for this purpose from the income from the vacant bishoprics (*vacantes*) of Peru and New Spain.[7]

A full century later the widow of Dr. Lorenzo Campins in Venezuela explained to the government in Madrid that her late husband, interim protomédico of Caracas, had spent so much time in the conscientious discharge of his official duties that he had not watched out for "his house and numerous family," thus leaving his widow in the greatest misery. The advocates of this widow could truthfully claim that Dr. Campins, through his learning and hard work, had made the practice of medicine flourish wherever he was. A native of Mallorca, he had taken the degrees of doctor of philosophy—called master of arts or philosophy in Spanish universities and doctor of medicine there. Once in Venezuela he became the first to hold the chair of prima of medicine in the Colegio Seminario de Santa Rosa de Lima, where he also became proprietary professor and doctor in the same seminary as well as in the royal hospitals. Indeed, it was his influence that led to the creation of a new tribunal of the protomedicato with the privileges of those already established in Spain and the other American provinces. The widow's plea was that in her "greatest misery" she might be given a pension equal to half her husband's salary, on the precedent of a military pension (*monte pío militar*). Unfortunately, Doña Juliana's advocates had neglected to put information in their documents on the number and sex of her remaining children. They did not even report the amount of her late husband's salary, half of which the widow sought. The governor of Caracas, who had supported this plea, should not have been surprised when the Council of the Indies called for a report on these obscurities.[8] It was the improper documentation, not the nature of the case, that delayed this application.

In 1811, on the basis of his "merits and services," the Lima surgeon, José Pastor Larrinaga, asked the government to make him head surgeon of the Callao garrison with the right to form a new central committee to regulate surgery (Junta Gubernativa de Cirugía). All the members would be surgeons of the bedchamber (*cirujanos de cámara*) and totally independent of the protomedicato, which—as might be expected—looked askance at the combination of audacity and superstition that marked Larrinaga's career. The best the pretender could do to counter criticism was to allege that the tribunal qualified some surgeons such as José María Falcón and Francisco Pacheco "without prior examination" and "certification" in surgical theory and practice. As there is no sign that the government in Madrid got the special report that it asked for in this case, Larrinaga's request apparently went begging, but his faith in the king's appreciation was typical.[9]

When the practitioner wished to evade the letter of the medical regulations, such as that requiring a formal medical education to practice, he generally tried to prove that "he was very beloved" of the people. This was, of course, the natural result of the extreme scarcity of legally qualified physicians and surgeons, but even those who could post all the certificates required still had higher honors they could seek. When well beloved or well connected, these might expect the viceroy to attend as a special tribute the conclusions they defended or the funerals they could not avoid.[10] It was conventional always for the viceroy and audiencia to lend the dignity of their presence to the annual lecture opening a "chair" in the royal university.

Despite the high-sounding phrases used by Spanish officials to show their admiration for the role of the physician in preventing "irreparable damages" to the public health, doctors had no room for expansiveness when they recognized how miserably in honor and preferment they stood below most classes of learned men. When there was a preference for the medical man, it was generally within the medical profession itself. Thus, in a sincere effort to entrust medical examination only to men of "science and experience" and in order to so elevate a post, the government made the professor of prima of medicine in the university in Lima also the chief protomédico of the realm. Begun in 1646, this practice was extended to the University of Mexico and eventually to other kingdoms of the empire.[11] There was, however, less difficulty in getting such "ancient and honorable distinctions" for the physician as the staff, the cap, and the ring set with precious stones.[12]

The first goal of a successful doctor was to be called "physician or surgeon of the king's bedchamber," an honor that sometimes carried with it an annual stipend. For example, in 1794 the full cloister of the University of San Carlos de Guatemala heard a communication from the captain general that Dr. José Felipe Flores had received the coveted title from the king as a reward for his wax anatomical figures, his achievements in medical instruction, and his general contributions to science. In this instance, at least, the title was not empty; it carried an annual stipend of twelve hundred pesos from community funds.[13]

But, beyond money, the colonial figure felt a jealously exclusive professionalism that would more than rival academic professionals today. Flores claimed that his anatomical figures were the first that could be disassembled. In such a mood he began to yearn for ceremonial treatment and to hobnob with foreign scientists. He pressed for it, too, or else why should Captain General José Domás y Valle (1794–1801) call upon the University of Guatemala in 1795 to advise him on the "mode of address" to be accorded this new physician of the king's bedchamber?[14] Before this advice could materialize, however, the news that Flores was leaving for scientific work abroad brought it to a halt.

This disposition did not mean, though, that Flores was a petty man. Dr. Narciso Esparragosa, his successor in medical education and experiment in the kingdom, felt the same impulse and in as marked a degree. He had developed an elastic whale bristle fillet to prevent the murderous and gruesome deliveries with iron forceps. He even published a memorial to publicize it.[15] Besides, Esparragosa taught a course in surgery at no expense to the crown and abandoned the barbarous "depression" method in removing cataracts in favor of new techniques. Thus, Esparragosa won the post of surgeon of the royal bedchamber with an increase in salary. This enabled him to approach the captain general for the right to wear the gold-embroidered uniform "lately decreed for all physicians and surgeons of the king's bedchamber." Though custom and law called for a long robe for all members of the cloister, the colorful new uniform, now seen for the first time in the university, the captain general argued, would "disabuse the public of the bad impression it had formed of surgery." Esparragosa thus won this grace with an unnatural promptness.[16] The seven-year delay that he had to suffer in his petition for the honor of being addressed as "Señor"[17] more than counterbalanced this quick victory, but Spain had been invaded, the Council of the Indies abolished, and the petition lost sight of. As it was, the authorities had to accord this impatiently awaited "mode of address" on their own authority.

To the very end of the colonial period, medical doctors in the Indies harbored many grievances against other professional men because of the humiliating place they took in universities. From the sixteenth to the nineteenth century, in any procession the newest theologian or lawyer in the cloister outranked the senior doctor.[18] First, the physicians might not become rectors of these institutions. They did begin well in Peru, for the first two rectors of the University of San Marcos in Lima were medical doctors, but these two cases, far from becoming precedents, were exceptions everywhere. Based upon Constitución IX and the royal cédula of May 24, 1597, for the University of Mexico, Viceroy Juan de Palafox (1642) excluded physicians and, of course, surgeons, from the rectorship. For two hundred years this complacent regulation prevailed, and organized signs of disaffection appeared only when the most original, learned professors turned out to be those with medical educations. Thus, in 1805 Dr. Luis Montaña, whose botanical research was famous even outside Mexico and whose reputation for learning was one of the highest in the whole cloister, raised the question of whether or not "it would be inconvenient to have medical doctors as rectors." This euphemism plainly meant that the medical profession was out of patience with this slight at a time that medicine was making spectacular progress and was, plainly, now the least static of all the disciplines. A meeting of the cloister heard a report on this problem and listened to a recital of all the names of medical doctors, duly listed in the record and entitled to vote for councilors who, in turn, elected the rectors.[19]

At a meeting early in 1819 the cloister of the University of Caracas endorsed the movement of the medical doctors to win the right to election as rector and to take their places in university functions on the basis of their seniority. Specifically, their complaint was that the doctor of medicine might not become rector under any circumstances, and that while those in the faculty of theology, canons, and civil law took their seats in university functions according to the seniority of their degrees, the medical doctor, regardless of the antiquity of his degree, had the humiliation of sitting behind the "least senior" of any theologian, canonist, or lawyer. Behind all these—even behind the physician—came the masters of arts—the Ph.D.'s of those times.

From these simple facts flowed many evils, if we are to heed the petitioners. These slights explained why the medical faculty was in such disrepute and did "not have all the splendor due it" as in all peninsular universities, and why there were so few properly trained doctors. In fact, the argument ran, in Venezuela General Pablo Morillo was obliged to recruit "apprentices and curers" to take care of the sick and wounded in his army. Under the humiliations imposed, young men had avoided educating themselves "in so useful a field."

When it was passed up to the king in the hope of a reform, the solemn act of the university cloister calling for reform of these abuses rested upon several telling reports. In fact, in his covering letter, the rector endorsed the view that Venezuela owed its lack of doctors, so keenly felt then at the height of the wars of independence, to this failure to raise the faculty of medicine to the high rank of the others. In his communication the chancellor stressed that the four petitioners were medical doctors enjoying the highest esteem and that the concession of this grace would be a great boon to the study of medicine.

Unfortunately, these were difficult times to obtain a decision from Spain. The Council of the Indies was "extinguished," the "Secretariat" harried with more immediate questions, and the Cortes appeared all but helpless. The Secretariat, whose duty it was to channel such overtures, agreed with the necessity of reform, but concluded that the step proposed was tantamount to annulling the articles involved—a function that remained the prerogative of the Cortes. There, between these administrative stools, this pressing matter fell down.[20] In fact, it took the six years after the Battle of Carabobo for the government of independent Venezuela to correct this ancient bias against medicine; in that year Bolívar enabled doctors and friars to succeed to the rectorship of the University of Caracas.

In almost any direction he turned, if he were sensitive, the medical man could feel a slight. His salary was lower—an ancient lament of scholars both failing and surviving. Toward the end of the eighteenth century the professors of medicine in the cloister of the University of Mexico protested[21] that the salaries of prima and vísperas of medicine came to three hundred pesos only, whereas the prima chairs of theology, canons, and laws enjoyed seven hundred pesos, respectively. Such chairs as method and surgery had salaries of only one hundred pesos each. The king acceded to the request for increasing the medical salaries to match the highest in the other faculties, but saddled the viceroy of New Spain with finding the most economical means to do this.[22]

Once the physicians braced themselves to fight for their dignity and, as they thought, for the health of the realm, they found injuries aplenty to complain of. When a professor of medicine fell afoul of the law and, perchance, into jail, the indignity was more an offense against the medieval "privileges and exemptions" of the university than against the less prestigious medical profession. Yet such a case is a good reflection of the grievances of medical men, now feeling the hurt and becoming more and more articulate. One day in 1754 the rector of the University of Havana got the news that a graduate of that institution and substitute professor of medicine in it had been "ignominiously arrested." At the request of the bishop adjutor, acting as ecclesiastical judge, the professor was in fetters in the castillo—treatment inappropriate even to the "vilest" criminal. To add to the jurisdictional outrage, the civil governor had cooperated by furnishing the picket of troops assisting the hangman in putting the irons on the professor.

This arrest was not only ignominious; it was outrageous on several particulars. The judge had contemptuously flouted the rector, who, under law,[23] had jurisdiction over members of the cloister. He had ignored the "public interest" by depriving the medical students of the lectures they were entitled to hear. Even worse, under the law a prisoner who was a university graduate or professor had to be jailed separately from other criminals, even if his offense called for the "public jail."[24] And his predicament, as the prisoner himself explained, was caused by some "marriage banns," from which we are allowed to deduce, but not to know, that María Gertrudis Cabrera had charged him with breach of contract.

The issue between the man and the woman was lost in the jurisdictional dispute between the bishop coadjutor and the University of San Jerónimo de la Habana. The rector and cloister of that institution quickly laid the case before the crown, bolstered it with affidavits, and begged that the coadjutor or judge take the "person of the said professor" from the jail to the "detention chamber [*sala de reclusión*]" of the university under adequate bond if necessary and refrain from such outrages.[25] With extraordinary dispatch, the king did all he could to reestablish the injured man's honor and that of the university by ordering him removed to a salon in the university—"more decent" and befitting a "graduate professor."[26]

The surest index to the prestige of an institution, person, or profession was its place in processions in honor of the king or in celebration of the arrival of a new viceroy. In one case in Mexico, though the king had rigorously prescribed the order of precedence in a royal cédula dated September 25, 1753, he had not fixed the place of the chapter of the Church of Our Lady of Guadalupe. In consequence, on the day of San Fernando, the royal protomedicato, with its hackles up, flouted the dignity of this church in a noisy fight about which group should come first. Some sensible functionary, apparently, saved the day by running the two in on the same footing.

The prospects of "dishonor" in the future, however, were very great, both for the protomedicato and the chapter, some distance from the center of Mexico. The protomedicato charged, sensibly, that frequent ceremonial excursions into the city required church canons and dignitaries to be away when they should be conducting the services of the "divine cult." The chapter then petitioned very reasonably to be excused from participation in all functions except those involving the "royal person" and the reception of a new viceroy. On these occasions the chapter of Guadalupe would be satisfied with a "place next to the metropolitan church," clearly above all secular tribunals. When the viceroy and his wife came to Guadalupe on Saturdays to worship "before the sacrosanct image of Our Lady, the canons and prebendaries would go out alternatively" to receive them. For all this trouble, the king agreed to give the chapter of Guadalupe precedence over the tribunal of the royal protomedicato, but nothing more.[27] The prestige of medicine was not rising.

Some slight indications that it might, perhaps owing to increasing alarm about public health, did begin to appear in the second half of the eighteenth century. The cloister of the University of Mexico refused to annex the chair of mathematics to the faculty of medicine, even though medical students were obliged to take mathematics. Upon the advice of Dr. José Bartolache, however, the university permitted a man with *only* the degree of doctor of medicine to become professor of mathematics.[28] Bartolache also mentioned problems of "accounting" and "machines" used in mining drainage as other justifications of mathematics. In this way, medicine was considered in juxtaposition with accounting (so important to the royal treasury), drainage of the Valley of Mexico, and the effective firing of artillery, all requiring mathematics. In 1787 as a culmination of this tendency, Charles III even commanded that medicine should have the same privileges and respect as other sciences, for "it contained in itself the noble quality of the scientific. . . ."[29]

Doctors might not, like other gentlemen, wear swords. When they came to the doctoral investiture they had to accept the spur instead of the more dignified insignia of the lawyer and theologian as the symbol of graduation. Accordingly, the physician was always tempted to wear side-arms. Whoever chose to ridicule him, if he could find him wearing a sword, could charge him with scientific as well as social sham.

The Disrepute of Medicine

Although the doctor of medicine tagged along in academic processions at the tail end with the masters of arts, this condition was fixed in law before the colonies were founded and did not necessarily mean that the people scorned the doctor. The truth, nevertheless, is that medicine as practiced did fall into greater and greater disrepute as time went on. The established system of overlaying classical and mysterious texts with reverent commentary, often used, no doubt, to befuddle the patient was getting to the point where, in the cliché, it had to get worse before it could get better.

The time for it to get worse, much less better, had not come in the seventeenth century when the poet of Lima, Juan del Valle Caviedes, punctured more than one swollen bladder of pomp with the point of his pen.[30] A doctor, forbidden to wear the sword, yet parading and preening himself with that emblem of prestige, was enough to throw Caviedes into a frenzy of biting but humorous poesy. On the subject of the doctor, however, his humor was more vitriolic than tickling, and very prolific. He even dedicated one of his efforts to "Death, Empress of Doctors." If his readers laughed at his blunt and cruel sallies, as surely they did, the public might also have shared his disdain for the medical profession.

A contempt for doctors bubbled over at every turn of phrase. His *Fé de erratas* gave him a chance to substitute for medical terms the damaging meaning that suited his cutting whim:

> And wherever the book says *doctor,*
> Be attentive, because you should read there
> *Executioner,* although the latter
> Is a little weaker.
> Wherever it says *prescription*
> You will say *sword*
> Because sword and executioner
> End up being the same.
> Wherever it says *bloodletting*

You should read *throat-cutting,*
And you will read *scalpel*
Wherever it says *medication.*
Wherever it says *laxative*
Read he finished off the patient
And where it says *remedy*
You will read *certain death.*[31]

For a dying man, Caviedes's Parthian shots had unusual vigor. In fact, he fired them, not on the run, but at the doctors, ruthlessly, systematically, one by one. When a cousin treated in Lima by Francisco Vargas Machuca, the professor of medicine, died, Caviedes gave that doctor an unenviable immortality:

A mi prima machucaste
Machuca. . . .
To my cousin you pounded
Machuca. . . .

When there was no name or word to play upon, Caviedes could play upon a man's distinctions. So he did with Dr. Barco:

Barco solo es eminente
y el primero en esta ciencia;
médico es de Su Excelencia
y matador excelente.

Barco alone is eminent
And the first in this science;
He is doctor for His Excellency
And killer par excellence.

Here was one figure of the late seventeenth century who never thought of doctors except as indirect, and frequently, direct killers.[32]

Caviedes was undoubtedly a rattlepate and an eccentric, but did he reflect a public contempt for medicine? It is difficult to say; his verses went unpublished until they were exhumed by Ricardo Palma in 1873. Yet it is quite possible that no censor would have passed his slanderous flippancies and that the public, convinced or not, might have been amused at his sallies. The public certainly could not and did not then look down upon medicine from a lofty scientific pinnacle such as every generation, including ours, imagines that it occupies. Untutored people kept innumerable curanderos in business, and the slightly more tutored urban population made more demands upon the licensed physicians than they could meet.

Why then should the Spaniard in the New World place so much odium on the physician, the healer—the most noble of human careers? Scholasticism, that great retarding element in intellectual advancement once it became anachronistic, must take first credit for this attitude. Besides, Spaniards were subjects of Ferdinand VII, who had the medical school of Madrid closed in 1825 in order to establish in its halls a bullfighting academy (*academia de tauromaquia*). Moreover, inherent in Catholicism was a tendency to create a saint for every trouble, and people inclined to look, for example, more to Our Lady of Succor (*Nuestra Señora del Socorro*) than to the succor of science when physical problems beset them.

The colonial doctor also wore clothes rigorously black throughout the seventeenth century, which it took difficulty to distinguish from the shrouds of their victims, and which Molière has laughed into ridiculousness in his *Médicin malgré lui* (1666), translated into Spanish by Leandro Fernández de Moratín as *El médico a palos* (Madrid, 1814). The collar was as indispensable an article to the habit of the doctor as of the clerk. As a stamp of infamy, doctors were not like other gentlemen permitted to wear swords, and when the medical doctorate was conferred, instead of offering the dignified insignia that went to other doctors, the medical candidate received the spur. As a substitute for the sword, however, and a practice that was preserved in Chile until well into the nineteenth century, doctors followed the custom of wearing green gloves and powdering their beards with a golden dust.[33]

Prices paid for professional services (an expression never used) were certainly no inducement to enter the profession. Francisco Javier Errazuriz, rector of the University of San Felipe in Santiago, prepared a memorandum for the regulation of the profession in 1781.[34] At that time when Chile was powerful enough and well populated enough to contest the arms of the mother country, there were only five physicians in the whole country, the same number that had been in Santiago two hundred years previously. With so limited a number of doctors, however, theirs was not to become a profiteering profession. The tariff of this humble walk of life went thus: a simple visit, four reales; a visit in the middle of the night, one peso; simple surgical operation, two pesos; a complex surgical operation, amputation of two legs, for example, four pesos, and for one leg, one peso. Visits to the country were charged by the league, one peso a league not too low, because they "were accustomed to walk a lot," or by the day, six pesos per diem. These "collateral ministers of nature" were obliged to attend the poor without charge, yet had to extend the cash to fill their own prescriptions in such instances. In the

Chilean Hospital de San Borga a physician's stipend was 150 pesos, a surgeon's eighty pesos and a nurse's fifty per annum. The porter lacked only four pesos a month of receiving as much as the most highly paid physician.[35] That the standing and reputation of the medical practitioner had not changed much by the wars of independence is not at all surprising.

S OME YEARS AGO, when World War II was billowing up to its dark-
est, a Spanish agent for a foreign drug firm in Maracaibo, Venezuela, stopped a passing group of friends to tell them with obvious
relish that he had just seen a pharmacist fill prescriptions for a single
patient that cost five hundred dollars. Among the listeners was at least
one historian who remarked wistfully as they walked away that the costs
of drugs—both useful and harmful—had been a pathetic tax on the
people there for three hundred years. Though illness is not a vice, the
sale of drugs has always been as sure and as profitable as the sale of
brandy or tobacco. In consequence, the clandestine regulation of drugs
was even more persistently difficult than the regulation of the manufacture and sale of alcoholic beverages.

Faith that medicines were among the supreme boons to man was
higher when the drugs in existence were as likely to be toxic as curative.
To satisfy so great and unsuspecting a call for medication, in the language
of Eugenio Muñoz, "God has prepared the boon of medicine in the three
kingdoms—animal, mineral, and vegetable." And, in America at least,
they remained classified in these three "kingdoms" until the viceroys
departed from the hemisphere. Here and there, though, mention of
drugs, "chemical as well as Galenic," indicated that in the capital cities
of the Spanish empire a new attitude was beginning to show late in the
colonial period.

General Qualifications and Obligations of the Apothecary

When at the end of the Middle Ages, Spaniards began their efforts to
limit the anarchy of medicine, everybody, including women, who got
"fame" as a "curer" might practice medicine or prepare a medicinal
brew. By the time the medical laws of Castile were transferred to America, however, any candidate for examination in pharmacy had to be a
male citizen. As he trained as an apprentice in an established apothecary's
shop and not in a school, he had to come armed with a knowledge of

Latin. Otherwise, the master who had received him was liable to prosecution, and the apprentice might not take the examination. At the end of four years the candidate for practice in the apothecary's trade had his certificate of apprenticeship notarized in the office of the magistrate of the town where his master had his business. For any infraction of these requirements the aspiring druggist was liable to all the specific penalties of his kingdom and one year's exile from it. Unlike the physician, who might practice as a "perfected" doctor when he finished his university education and passed his examinations, the apothecary had to be twenty-five years of age,[1] and just as the physician, had to establish his blood purity.[2]

Among all the restrictions upon the apothecary, the one that the office might not be held by a woman is the most inexplicable. Although women were constantly falling heir to such shops, after 1593 they could not operate them "either publicly or secretly," even with a "licensed master" filling prescriptions in them.[3] As adamant as was this position, during three whole centuries the documents left behind do not turn up a single explanation, much less a justification. The prejudice against women in the professions must have been something like the bias against them in the ballot box in far more recent times. The incisive and severe nature of this law seems especially strange, since Roman law did not exclude women.[4] Moreover, the laws of Ferdinand and Isabella promulgated in 1477 required the protomédicos to examine physicians and surgeons— "men as well as women."[5] Here is an excellent example of a bias, unintelligible today, yet so clear then that it needed no justification. Aside from the normal historical bias against women in the professions, the economic factor had an unrelenting part. Competition in the drug business, except in the villages where nobody could make any money from it, was always keen. An apothecary who waited thirty years for a prestigious competitor to die could not rejoice, when that happy event occurred, to see his widow stepping in, hiring a manager, and retaining her husband's clientele and business.

Spanish kings were not slow to discover that greed could lead to conspiracies between physicians and druggists to fleece the public. One corrupt practice was that of the physician who wrote prescriptions to be filled in an apothecary's shop operated by his son or son-in-law or prescriptions written by sons and sons-in-law who were physicians to be filled in apothecary shops of their fathers. As early as 1537 there were many instances of such working arrangements, which forced the government to forbid these combinations.[6] At this juncture, however, the enforcement of this prohibition was left not to medical but to civil officers, the corregidores and magistrates.[7]

The temptation of physicians and surgeons to use their own houses to compound and sell medicines was never very successfully resisted. The severity of the penalty for violation conveys some idea about the prevalence as well as the seriousness of this dereliction—10,000 maravedís for the first offense, 20,000 for the second, and 20,000 for the third along with banishment five leagues beyond the town or place where the infraction occurred.[8] Such legislation meant, naturally, that no man could set up—even though he could qualify—to be both physician and druggist or surgeon and druggist, whether he filled his own prescriptions or not. Such a man had the option of deciding to practice whichever of these two professions he preferred.[9]

Druggists had such an awesome obligation to be available when the lifesaving drug was necessary that they could leave town only under the most special circumstances. Early in the eighteenth century (1711) the protomedicato in Madrid ordered apothecaries both inside and outside the city not to depart their shops without leaving a qualified druggist on duty on pain of a fifty-ducat fine.[10] Mere legislation and threat of a drastic fine, however, did not prevent the practice from becoming so prevalent that three decades later the crown authorized the inspectors to take even more drastic steps. Even if the pressure of other affairs kept the druggist away from his "primary" business, he was liable to a fine of six hundred maravedís, and, not mending his ways, he might see his shop closed. And the judges who delayed or failed to enforce the law, either because of the influence of the druggist, or, to be more cynical, because they received a bribe, themselves became liable to pay the damages.[11]

Having more than one shop, the regulations assured, might distract the druggist from "his primary business" in the other. In 1694, for example, the protomedicato in Spain issued an order to all druggists of Madrid requiring them on pain of a fine of one hundred ducats not to have more than one store. Five years later the practice was still so persistent that the protomedicato had to menace two obdurate apothecaries with fines of 30,000 maravedís to limit their business to one establishment. Much less might a man operate a shop in two different towns. The inclination to get chain drugstores going was so persistent, however, that the comprehensive instructions for the guidance of drugstore inspectors in 1743 expressly warned visitors to be on the lookout for it,[12] still another of the many laws and restrictions governing the activities of the apothecary in Spain and the Spanish Indies.

Pharmacopoeias

The development of a Spanish pharmacopoeia clearly illustrates the consistent inclination of the Spanish crown to systematize as well as regulate the drug business. The legislation of Ferdinand and Isabella indicates that this concern was fully developed before 1477, but it does not take a great deal of imagination to understand how the lack of a uniform, approved method of compounding medicines resulted in gross errors that injured further or killed patients the physician intended to help. In the Ordinances of 1593,[13] Philip II required that within three years a commission composed of three physicians and three pharmacists be appointed to draw up a general pharmacopoeia by which the pharmacists of Spain might compound or prepare medicines and other things necessary in their stores. Moreover, the king required that these shops be inspected and the druggists punished who did not have this book and the drugs it required.[14]

This same pragmatic also called for preconizing a new, standard set of weights and measures in all apothecary shops. The chief change was substitution of the Castilian mark for the Salerno mark.[15] In other cases, such as "syrups and waters, or decoctions," the physician and pharmacist might use whatever measure they preferred. If the physician did not stipulate the measure, however, the druggist took him to mean measure and not weight.[16] By implication, these new laws made it plain enough that the public had suffered for want of method and honesty among apothecaries. These druggists, for example, might not sell any "waters" to be taken by mouth unless they had been distilled "in an alembic glass in a water bath."[17] At the same time Philip II gave the protomedicato in Madrid the authority to seek out and punish any "physicians, surgeons, bonesetters, apothecaries, and dealers in spices and aromatic drugs [*especieros*]" for using false measures.[18]

Philip II, however, did not get his pharmacopoeia within the three years ordered. In fact, it took 146 years and repeated orders from Philip's successors to pry a pharmacopoeia out of the protomedicato. Finally, in 1739, the royal protomedicato of Madrid presented the Council of Castile with the famous *Pharmacopoeia Matritensis,*[19] whose purpose was to fill and make all prescriptions, "Galenic as well as chemical," according to set formulas in all the pharmacies of Spain.[20] The protomedicato boldly proposed that the government require all druggists to have this work within six months and that henceforth every successful candidate examined in pharmacy be handed the book with his license—at the prevailing price, of course. Not having a copy within six months after the Council of Castile endorsed the proposal became a crime. The penalty for failure to follow its particulars cost the druggist a fine of two hundred ducats and revocation of his license.[21]

Prior to the *Pharmacopoeia Matritensis* the accepted pharmacopoeia had been a standard work by Félix Palacios, the *Palestra farmacéutica,* almost all of it incorporated in the new official *Matritensis* pharmaco-poeia.[22] This work appeared in at least nine different editions and re-printings in the course of a century and sold seven thousand volumes between 1706 and 1723, the dates of the first two editions.[23] This was enough to provide a copy for every licensed pharmacist in Spain and the empire with many left over for physicians. Palacios defended "the mod-erns" and "the chemists" with ardor, but since there was no scientific testing of medicines, he clung tenaciously to all the oddities that centuries of Galenism and folk medicine had deposited in the Spanish pharmaco-poeia. He was careful, though, when presenting such a strange thing as a "unicorn's horn" to explain that though the ancients believed there was a "true unicorn," the moderns had found that there was no such animal. Specifically, the London College of Physicians had declared against the existence of any unicorn beyond the rhinoceros. It was the tusk of the narwhal, he explained, that the ancients confused with unicorn's horn. The horns actually sold, furthermore, were those of this "marine uni-corn." As Palacios looked upon himself first of all as a man of modern science, he could not accept point-blank the "view of the ancients" that this "horn" was an antidote for poison. He explained in a manner typical of the whole work that "it abounds in volatile salts and oil"; hence, that justified prescribing "from a half to two scruples" for such afflictions as smallpox, pest, and measles.[24] Thus, cochineals, crawfish, tumblebugs, toads, and frogs, because they had their "saline-sulphurous" parts "most fixed," were diuretics and blood-purifiers. In the same manner, crawfish, vipers, serpents, deer antler, human craneum, hoof of the tapir, and blood of a he-mule or goat, because their saline-sulphurous parts were volatile, diaphoretic, and cephalic could be used as a cure for morbid drowsiness, palsy, and apoplexy, as an antidote for poison, and as a coagulant.[25]

Though Palacios was quick to spurn the superstitious and embrace the scientific, he often embraced the superstitious nevertheless. On the one hand he explained that water from Chinese-made vases of rhinoc-eros horn would not cure any poison as generally believed and that Chinese doctors, "to be politic, and win the goodwill of the owners," sanctioned the superstition. No sooner had he made this observation, however, than he entered in his book the "virtues" of rhinoceros horn as a man of science saw them. In short, in powder form it would stimulate and fortify the heart, provoke sweat, and cure malignant fevers.[26]

Compiled before experimentation on the effects of drugs began in earnest, the Palacios *Palestra*—by modern-day standards—propounded a host of outrageous remedies. Crawfish eyes—or at least what looked like crawfish eyes (the small white stones growing below the head toward the stomach)—in powder form were good for kidney stones, bladder contusions, hemorrhoids, and side aches. Dried frog intestines when taken internally would dissolve such things as kidney stones. A wolf's liver and also his intestines, when dried by fire, were good for windy colic. Young swallows (pity the poor *golondrinas*!) when killed should first have blood put on their wings, then the wings pulverized with a little common salt and some "powders." Such a concoction "excited the urine" and helped to throw off bladder infections. For epilepsy, paralysis, apoplexy, and other ailments of the head, one could take powders made from the ground-up cranium of a person recently dead by violence, but the cure was only good if the powders came from one who had perished violently, not benignly of mortal sickness in bed. Fox lungs that were washed, cut in pieces, dried in the sun, and made into powders were useful for chest ailments and lung problems such as asthma. Tapir (the great beast) fingernails were good for epilepsy, trembling, convulsions, and nervous disorders of all kinds. These could be taken internally in powder form or applied externally as an amulet; Palacios recommended the amulet as the best way to get results. Pathetically eager to be scientific, Palacios wanted to produce only natural and physical justifications for his medicines, but the outrageous medicines crept in nevertheless. A good example was his solemn retention of the urine and excrement of various animals as medicines, particularly of the goose, ass, peccary, ox, cow, goat, stork, serpent, horse, chicken, man, sheep, sparrow, turkey, and dog. These medicaments could be used to bring out the "humors" through the skin by perspiring and to control "fat or oily humors" that cause obstructions producing epilepsy, apoplexy, paralysis, and palsy.[27]

Palacios not only tried to give a natural, chemical explanation for even his "Galenic" drugs but also turned with inveterate persistence upon those who tried to defend "the ancients" at his expense. Seven years after the first appearance of his *Palestra farmacéutica,* he devoted a whole work to annihilation of the "calumnies and impostures" that Miguel Boix published in *Hippocrates Defended* (1711).[28] However, the work of this type that cut Palacios to the quick was a book brought out by a Jorge Basilio Flores defending the Arabic physician in Spain, roughly titled *Juan Mesue the Elder against Palacios.*[29] Since this was two years before the appearance of the second edition of the *Palestra* in 1723, Palacios must have devoted all of his spare time to a rebuttal before he turned in his copy to the printer, for in a work of about 700 pages he devoted 108 pages of his "preliminary discourse" to what was, essentially, a defense of himself against Flores's book, which anybody but a proud Spaniard might have chosen to leave in oblivion. Neither was the task so difficult as to justify the use of so much space, for Flores

was distinctly vulnerable. He had even said, Palacios claimed, that anything not done according to the rules of Mesue was in error—a great
deal to claim for an Arabic physician who lived in Baghdad. Flores, for
example, confused deadly carrot (*tapsia*) with turbith. In the same vein
Flores, as did many other people as late as the eighteenth century, claimed
all spiders were poisonous, whereas if he had read the proper authors
such as Lemeri, he would have seen that some spiders such as the taran-
tula were poisonous and others were not.[30]

This *Palestra,* the most formal and formidable Spanish pharmacopoeia up to the eighteenth century, was the work of one man. It was
dedicated to the protomédico of the royal armies, Dr. Juan Higgins, and
carried the nihil obstat of Presbyter Dr. Joseph de Losada of the Congregation of the Oratory of Saint Philip Neri and the license of the "inquisitor in ordinary" and the physician of the king's bedchamber, Dr. Joseph
Suñol, who endorsed it because it contained nothing against the "purity
of our Holy Faith, good customs, and decrees of His Majesty. . . ."[31] It
must not be imagined, however, that Palacios was a mere superstitious
herbalist; he was a member of the Royal Chemical-Medical Society of
Seville, druggist in the court at Madrid, examiner of the royal protomedicato, and visitor-general of drugstores in the bishoprics of Córdoba,
Jaén, Guadix, and the Abadía de Alcalá la Real. What he put down
must, therefore, be taken as representative of pharmacology in Spain
during the early and mid-eighteenth century. Besides, this was the man
who, with the greatest catholicity, had prepared, by both the chemical
and the Galenic method, "compositions" not only from Madrid but also
from all over Europe written down to that moment. In consequence, the
bringing together of medicines from all parts and all ages, as long as
there was no experimental method to eliminate the inert and the dangerous, led to such a possible accumulation as to make the shelves of drugstores in America, where nature was prolific, look discriminating if
anything.

It might be pleasant to the historian who must have everything fit
his pattern to believe that the *Pharmacopoeia Matritensis,* which after
years of waiting appeared in 1739,[32] launched Spanish pharmacology
into the modern age. This compilation, however, was no more scientific
than Palacios and included much that was in the *Palestra.* Moreover, not
only did Palacios scour Europe for the latest medicines to include in his
Palestra, but also there was no bar to the publication of other pharmacopoeias, which did appear in Spain and the Indies.[33] Thus until the end of
the Galenic age and until experimentation and testing of drugs became
the rule, the *Palestra* and the *Pharmacopoeia Matritensis* and their proto-
types remained the guidebooks for Spanish and Spanish imperial apothe-

caries and physicians. As outrageous as the remedies and simples may seem by modern-day standards, the Spanish pharmacopoeia was not that much different from those being used elsewhere in Europe or America.

Outrageous Drugs

The Spanish empire was an almost perfect place for the encouragement of outrageous drugs. They ranged from the drugs of Moslem and Christian Spain to the sorcery and medicines of the American Indian. In time it ran from the "Galenic" to the "chemical" period in the history of drugs. In fact, in the three hundred years that followed the discovery of America there were few places on earth anywhere that had the learning and the facilities to determine whether drugs accomplished the purpose they were sold for. Three centuries are a long time to allow superstition and European pseudoscience to intermingle. And yet in 1739 when the proto-medicato endorsed the Madrid pharmacopoeia and thrust it upon druggists in Spain and the empire as standard, it included legitimized and dignified medicines that seem incredible two hundred years later.

In the "decadent" phase of the Galenic epoch, many weird simples and weirder compounds found their way up from folk medicine to the most reputable and even renowned pharmacopoeias. Anyone who has ever read Bernal Díaz del Castillo's account of the battle of Tlascala, where Cortés's men dressed their wounded with the grease they took from a fat Indian, will make some kind of surmise on the state of medicine in that "Golden Century." Grease from animals so strange and unexpected as to suggest occult powers enjoyed the highest preference. Spanish hospital books contain entries of the petty cash paid for "man, lion, heron, and bear grease" to put in the apothecary shop.[34] Even the College of St. Peter and St. Paul in Alcalá de Henares paid out its money for grease of buzzard, gander, and serpent.[35]

The practice of applying live creatures or exotic parts of animals to certain places on patients' bodies required the hospital apothecary shop to have cow bladder "to put on the breasts and one side of a sick woman."[36] Pups were bought to put on the head of a male patient and buzzard wattles to put on the stomach of another "who had little heat in him."[37] Squab pigeons, "to put on the head" of a female patient,[38] were also used to stanch the flow of blood in miscarriages. In like manner the caul of a sheep was put to the belly of the sick.[39] In such an atmosphere what was more natural than for a hospital pharmacy to buy scorpions or frog salve[40] for the pharmacist? The Hospital del Pozo Santo in Seville bought foxtails in the sixteenth century for its apothecary shop.[41]

Many simples were so hard to imagine that their very mystery made them occult and, somehow, healing. Though in the late eighteenth century simples were less likely to be placed upon the pharmacist's shelves under "animal, vegetable, and mineral," the pharmacopoeia called for many, and there were still enough "animal" to yield passing strange items. Horny excrescences reposing upon these well-stocked shelves included the hoof of the tapir,[42] stag and human craneum—this last one in all but universal use. Other types were lizard excrement, spider webs, peacock and gander dung, urine of the cow, and afterbirth of a woman. The irresistible mystery of sex had placed in the list the penis of bull and of deer. The occult property sometimes sprang from sex difference, and when it did, the male was most often singled out. From the internal organs, especially the more puzzling ones, came wolf's liver or lungs of the vixen. It was not enough to get a strange part, but the animal itself had to be rare and hidden if not actually occult. Thus, horse fat was not enough; there had to be bear fat also. These creatures were strange enough in their general right: earthworms, toads, frogs, vipers, and swallows. The *tlacuache,* an Aztec contribution, which added its tail to the pharmacopoeia, was as strange as its tail was esoteric—two commendable pharmaceutical properties.

But how did the apothecary keep these organic items in his shop? Needless to say, all these items that were not already dried had to be processed and dried. Spider webs, for example, could be rolled or pressed into pills or put in "papers" and taken internally. Earthworms were dried and ground into powder, whereas toads and frogs were pickled and kept in this way. As in good cookery, the apothecary washed some parts in wine before drying them, as with the liver and intestines of the wolf, lungs of the vixen, and penis of the deer. As a special turn for dogs, learnedly dubbed *canina* or Greek White (*album graecum*),[43] the apothecary washed them on a marble slab with juice from the plantain and, at the right consistency, cut his handiwork into cakes and completely dried them. The droppings of the peacock and the gander he prepared in the same way, except that he mixed the first of these with peony water and the second with chicory water. The blood of a male animal, especially of the mule, he gave special treatment, but inevitably he dried it, for it went on the market as "powders *ad casum.*" From the swallow he took the feathers for poultices. The apothecary alone could keep vipers and other venomous creatures. As vipers inspired religious awe, if not some religions themselves, they were bound to suggest themselves as medicine. Thus, the apothecary took their blood, trunk, heart, and liver to mix and cut into cakes. No one had the idea, naturally, to use their venom as an antivenom.

If these were the simples, what of the compounds that contained them? To make *agua polycresta,* the apothecary used a formula calling for 127 different substances, one of them "viper broth." Into the making of "frog plaster" went the fat of vipers, earthworms, and live frogs. The apothecary dubbed it "frogs without mercury." Oil of earthworms and of the she-fox were a specific balm to troublesome joints, while oil made from live scorpions served as a diuretic remedy. "Tincture" of the human skull with alcohol as the solvent was designed as an antiepileptic and antihysterical and would have met a great colonial need—if it had had any properties that were not purely and accidentally psychological. Likewise, a mixture called powders of Guttera (*polvos de Guttera*), which, in addition to the undried human craneum, contained bits of marble, deer antler, and hoof of tapir, came even more highly recommended for epilepsy and hysteria.

When drugs were legitimized in such an unscientific way, among those that would horrify the modern physicians were bound to be some that, properly handled, could serve a useful purpose. Thus, Palacios, whether by chance or not, had in human urine enough sodium sulphide and uric acid to arrest certain types of eye infections. Opium was another. Palacios described opium as "a gummy teardrop from the heads of poppies," which, though cultivated in Greece and Turkey, the Turks monopolized for their own use. He hastened to explain, however, the process of pressing and evaporating the juice to make a hard substance which, wrapped in leaves, could be transported. He does not appear to have been concerned about opium as a problem, probably because the supply was too small to lead to addiction. He warned casually, however, that the drug should be administered with the "necessary precautions." He understood well enough the effects of the drug, though, for he listed its virtues as "calming turbulent humors," including sleep, provoking sweat, arresting the flow of blood, and other effects. The dose he recommended varied from a half to a whole grain.

On other matters though Palacios belonged with his age. Feijóo's modern outlook, it is sad to relate, did not make its mark on Palacios, who did not hesitate to include gold filings treated with ammonia acid and water to purify the blood, to treat epilepsy in children, and to cure colic, smallpox and other diseases. Over the efficacy of this medicine, Palacios approached ecstasy. At least gold, when reduced to powder, did not strip the lining of the esophagus. On the other hand precious and semiprecious stones and other hard substances had their honored place among drugs. Pearls, mother of pearl, coral, burnt ivory, sea shells, hematites, and the Iman stone (magnet), garnets, amber, emeralds, and topaz might all "absorb sour and acid humors," cure hemorrhages and gonorrhea, and control the flow of blood.[44]

Indian remedies of little worth also found their way into the Madrid pharmacopoeia. The bezoar stone, taken from the stomachs of certain ruminant animals of the Andes, was at one time an antidote for syphilis, reputed to have been prescribed for the kings of Spain. Ground up and mixed with water, it "made the heart glad." The bezoar stone was extremely expensive, half as much as the yearly salary of a highly paid university professor, and this no doubt recommended it at a time when the most costly elements were likely to be prescribed for princes or anybody else who could afford them. Feijóo said that he for one thought the least virtuous plant of the fields more useful in medicine than all the emeralds of the East. To be sure gold made the heart glad, he said, but in the pocketbook and not poked into the stomach. To him the bezoar stone, which entered into nearly all the cardiac prescriptions, was a pure fable. Though bezoars belonging to princes and potentates were prescribed for Charles V, they did not produce the slightest improvement in his condition.

Poisonous Drugs

One of the great dangers in the primitive stages of medicine was administering mortally poisonous drugs to patients. In the thirteenth century the law stipulated that any physician or surgeon who, out of ignorance, gave a drug resulting in death was liable to a penalty of five years' banishment on some island, though death was the penalty for knowingly or maliciously dosing with a fatal drug. The apothecary who gave scammony or other strong medicine to a man or woman to "eat or drink" without a doctor's prescription was guilty of homicide.[45] And even more so, the physician or dealer in aromatic drugs knowing that the buyer intended to kill another person with them, was as guilty of murder as the buyer. In case the victim died, the "killer" died dishonorably. Dying dishonorably meant that he was thrown to lions, dogs, "or other wild beasts."[46] And there was, apparently, no shortage of extremely dangerous chemicals when Spanish hospitals in the sixteenth century were buying orpiment, trisulphide, or arsenic "to kill flies in the refectory."[47]

From very early times the government of Castile forbade the sale of venoms, poisons, or herbs known to be mortally toxic. Some, such as scammony, however, might be sold because they lost their poisonous quality when mixed with other drugs.[48] However, the proper restrictions on the sale of poisonous drugs were still under litigation in Madrid, where the wholesale druggists (*drogueros*) often sold poisonous simples and compounds. In 1751, for example, licensed pharmacists (*boticarios*) had a suit pending to stop this dangerous practice.[49] Yet it had been the law since 1537 that no apothecary or wholesale druggist might sell corrosive sublimate (*solimán*) or "other poisonous things" without a physician's prescription.[50]

America inherited the same problems of food, brews, and poisons. Juan Antonio Suardo, the Lima diarist, solemnly made the entry on March 10, 1631, that the criminal section of the royal audiencia had sentenced a person to two years' exile from Lima for selling a fermented drink made from carob beans (*alojas*) because great pieces had been "thrown into the liquor that could have resulted in very great harm to the republic."[51] Neither the civil courts nor the protomedicato, in America or anywhere else, could tell when a strong or spoiled drug that might be fairly tolerated by one might kill another, but they occasionally put their heads together to resolve the difficulty. In 1724, for example, some Mexican court—which, record does not say—fined a physician 6,000 maravedís and completely barred him from practice after a purgative he had administered "killed the daughter of Cristóbal Pérez."[52]

The imputation that a practitioner was administering dangerous drugs could be well nigh fatal to his practice. In 1795 Dr. Pedro Carbajal, a ship's surgeon recently arrived in Mexico from Spain, complained bitterly to Dr. José Ignacio García Jove, president of the protomedicato, that he was suffering from the charge of the inspectors, José Villaseca and José Inza, that his patient died because he was given "excessive quantities of opium" and "purged against every rule." The first consequence, he feared, was that the druggists would be afraid to fill his prescriptions. He attributed his plight to the envy of a peevish and ungovernable rival. Though, on the advice of the intendent, he restrained himself, he leaves the impression that he was envied as a competitor, a peninsular competitor.[53] Carbajal, a surgeon, emphasized that there was no curandero whose prescriptions of emetics, purgatives, and narcotics were not filled. The success of the omnipresent curandero in getting his prescriptions filled, however, was nothing to bolster his spirits or his argument either. Indeed, Dr. Justo García y Valdés wrote the Marqués de Sobremonte in 1806 that in less than a month in Buenos Aires he had treated fourteen persons poisoned with toxic substances ingested upon the advice of charlatans and curanderos. And, as was usual in such cases, Sobremonte ordered Protomédico Gorman to take drastic steps to see that apothecaries did not sell through these quacks but by prescriptions of licensed physicians.[54]

Prevalence of Drugstores

How many drugstores existed in the Spanish empire in America there is no way to tell because many sprang up in towns and villages where the sway of the royal protomedicato was never felt and where an unlicensed practitioner ran less risk. Many of these were too insignificant to be called drugstores. Besides, some legitimate ones were always being closed or fading away while new ones came into being. Also some drugs that, according to law, only licensed pharmacists could sell were sold in grocery stores, toward the end of the colonial period a steady complaint of the licensed pharmacists. Some places were too remote not only from the capital but also from the headquarters of the delegated inspectors ever to undergo official examination.

Not surprisingly, then, not even the royal protomedicato in New Spain could be absolutely certain how many pharmacies there were in the kingdom.[55] By a "prudential calculation," however, it concluded in 1788 that there were between 100 and 110 legal establishments in the viceroyalty.[56] Of these, thirty-four were in Mexico City, though there were only twenty-nine towns in the whole kingdom that had any place where a man could buy drugs legally. Of these twenty-nine places with pharmacies, twenty-seven had seen decades pass—and some of them centuries—without the biennial inspection required by both the laws of Castile and those of the Indies. Since there were twelve towns among the twenty-nine that had drugstores with only one licensed pharmacist, whom the delegated inspector, usually a physician, could delegate for inspecting that particular store is not clear, since the lone druggist could not serve as the expert to detect his own malfeasance.

Inspections and Jurisdiction: The Spanish Model

Toward the end of the colonial period a judge of the royal audiencia asked the royal protomedicato in Mexico what "ordinances" governed its organization and conduct, for the guild tradition had invariably left every successful corporation with its set of rules duly sanctioned by the king. He must have known there were none, even though the protomedicato did reply without qualifications that the Muñoz *Recopilación* of 1751 guided its activities. In fact, the protomedicato had been acting upon scattered Spanish law and upon a very brief section in the laws of the Indies. The *Nueva recopilación* (1640), in a law springing from Philip II's decree of 1588, required the protomédico and examiner in Spain to visit the drugstores in Madrid in person and also to inspect the drugs the merchants sold wholesale. Within the five-league limit around the capital, the protomedicato appointed one of its own examiners to conduct inspections. In case it became necessary to pass sentence, however, he had to bring the culprit before the protomedicato itself. Inspections farther away from the capital than fifteen leagues fell to the senior examiner. If the protomédico did not duly appoint this examiner, he forfeited a third of his salary, and if the examiner did not accept appointment, he lost a year's salary. All penalties, in three equal parts, went to the man reporting the delinquency, to the fine chest for the king, and to the hospitals of the capital.

The law required inspections in the court city and its surrounding district every two years, but in all other towns and cities of Spain it required them every year—just as the corregidores, in the company of local physicians, had formerly done. No specific days were set; they merely had to be carried out within the specified term. Though inspectors might return to check up on a drugstore before the expiration of the term, they might not receive extra pay or inflict monetary punishment for a second visit.[57] For each day of work the examiner collected 748 maravedís, the druggist accompanying him as expert 500, the fiscal 300, the clerk 300 plus notary fees, according to the established tariff. By the reign of Philip III the examiner drew over 1,000 maravedís, the clerk 500 maravedís, the tipstaff 500—all derived from fines or, if there were not enough of these, from the chest of the royal protomedicato.

The protomédicos of Spain were first called examiners—examiners of the preparation of candidates to practice the medical professions and examiners (inspectors) of apothecary shops and wholesale drug houses. In time, as these officials became more important, they delegated examiners of drug establishments. This process of passing the work on to a lieutenant could go on, with each man taking a share of the fees without doing the work, until there was nothing legitimate left to pay the man who in the end made the inspection. The examiner, though, could find ways to make his assignment worth his while. Thus, between 1523 and 1593 Charles V and Philip II took into account an increasing number of evils, including this one. Civil law required the inspection of wholesale houses and demanded that examiners do their work personally and not through a substitute. At court, however, the examiner presented his evidence of malfeasance to the tribunal for sentencing. Outside five leagues, corregidores and local magistrates, after naming an "approved" physician of the place to accompany them, took responsibility for the inspections.[58] These passed sentences, levied penalties, and collected fines regardless of appeals.[59]

The fear of fraud lay behind the requirement that inspections come as a surprise. Thus, Philip II's pragmatic of 1593 stipulated that they come "irregularly and on no set day." What troubled the government was clarified when Philip III repeated this law and defended it by saying that "experience had shown" that an apothecary, if he knew he was about to be visited, merely borrowed the "good medicines" he lacked, hid the "bad" ones, and put everything into order.[60] What Philip III did not say was that "experience had shown" that no amount of repetition of decrees and statutes eliminated a fraud or curtailed a profitable abuse. In the eighteenth century, when the medical tribunals had been in existence for more than two centuries, graft, if anything, was increasing. Whereas in the time of the Habsburgs appointment as inspector had to be made every two years, under the Bourbons the crown began in 1704 to assign this profitable duty in bishopric after bishopric on a virtually proprietary basis. Complaints against "abuses and excesses" arose on every hand, and, as there were no reports, lawyers and judges found themselves foiled in establishing even the facts of a case. The petition of the protomedicato in Madrid requested that the commissions of "lieutenant" examiners be taken up and that the proprietors do their own work. In the case of a vacancy among the proprietary examiners, the royal protomedicato would select a qualified person. The Council of Castile agreed.[61]

The king apparently issued no covering cédula, and the ancient abuse of appointing lieutenant inspectors went blithely on until 1750. By then, Dr. Joseph Suñol, president of the protomedicato in Madrid, reported to the king about "the great clamors and repeated suits, of towns as well as druggists in these kingdoms of Castile . . ." on account of the "prejudices and continued excesses" flowing from the method of conducting inspections of drugstores. Not wishing to take the trouble to meet the terms of their commissions personally, it seems, the proprietary visitors approached the royal government and, "under various pretexts," got the right to name substitutes from whom they would collect "half or two-thirds, when not all," of the fees. Moreover, it was not to be presumed that the lieutenant inspectors left the greatest excesses without punishment, took the slightest offenses as the gravest crimes, except to recompense themselves, or recorded some drugstores as inspected because the trip was too uncomfortable. In point of fact, instigated by individuals, two cases against lieutenant inspectors were pending, while the rest were not indicted because many druggists were afraid to institute suits and the justices adamant against hearing them. This time a royal cédula in concrete terms was the issue. This document[62] ordered the commissions of substitute inspectors taken up, required the proprietors to make the inspections personally, and, in case they were unable to do so, ordered them to notify the protomedicato so that it could appoint persons of ability and character. This was not to say, though, that the king might not make whatever arrangements he saw fit for the conduct of drugstore inspections.

Inspections and Jurisdiction in the Indies

In America as with any other deep-seated and necessary custom, the inspection of drugstores might be said to have been planted with the conquest itself. In 1540,[63] when there was not a handful of physicians in Mexico City, the situation was ripe for excesses of all kinds. As there was still no protomedicato in the Indies, the town council, which never gave up its role in medical matters, intervened to arrest a number of growing evils. The people had complained that they were sold either spoiled drugs or those improperly made in the first place. The cabildo attributed this development to the fact that "so much time has elapsed since they were inspected" and accordingly ordered that the rounds be made. Because when one branch of medicine degenerated all seemed to fall into decline, they gave instructions for gathering information on the physicians and midwives charged in the same complaints with demanding excessive fees.[64] The town council even assumed the right to name those charged with "examination" and inspections of drugstores and related matters.[65]

It is a sad but typical commentary that Spaniards in the Indies after these early days, though faced with the problem every few years, should have floundered through the whole colonial period without really clarifying and fixing jurisdiction in medical matters, especially the inspection of drugstores. Formulated a priori, the first laws set up a type of organization that was completely outmoded before the crown authorities even understood the type of problem that time was inexorably giving them. Established in the first medical statutes, the protomédico general plainly imitated the appointment of such men as Francisco Hernández as protomédico of New Spain and Sepúlveda as protomédico of Peru, a type of office that did not endure as a bureaucratic institution. It is the protomedicato, which came later, that made the bid for jurisdiction.

Until the protomedicatos were formally organized—and these had no prolonged existence anywhere except in Lima and Mexico City—individuals got appointments as individual protomédicos to enjoy the sheer preeminence the appointment gave them, to collect fees for inspecting drugstores, to drive out competition, and lastly to preserve the purity and integrity of drugs by the standards of Galenic medicine and, at the end, those of modern chemistry. Most conflicts of authority arose over jurisdiction in the provinces. In the very early days, before a formidable tour of inspection was profitable and feasible, the contest was nonetheless joined. About 1625 the protomédico general of New Spain, Dr. Jerónimo de Herrera, also senior member of the faculty of medicine, superannuated (*jubilado*) professor, and "perpetual examiner" of the university, made it known in Spain that though he was "in good, robust health" and qualified to fulfill his duties as protomédico, the viceroy, the Marqués de Gelves (1621–24), in order to favor his own physician, had given a private commission to Francisco Ortiz de Navarrete to inspect drugstores in violation of Herrera's title. In fact, Ortiz and a Dr. Rodrigo Muñoz even pretended to be partners and coadjutors in the protomedicato. The viceroy, however, got instructions from Spain to leave this office exclusively in the hands of Herrera without encumbering him with an "associate [*acompañado*] or coadjutor" in inspections of drugstores or anything else and to let him enjoy the privileges accorded him in his title.[66]

When riots and turmoil in Mexico ultimately forced the king to recall Gelves, the new viceroy, the Marqués de Cerralvo (1624–35), far from putting Herrera's cédula in force, instead appointed two more protomédicos to serve with him "in the manner of a tribunal," setting up two new salaries for these men. How could these men be paid, Herrera protested, when he had served at a salary of 300,000 maravedís for twenty-two years and, by the end of 1626, had failed to collect 15,000 maravedís of this sum? (The truth was that the tribunal had taken in only four pesos since its establishment and that it had no hearings because of the lack of business.) Thus, pending a report from the viceroy, the king restored Herrera's exclusive authority.[67]

Once formed as a tribunal in the 1640s, the protomedicato soon developed the "custom and style" of inspecting drugstores in Mexico City and "five leagues round about" or of appointing acceptable and qualified druggists to do this work for them, as was done in Madrid and other kingdoms and cities of Spain, where the same laws and regulations were in force. Beginning in 1674, however, Viceroy Payo Enríquez de Rivera (1673–80) three different times named three judges of the royal audiencia to "reinspect" apothecary shops. The first time the three protomédicos received notice of the inspections and went along; but the second and third times the viceroy did not notify the protomedicato at all, and the civil judges appointed a doctor and an expert druggist of their own, completely bypassing the protomédicos and denying them their precious jurisdiction. The protomedicato very boldly charged that the viceroy should not meddle or violate their privileges unless he found "omission or collusion" on the part of the protomédicos, and then he should proceed against them according to the offense. They were willing, they said, to have an oidor accompany them in their inspections, but without fees and merely to see that the procedures were legal. The audiencia and the

viceroy were accordingly ordered not to interfere on any pretext whatsoever pending a report on the situation from the royal audiencia.[68]

There were many classic tricks to deceive the inspector of drugs, but
the authorities recognized and effectively countered them. There were,
however, always new devices. In Mexico apothecaries refused to show the
medical stocks they had bought from merchants of the trade fleet. This
claim so alarmed and enraged the protomedicato late in the seventeenth
century that it petitioned the king not to allow merchants to sell drugs
shipped from Castile until they were inspected and, if found unacceptable,
burned by the Mexican protomedicato. The crown summarily rejected
this plea, but after the drugs passed from the hands of wholesalers and
intermediaries, they might be inspected in individual shops just like any
other drug.[69]

If the medical laws of Spain itself were scattered around among the
codes, among occasional pragmatics, and among royal cédulas without
order or method for a span of three centuries until 1751, they were even
more unorganized in the overseas empire. Since most corporations in the
eighteenth century had their "ordinances," the slowness in bringing laws
respecting medicine together is not easy to explain. When these laws did
appear, however, it was not just with the usual imprimatur, but with the
express license of the king and the Royal Council. In fact, the endorsement of the Council of Castile, drawn up by a criminal judge of the
Audiencia of Valencia, went so far as to state: "The sublime, happy state
in which the Royal Protomedicato of Spain finds itself is publicly
known."[70]

One of these scattered pieces of legislation was a cédula of 1743
setting up the conditions for inspecting apothecary shops in Spain—over
two-and-a-half centuries after decrees of Ferdinand and Isabella had
made drug inspection the most urgent matter in the regulation of the
medical professions.[71] Yet, as late as 1790, the protomedicato in Mexico
City, because, as it professed, there were great abuses brought on by the
improper handling of drugs and the practice of medicine without a
license, needed to repeat this forty-seven-year-old cédula verbatim.[72]
Without doubt, the real motive was that because of the "innumerable
and grave injuries" done in the past, this cédula absolutely forbade any
town council or commissions to interfere with the work of the inspector.
The inspector also had to do his work in person in the presence of a
royal secretary.

The note of distrust of both apothecaries and medical practitioners
that ran through this document restricted the inspector as much as the
apothecary under scrutiny. Though it might never reach the stage of

conspiracy to defraud, collusion was a constant danger. For example, outside Mexico City and in provincial towns such as Guadalajara and Querétaro, there was rarely a public house suitable for the entertainment of the visiting inspector. Hence, the cédula of 1743 ordered the inspector not to stay in the house of the druggist about to be inspected or in that of any of his relatives. Instead, he had to lodge in a private house selected by the local magistrate and pay his own expenses. Neither could the poor inspector accept any present or gratification from a druggist, directly or indirectly.

Once in town the visitor proceeded according to a fixed scheme. He presented his commission and viceregal exequatur to the ayuntamiento and, certainly in smaller places, put himself in contact with the local magistrates to ask for their help. He then sent a notice to all apothecaries not to leave their establishments before ten o'clock in the morning,[73] for had it been known upon which shop the inspection might fall, that particular one would have opened with a complete stock of simples, compounds, and every other item needed. The doctor or surgeon expected to participate with the inspector had to be present at the hour designated for a visit on pain of a fine of six thousand maravedís.

As the very first item of business the inspector asked the apothecary for his license. In the next step the notary administered the oath to the apothecary, who swore not to hide any medicine asked of him or to display as his own any items lent to him by someone else. If he failed to produce his license, the inspector was to close the shop immediately, levy a fine of six thousand maravedís, and warn the operator that either "public or secret" operation of his store would result in a fine of five hundred ducats. Any serious defect or negligence in operation of the shop was in itself sufficient cause for an inspection, whose papers and decisions went directly to the protomedicato in the capital for a definitive decision. However, should the case against a druggist arise from the accusation of a private party, the accuser was obliged to post bond. Thus, in case his charges were false, he could assume the costs and penalties—as the law required. Should the "fault," such as not having a minor ingredient, not be "very serious," however, it was the duty of the visitor to warn the operator and require him to obtain the necessary drug in a short time.

One of the duties of the inspector was to determine whether medicines were "corrupted or altered," either on account of the "defective keeping in vessels or for any other cause," and to pour them out or burn them. The first fine for not sorting out and correcting this situation was six thousand maravedís, but if this proved insufficient to uproot the abuses, the inspector in consultation with the protomedicato closed the shop on pain of a fine of five hundred ducats. The inspector also had to look into the ownership of a shop. If he found any "deal," or simulated sale, he had to close it and make a report to the protomedicato.[74] In these tours of inspection it was not necessary to determine whether the druggist had pure blood or was an old Christian, as Castilian law required,[75] for the applicant had to comply with this formality previously when he went before the royal protomedicato to be examined for his license.

Once these preliminaries were over, the inspector faced several problems, all petty if not paltry. The first of these was fees. Since fees were on deposit, the inspector collected for his work without trouble, except when the apothecary was too poor. Though fees were fixed in Spain, in Mexico the inspector outside the capital sometimes varied the fee of thirty-five pesos—always upward. Then the inspector, to be strictly legal, had to present the druggist with a "petitory," a printed official list of the articles a druggist was expected to have.[76] This, or some kind of list, was drawn up and fixed by the protomédico in conjunction with two licensed pharmacists freely chosen by him.

How inspections actually worked can be seen in the case of Blas de Naveda, an apothecary in Mexico late in the seventeenth century. On January 21, 1693, presumably in the morning, Dr. Francisco Antonio Jiménez, professor of prima of medicine in the Royal and Pontifical University of Mexico, with Joseph Montaño, professor of surgery in the same institution, both members of the protomedicato, appeared in the drugstore of Blas de Naveda to "reinspect" it—plain indication that they had already found it wanting. After they took Naveda's oath to show all his medicines and wares and to hide nothing, they swore in Joseph Gallegos de Velasco, the druggist selected to accompany them to examine the drugs and declare which were good and which bad. A scribe, Pedro Castillo Grimaldo, took down the record of inspection.

The routine inspection that followed was instructively typical, especially of cases in which the authorities suspected some serious dereliction. He was first asked to produce the "books the masters go by," meaning, apparently, the "petitories," though exactly what these were is hard to say. When they next asked him, as they should have done in the first place, to produce a certificate that all his drugs had been inspected and passed, he replied that they had, but could not produce a certificate to that effect. His scales and weights, however, they found in order. When they asked for his oils, he could show nothing but a little rose-colored oil. The rose-colored honey (*miel rosado*), which he had just made in a kettle, they passed. Of abstergents and the "usuals," he could only show endive, borage, and roses. When asked to produce unguents of gourds, lead, tutty (a sublimate of calamine collected in a furnace), and sandalwood, he could not do so. As for seeds he could only come up with fenugreeks, linseeds, and broad beans. Among other things he was asked to produce and could not were bees and vinegar of Castona and a kermes-colored alcoholic confection. Of powders he could not show that of the huisache tree and two others. Among the electuaries, he did not have that of Temis, simple or compound. His "conserves" had lost their virtue, were hard, and would not ferment. For *diacatholicon,* a "universal purge," he showed some simples, but did not have senna and licorice. He also lacked most of the purging electuaries. Of lids for his alembics, he had only one—that of lead, but none of a copper-tin alloy required. Having declared that he supplied medicines for the Convent of Regina Coeli and the royal hospital, he was asked where he got those needed by those two communities in his charge. He replied that what he lacked he bought in order to meet their requests.

This inspection sealed the case against Blas de Naveda. The protomédicos found him guilty of lacking the usual and common medicines and the purgatives he needed to take care of the two communities in his charge. The case was strengthened and confirmed by reports coming to the protomédicos of his bad "preservation" and preparation of his drugs. Despite repeated inspections and reinspections that had preceded this one, Blas de Naveda had not mended his ways in the slightest. Moreover, Naveda was a miserable diplomat. He showed little respect for the inspectors, delayed following their instructions, and insolently slapped down on the counter the earthen vessels and jugs demanded of him. When added to his patent failure to fill the obligations of his trade, this impression led the protomédicos to call for Naveda's arrest and imprisonment and the closing of his shop. They took care at the same time to notify the two communities that depended upon Naveda to make arrangements to purchase drugs from other apothecary shops.[77]

Naveda showed his contempt, however, when "somewhere around eight" the following morning he blithely opened his shop to do business again! Thereupon, the outraged protomédicos Jiménez and Montaño ordered their functionaries to go immediately to the shop and padlock the door. On the main one, opening into the principal court, the bailiff Juan Beltrán put a padlock and new staples and turned the keys over to Diego de Salcedo, the fiscal of the protomedicato—all of which he carried out in the presence of three witnesses. The next day the two protomédicos issued a request for Licentiate Manuel de Figueroa, an attorney of the royal audiencia, to give an opinion. Figueroa apparently advised that a confession be taken on the points raised and that Naveda be required to state from whom he bought the drugs he lacked when fulfilling his obligations to the Convent of Regina Coeli and the royal hospital.

Two days later on January 28, Dr. Montaño went to the jail in person to take Naveda's confession. When Naveda asked why he was in jail, the questioner told him that he was there because of a shortage of necessary medicines in his stock. Naveda replied that this lack was owing to his having a lot of business early in the day he was inspected. In fact, when the "master" druggist called in by the protomedicato arrived to tell him that the protomédicos were on their way to inspect his shop, he was "just about to go out" to buy additional stocks. Declaring that he did not "send out" to particular stores to buy what he needed, he had given money to his handyman, Juan de Padilla Colmenares, to purchase them. On one occasion, he remembered, he sent Padilla to the shop of Francisco Cornejo for a bottle of oil of Aparicio and almond seeds because he did not have these supplies. A journeyman in the Cornejo shop testified that Padilla did appear to buy a bottle of almond oil and that later an Indian, whose name had escaped him, appeared to get the same thing.

The protomédicos then turned this record over to Diego de Salcedo, fiscal of the protomedicato, for his disposition. According to rigorous legal and clerical procedure, Licentiate Manuel Figueroa, a judge of the royal audiencia, and Drs. Jiménez and Montaño signed the order to burn without delay all the "spoiled, damaged, or aged" medicines in the "Plaza Mayor of this city next to the gallows there." In addition, the protomedicato ordered Naveda's license to be suspended for four years and for him to pay the costs of his case. Thereupon the notary Castillo Grimaldo, promotor fiscal of the protomedicato, Licentiate Diego de Salcedo, and the bailiff Juan Beltrán went to the shop, opened the doors, and took out the spoiled articles. Salcedo then locked the shop and went to the Plaza Mayor, where he "ordered an Indian" to build a fire next to the gallows. When it was burning strongly, he broke and cast in two jars of mint syrup and other bottles containing spoiled drugs, feeding the fire until they were all consumed. On January 31, 1693, only ten days after the date of the inspection, the drugs were burned and Naveda formally released from jail.

Delegated Inspections in the Provinces

Inspections outside of the capital cities caused problems. Spanish law at the time protomedicatos began operation in America assigned the inspection of drugstores five leagues beyond the bounds of the court city to corregidores and magistrates who, in company with two aldermen and a licensed physician, carried out the actual work. In fact, if the protomedicato sent "commissaries" beyond these limits, the justices had the power to arrest and throw them into prison. Moreover, the protomedicato had no power to summon or bring any person from beyond the five-league boundary.[78] In 1751, however, Muñoz insisted that these laws did not derogate those laws giving the protomédicos and their examiners power in all "the kingdoms and dominions" and that the protomedicato had "universal jurisdiction" over all "practitioners of the medical and auxiliary faculties." Besides, since the senior protomédico had the power to select the examiner and all other personnel for an inspection, and since no one could legally practice without the legal approval of the protomedicato, there was no question about the authority of the tribunal. In addition, the corregidores had no power to punish physicians, surgeons, and druggists for their professional transgressions, merely to prevent them from practicing without a license—something, Muñoz said, that "endures today." His conclusion was that none of "these legal dispositions" altered the fundamental law that the protomedicato had jurisdiction in "all the kingdoms and seignories of the crown" and that to fulfill the obligation thus involved, the protomedicato would have to appoint and use subdelegates.[79] This, nevertheless, created still another uncertainty fraught with promise of trouble in America.

As it was bound to be, the protomedicato in New Spain found itself involved in quarrels and litigation nearly every time it appointed and dispatched delegates to investigate medical practitioners and inspect drugstores outside Mexico City. For a century and a half, however, the protomedicato had established the custom of appointing delegates to do this work of inspection in the cities and bishoprics beyond the capital. When in 1775, after the retirement of Bachelor Tomás Bernardo de Otáñez from this laborious post, the tribunal in Mexico City appointed Dr. Bruno Francisco Sánchez Sueiro as "commissary-inspector" of Puebla and its environs, it also authorized inspections typical of those designed for the regions important enough to justify the trouble and with enough drugstores to provide the fees necessary to pay the inspector and his assistants. Also armed with an exequatur from the viceroy that served both as sanction of the commission and as a passport, he could show it to local town councils and magistrates to get the required authority and, the protomedicato realized, prevent much petty hindrance.

The instructions the protomedicato drew up for the guidance of Sánchez expressed the best aims and worst fears. (His first assignment was to go to Puebla and visit all drugstores not visited within the last two years by the outgoing Otáñez.) Whereas the authorities confined most general or itinerant inspections to the examination of drugstores and the suppression of quackery, this one required the visitor to keep an eye out for any "plant, fruit, flower, stone, or earth, animal, or anything else" that might possess a particular virtue for some sickness. It thus became his duty to investigate and remit the item and accompany it with a written statement distinguishing it as a tree, herb, or vegetable, explaining where it grew, what illnesses it could be used for, and how it should be dispersed. At the same time he took such care in the "vegetable" kingdom, he was to watch for animals, "minerals, and stones" that might have similar properties.

The protomedicato was especially careful in its instructions to Sánchez covering the apothecary. Prescriptions had to be written and filled according to the pharmacopoeia of Palacios, except those drugs declared by the protomedicato as "of little or no use." Thus, in the course of an inspection, Sánchez must require druggists to have the Palacios pharmacopoeia and examine their shelves in accordance with it, except in the case of scarce medicines coming "from the kingdoms of Castile." Otherwise, the druggist might expect to be fined if he did not have the ones listed by Palacios or if those he had were spoiled, beginning to rot, or in any kind of disarray. The penalty was two-pronged: the druggist had to agree to pour such tainted drugs into the streets and then had to pay a fine that the inspector, with the others he had collected, duly sent on to the protomedicato in Mexico City.

All the care and suspicion of the protomedicato in Mexico City, however, never succeeded in putting these inspections on a businesslike basis. With delegated authority, Sánchez was ready enough to report and to account for fees taken in, at least at first, for he found a situation that required support. He wrote that in Jalapa, Córdoba, Orizaba, and even in Veracruz there was no one with the authority to conduct inspections. Some local inspectors had vague, out-of-date commissions or they simply had none at all. When his case was looked into, one man claiming the right to inspect and collect fees did not have a license to practice, much less inspect.[80]

The death of Dr. Sánchez in 1777 did not change the makeshift practice of delegated inspections in New Spain. Appointed by the protomedicato for a two-year term to replace Sánchez, José María Torres seemed a worthy successor and visited drugstores in Puebla, Cholula, Huejocingo, Tlascala, Atlisco, and Puebla de Azúcar. With viceregal authorization he won the approval of all the local town councils who supported his inspections.[81] In May 1779, therefore, the protomedicato renewed Torres's appointment for two more years, and to the end of the year he made fourteen visitations outside of Mexico City. Early in 1780, however, he was discredited by a scandal involving his brother-in-law, who was charged with murder, and Torres was relieved of his post. On March 4, 1780, the protomedicato replaced him with Dr. José Ignacio García Jove, charged with going to Puebla to inspect physicians and drugstores in that province. Unlike Torres, however, García Jove had no authorization from the viceroy, and a jurisdictional dispute broke out, a dispute that showed how jurisdictional problems constantly intruded on the consistent inspection of drugstores.

In the controversy many evils emerged that might otherwise have remained obscured. According to the viceroy's fiscal, an investigation conducted by the governor of Puebla revealed that Dr. García Jove had come to the district and exacted higher fees from the drugstores inspected than the established tariff allowed. For his part García Jove admitted the charge but defended himself on the grounds that since he had come from Mexico, his expenses were greater than those of a local doctor, justifying the higher fee charges. Since García Jove was operating without viceregal authorization, however, the fiscal advised that he not be reinstated as inspector and be required to deposit the fees that he had collected so that these could be returned to the Pueblans who had paid them. Since Torres still had viceregal certification, the fiscal believed he should be allowed to finish the second biennium of his inspections. Likewise, the fiscal advised that in the future the protomedicato not initiate such inspections without initial certification of the viceroy.[82] Whether Torres was able to continue his inspections is not clear, but probably not. Ignacio Cruz seems to have replaced him in 1782 as delegated inspector but without viceregal approval, once again creating tensions between the viceroy and the protomedicato over jurisdiction.

Thus, in practice, the king's legal advisers and civil officials everywhere clung to the idea that it was the responsibility of viceroys and governors to initiate inspections of drugstores. In fact, though, the initiative usually came from the protomedicato, and crown officers merely gave the inspectors legal sanction after the fact. Jurisdictional disputes, however, could always arise—and did—between the protomedicato and viceregal and local officials. This made delegated inspections of apothecary shops in outlying provinces problematical and haphazard. Without the support of the viceroy and local town councils, the protomedicato simply could not establish provincial visitations of drugstores on a permanent or regular basis.

Insurance and Drugs

In the Spanish colonies poverty was accepted as natural. The conscience was salved, even if amends were not made, by a universal recognition that charity was commendable. Time after time men under arraignment for practicing medicine, surgery, or pharmacy without a license sought to soften the rigor of the law by proving that they treated the poor without pay and, as an added fillip, even paid for the drugs themselves. When the problem reached critical proportions, as during a grave epidemic, the viceregal government and the ecclesiastical hierarchy sought to avoid catastrophe at this very last moment by suddenly expanding the charitable role upon which colonial society prided itself so much. In normal times, though, the poor and helpless had to depend upon individual charity—something that did not remotely meet the need. Thus, while the government did not hesitate to take authoritative charitable measures in a crisis, its very nature made it veer off from spending anything except for absolutely essential expenses. Still in 1815, when five years of revolution had brought Mexico City to near-collapse and "obstructed all charitable resources" and when refugees had overrun the poor quarters of the city, Rafael Ceballos, the pharmacist of the Royal Indian Hospital, proposed a charitable establishment for the "succor of the sickness of the unhappy ones of this capital."

His plan was unique. Instead of depending upon inadequate conscience-soothing personal charity, he boldly proposed a plan of health insurance. Working in the drugstore of the hospital that treated indigent Indians, Ceballos had ample chance to see how hard it was for the unhospitalized native to get medicines or for the druggist who furnished them to get his pay. The provisions of Ceballos have a curiously modern ring. In the first place any individual, regardless of class or wealth, who was not already sick, pregnant, or over fifty years of age, could get his or her name entered in the books by paying two reales. By paying three quarters of a real promptly every week, he could remain in good standing. After two months a member could begin to draw upon the benefits of the cooperative arrangement, although he could draw nothing when in arrears. When he became sick the "shareholder" went to the treasurer who gave him a signed ticket so that he could go to any doctor he chose. If too sick to visit the doctor, the doctor would come to his house and treat him there until he was well. The attending physician would write the name of the insured patient and the street and number of his house at the top of any prescription he wrote. Then the patient would go to the drugstore of the Royal Indian Hospital to have his prescription filled, though it must be said that Ceballos expected other stores to be added later, when it could be determined which of these were most suitable.

Ceballos also catered to the protomedicato in his proposal when he indicated all pharmacists had to satisfy the requirements of the protomedicato. Regardless of "how much" or "how costly," the medicine ordered would be supplied "with all conciseness, cleanliness, and interest" in full compliance with the stipulations of the protomedicato. An insured patient might change doctors by giving notice to the treasurer, and if a consultation became necessary, the patient could get it authorized in the same way. In case of the death of the insured of at least one year's standing, the treasurer provided one-half of a death shroud or its equivalent.

Ceballos sent his plan to the viceroy with a forceful argument for its adoption. He felt that since hospital care, such as it was, had virtually disappeared, the only way left to prevent a plague was to treat the poor at the beginning of their illnesses. His plan, he thought, was the only way left to do that. As for his motives, his only concern was "charity for the unhappy people in need, whose wants lacerate my heart without my being able to help. . . ." Viceroy Calleja sent the petition to the protomedicato for a report,[83] but apparently no record of any response has survived. It was not in the nature of the protomedicato as a bureaucracy to respond, and conditions were becoming even worse in New Spain.

Sad Plight of Pharmacy and Attempts at Reform

In the forty years before independence there were regular outcries against the sad plight of pharmacy and the neglect of surgery. These two plaints seem almost to alternate in a kind of orchestration. The criticisms, however, were more likely to come from private sources than from the royal protomedicato, which was touchy about shortcomings where it was even indirectly responsible. The protomedicato, too, enjoyed the "reverent awe" of other doctors and druggists. Druggists were not likely to forget that this reverend body inspected their stores, but one of them, when sorely sick, if not on his deathbed, did at last feel free to involve the tribunal in the malpractices of the drug business.

Joseph Mariano Pino, finding himself in the early 1790s so near death, he said, that he had to relieve his conscience, wrote the viceroy that many shops in Mexico City were operating without examined and licensed pharmacists. Others, approved by relatives or "interested parties"—the protomedicato—did not even know Latin and hence put one medicine in the place of another. He concluded this bold assault with the blunt charge that the protomedicato was careless.[84] The viceroy accepted the advice of his fiscal to demand a report from the judges of the eight wards of the city requiring them to submit a list of all the drugstores in their jurisdiction that were managed by an approved pharmacist and those that were not, asking at the same time for a statement of the owners or other "interested" people in each case. Beginning the next day the reports began drifting back to the government. Mexico City had thirty-four stores. Of the thirty-four the owner and operating pharmacist were the same in twenty-four cases; the remaining ten were the property of others. Among these owners, two were widows; one was the "heir" of the denunciator, Joseph Pino; and five could not show a license. Two of these said they paid the half-salary tax to the viceregal secretary, but the scribe had not sent back the certificate, while the third stated that the clerk died before getting the certificate to him. A fourth was waiting for his baptismal certificate from Spain, and the fifth, Manuel Sevilla y Tagle, preferred the classic explanation: he had lost his.

In the midst of this canvass, word reached the protomedicato that one of the judges of the audiencia, Pedro Valenzuela, had summoned all the pharmacists in his district to come to his house to show their licenses. Valenzuela acknowledged not only that he had summoned them but also that he was asking the owners and assistants to provide additional information.[85] Although in 1794 the protomedicato reminded Viceroy Revilla Gigedo that everything, such as checking on licenses and correcting excesses, fell under the authority of the protomedicato,[86] it was not until 1796 that it finally salved its sensitive honor by putting to rest the charges attributed to the late Joseph Pino. The tribunal first required all pharmacists in Mexico City to assemble on August 3 to state whether the protomedicato had ever passed and licensed an unqualified person as a pharmacist. At this meeting the thirty-two apothecaries present appointed two of their number to draw up a report, which insisted that the protomedicato efficiently made the regular biennial inspections and that this breath of scandal was a surprise to all. Moreover, the two investigators said, the document attributed to Pino was not in his handwriting, and members of his family could not recall ever hearing him make any comments bearing out the charges. When the protomedicato had assembled all this favorable evidence, it informed the viceroy that a thorough inspection had not located a single drugstore without a "master" and not a single master without a license. The protomedicato then intimated that the spurious Pino accusation was the work of some disgruntled person, perhaps filled with hate, because they had neither passed examinations for which they were inadequately prepared nor been able to practice illegally. At last, the viceroy closed the matter by informing the protomedicato that he regarded the Pino document as a forgery and the charges unproved.[87]

There was, nevertheless, a constant murmuring against the druggists that varied only in its intensity. In 1809, the very last year before everything in Mexico City began to collapse, three physicians and scientists, at least two of them of some renown, addressed a letter to the protomedicato,[88] saying they had heard daily of cases where drugs rotted and moldered in vessels, and druggists, because of their ineptitude, made them worse by the way they prepared and filled prescriptions. The solution they suggested was more frequent inspections. Since they thought the delays were owing to the difficulty of assembling the three required inspectors, they proposed that inspections be undertaken by one only, the three taking turns, and that all three foregather only in case of doubt or need of consultation. In a tone unmistakably that of Dr. García Jove, the protomédico reminded his critics that the consent of the Superior Government was necessary; that it was no trouble to the protomedicato, as these critics had stated; that it was not their function to press administrative changes of this kind; and that if any of the cases they heard of were brought officially to the attention of the protomedicato, that body would proceed promptly against them.

The nervous reorganization of medical tribunals in Spain during the last half-century before independence had practically no effect in America, but it did encourage a number of ill-fated efforts to reorganize the management of the drug business in the New World. In 1802 one of these newly created organizations in Spain, the High Committee for the Regulation of Pharmacy (*Junta Superior Gubernativa de Farmacia*), did ask for authority to conduct the biennial inspections of drugstores in the overseas kingdoms[89] and with the fees, to establish chairs for public teaching of pharmacy in the capitals.[90] The contention was that since the days of Charles I, when the inspection of drugstores was committed to viceroys and governors, there had been no other royal directive on the subject. According to the petition, this was sad because outside the capitals "there were no drugstores, or if there were, these were harmful" because the pharmacists were ignorant men "not even holding certifications of examination." The druggists of Puebla bolstered this request by petitioning for the extension of the rules and authority of the Junta Superior de Farmacia to their district.

The Mexican protomedicato, however, got word of the Puebla druggists' efforts to throw off its authority and came back with arguments that the fiscal of the Council of the Indies found hard to dispute. The druggists, said the report, clearly recognized the efforts of the protomedicato to hold them up to standards that would protect the public health, but freeing them from the protomedicato would inevitably bring greater "disorders" to the drugstores. They said flatly that a junta of pharmacy made up of the druggists themselves would not improve dispersing of drugs, for the druggists would favor their own kind in their shops. Moreover, drugstores would not be inspected; the vices of the stores would be indulged in with impunity; ordinary citizens would have to bow their knee to them in their business deals; prices of medicines would be set by whim; and the public health would suffer the consequent ravages.

The Council of the Indies then decided that the new laws proposed for the regulation of pharmacy in America be sent to the viceroys and presidents of audiencias for their assistance. These officials were ordered to establish a junta composed of the regent, oidor, and fiscal of the civil section of the audiencia, the senior regidor, the viceregal attorney, and a member of the ecclesiastical cabildo. This junta would hear the arguments of the protomedicato or any other body or individual thought necessary in order to adopt what would be best suited to the needs of the country. Meanwhile, the junta might not put its findings in force until it got permission from the king to do so. In the end nothing came of this effort. The United Faculties of Surgery, Medicine, and Pharmacy were abolished by 1806 and once again were replaced by the royal protomedicato in Spain before the juntas could take action and make changes in the regulating of pharmacies.

Unfortunately, the indecisiveness of Spanish medical reform meant that whatever evils existed in pharmacy in America in 1804 continued into the wars of independence and then got even worse. In 1813, sponsored by the druggists of Havana and Lima, José Antonio Jiménez Salinas, professor of pharmacy and chemistry in Cádiz, made an overture to the government that reads like a rewrite of the petitions made from 1800 to 1804. The faculty of pharmacy and chemistry, he said, was "almost" ruined in America because the people could not tell the bad and unqualified druggist from the honorable and competent one. Consequently, pharmacy was all but abandoned by serious people in Cuba and Peru. This near disaster, he said, came from not putting into force the new ordinances of 1800 which provided that a candidate for a license to practice pharmacy who had the degree of bachelor of arts could, after two years in one of the colleges set up for the "united" medical faculties, be examined in the college itself. Jiménez therefore reduced his plea to three points. (1) The ordinances of 1800 should be observed, with the limitations that the circumstances in America made necessary, and colleges of pharmacy in Lima and Havana should be immediately established. (2) He next recommended setting up a protomedicato in each capital, modeled upon that just created in Spain, combining in its personnel representatives of medicine, surgery, and pharmacy. (3) If such a tribunal were not suitable, he proposed the creation of a "subdelegation" to represent individuals of the various medical faculties—not just medicine.[91] Nothing came of this facile petition, however.

The rumors that reached Spain of the terrible plight of pharmacy in America, though exaggerated by interested parties, came simultaneously with reports of equally sad conditions in surgery. Though some concrete results were achieved in the reformation of the education and practice of surgery, there was a kind of tacit admission in Spain—and

BEFORE THE MIDDLE of the eighteenth century surgeons in Spain enjoyed a status very inferior to that of physicians, and in America a full quarter of a century had to pass before any effective voice was raised for the man with the scalpel. Except that he might pull teeth, deliver babies, and let blood, the surgeon stood no higher than the phlebotomist or the algebraist. Scarcity and necessity, however, gave the surgeon a dignity with laymen that professional rivals in medicine never willingly conceded.

Qualifications, Training, and Status of Surgeons

If there were no legally qualified surgeons with the conquerors, the conquest itself threw up its own practitioners. A surgeon called "Master John," who came with Pánfilo Narváez, "treated bad wounds and made up for it with excessive prices."[1] So great was the demand that surgeons flourished, and flourished without being examined. In 1610, exactly three years after it began appointing physicians to work with the indigent, the Mexico City cabildo also began to appoint surgeons.[2] Fourteen years later the viceroy himself, the Marquis of Cerralvo (1624–34), named Diego Ruiz de Estate "surgeon and barber of the court jail in Mexico" at 160 pesos a year without privilege of charging fees "to do the bloodlettings" there.[3] In 1620 the Marquis of Guadalcázar (1612–21), recognizing the obligations of the town of Xochimilco, had even gone so far as to order that it furnish the surgeon Martín de Valderas two Indians, "to be paid every week," while he attended the wounded and supplied the poor with drugs.[4] Surgery, however, did not have enough dignity in the seventeenth century to attract men qualified and willing to go before the royal protomedicato for examination. In consequence, while forty-seven candidates to practice medicine came before that tribunal between 1659 and 1700, only one surgeon—in 1695—took the trouble to do so.[5] The members of the protomedicato spurned surgery, and even if they had not, they had no money with which to enforce the laws.

Almost any fact of any law relating to surgery, in some oblique way, reveals the disparagement felt for the profession in Spain and in America. In Spain, for example, the price for shaving a man in a hospital was one real[6]—the same as the surgeon's charge for setting an arm. A surgeon might not even "execute any kind of evacuations" or bleed a patient on his own judgment, but, like a lowly phlebotomist, he had to await the consent and signed order of the physician.[7] When in 1621 Dr. Cristóbal Hidalgo Bendaval reminded the king that there was no chair of surgery and anatomy in Mexico City, he might have added that neither was there one in the whole viceroyalty. The king answered his plea for appointment as professor of surgery by asking the viceroy for a report on the matter.[8] When the University of Mexico finally acquiesced in the creation of the chair, it insisted on Bendaval's stipulation that he would serve without any salary.[9] The chair of medicine thus came into being forty-three years before that of surgery with a salary of 150 pesos, while the chair of surgery paid nothing. After a lapse of thirty-four years the viceroy intervened. Because of "the importance of surgery to this kingdom" and in the full realization that no one would take the chair of surgery without a stipend, he appropriated one hundred pesos from the annual salary of the professor of Mexican language for that purpose. No one had taken the course for years, and, at the moment, only one lone student was registered. As might be expected, this raid upon his salary was altogether unpleasant to Dr. Antonio de Tovar Montezuma, the proprietary professor of the "Otomí tongue."[10] Over a century later in Peru, even at a time when Dr. Hipólito Unánue had reached an almost frenzied peak of enthusiasm for anatomy and proclaimed it as a panacea for the handling of human ills, the chair of anatomy established in the Hospital de San Andrés drew a salary of only five hundred pesos[11]—850 pesos lower than the top salary in San Marcos de Lima at that time.[12] But to establish a contention such as this is gratuitous. Surgery was a profession that dealt in manual and mechanical operations for which no learned man who dealt in words, as Martín Martínez said with so much disdain, would have much to do.

The lack of "approved" surgeons plagued the Spanish colonies just as did the lack of physicians. As late as 1766 the city attorney of Guatemala, in an effort to get relief, declared that of the three qualified surgeons in the city, two were very old.[13] Also to find any surgeon at all in towns away from the capital cities was a very rare thing. One reason for their scarcity was that surgeons passed over into the practice of medicine in the capitals because medicine was more prestigious and remunerative; and they were bound to practice medicine in the towns, or no medicine would be practiced at all. Even in Lima, where both Latin and especially romance surgeons seemed literally to swarm, the physicians could not hold their own. As a result, in the 1760s Dr. Hipólito Bueno de la Rosa, first protomédico, undertook to keep pharmacists, phlebotomists, and especially surgeons within the confines of their profession. In fact, so common had the instruction of the predominantly black surgeons become that some physicians no longer regarded it as an indignity to hold consultations with surgeons. The prosecutor agreed with Dr. Bueno de la Rosa and asked that the bailiff notify both romance and Latin surgeons that henceforth the practice of medicine by surgeons would bring quick penalties—a fine of 6,000 maravedís for the first infraction, 12,000 for the second, and exile and discretionary punishment for the third.[14]

Qualifications and Examinations for Latin and Romance Surgeons

No sign of real dedication to surgery in New Spain was in evidence before the establishment of the chair of surgery in the University of Mexico in 1621. It was not, however, until 1665 that Viceroy Marqués de Mancera gave the subject a boost by ordering the protomedicato not to admit bachelors in medicine to examination without a certificate that they had had the course in surgery.[15] No serious evolution in the attitude of the government toward surgery, however, took place between the pragmatic of Philip II in 1593[16] and the foundation of schools of surgery in America in the eighteenth and early nineteenth centuries. Thus, it is logical to suppose that candidates could qualify in America under the same terms, but there were so few universities in America with medical chairs enough to provide this prerequisite, and, where these did exist as in Mexico and Lima, records of examination of Latin surgeons have not survived to show what the practice was. There is much reason to believe, however, that very few physicians cared to bother with formal examination in surgery, especially if this step meant fulfilling the requirement in Spanish law that the candidates commit to memory the compilations put together by the protomédicos on tumors and all kinds of sores and their proper treatment. Only after the examiners had determined whether the candidates had these digests by heart might they proceed with the examination.[17]

If surgeons in Mexico City conducted a running fight to participate in the examination of their kind, in the remote towns and provinces of the empire the surgeons were lucky to get anyone to examine them legally. Julio César, who came to Havana about the last year in the sixteenth century, dubbed himself a surgeon, effected many important cures, and having practiced the four years "required by the ordinance,"[18] now wanted a license to practice. He therefore appealed to Captain General

Pedro Valdéz (1602–8) for permission to leave the city to take the requisite examination. It is an indication of the desperate straits of medicine and surgery in Havana that the governor refused this permission, even though the services of the applicant were so urgently needed in the city. Because there was then no protomédico in Havana, the governor appealed to the Council of the Indies to allow some physician there to conduct the examination. The crown then authorized the captain general to stage the examination in Havana under a physician or naval surgeon, and in case César passed, to issue the proper license.[19] In Buenos Aires as late as 1779 Matías Grimau had to have a special order of the protomedicato in Madrid and the agreement of the Council of the Indies in order to take an examination in surgery.[20]

Much confusion and obscurity have surrounded the question of qualifications to practice as a romance surgeon. The very designation under which he suffered—*romancista*—indicated that he had never loitered in a university and had taken his instruction secondhand, and not in Latin. Moreover, after 1770 the prerequisites underwent a number of changes growing out of the establishment of the colleges of surgery at Cádiz (1748), Barcelona (1764), and Madrid (1787). In turn, these institutions themselves were the result of the Spaniards' uneasiness about what they knew to be the unsatisfactory state of surgery aboard ship and what they feared was the decadence of Spanish surgery in general.

Five-sixths of those practicing surgery with a license during the colonial period had at least four or five years' apprenticeship in a hospital—the sole preparation required of them[21]—or lacking that, under some "approved" surgeon who, more likely than not, got his instruction in the same way. Before he could claim the right to be examined, the aspiring surgeon had to produce documents establishing his blood purity, a certificate of baptism, documents of good character and habits, and an affidavit from a surgeon testifying that the candidate had had a five years' apprenticeship.[22] After the establishment of the School of Surgery (romance as well as Latin) in Mexico City, Viceroy de Croix in 1770, in order to unite "the principles and knowledge of the art of surgery, those of practical anatomy, and the method of operating with perfection," ordered the royal protomedicato not to admit any candidate whatsoever to examination unless he first submitted a certificate from the "professor of the Chair or School of Practical Anatomy and Surgical Operations" that he was qualified.[23] Henceforth, candidates for examination would bring proof of having four complete courses in the school. Those who had already passed time as apprentices were obliged to finish the time prescribed in the school, and during that time the professor would decide whether or not to certify them. Those who had qualified under the "royal pragmatics," even if they were found in hospitals and other towns of the viceroyalty, had to have the professor's written endorsement or come to the Royal Indian Hospital for the four courses specified. Any license obtained after the date of this order would be declared void and taken up while all other penalties prescribed by law would be imposed.[24]

Very soon, however, the old interests began to operate against the modernization and improvement in standards implied in the requirement that all surgeons have the certification of the professor of surgery in the Royal Indian Hospital. For one thing, the chief surgeon (*cirujano mayor*) in the Hospital de Nuestra Señora de la Concepción y Jesús Nazareno in Mexico City found that his "interns" (*practicantes*) could no longer qualify for examination before the royal protomedicato. Accordingly, in 1781 the Duke of Terranova y Monteleón, patron of the hospital, had represented to the Council of the Indies that this training had been going on since time out of memory and that the protomedicato received, examined, and licensed the candidates from the Hospital de Jesús Nazareno. In 1782 the king, upon the advice of the Council of the Indies, then instructed the royal protomedicato and the juez conservador of the hospital to continue this practice.

Surprised, the tribunal for once wrote a document favorable to the School of Surgery. Indeed, the practice was immemorial, but since the establishment of the School of Surgery, candidates had actually been taking courses in the school, although they might intern under surgeons in other hospitals. The professor of surgery in the School of Surgery would certify that the candidate had taken the required courses, and the surgeon of the Hospital de Jesús Nazareno would certify that the candidate had served his internship there. The protomedicato continued that it believed such a privilege should be extended to the hospitals of San Juan de Dios and San Andrés. In all of this the protomédicos could see no conflict with the ban of Viceroy de Croix. On the self-assured legal advice of the fiscal of the Council of the Indies, the crown in 1783 dispatched new cédulas to the viceroy, who had not replied to the first ones, requiring that the custom prior to 1770 be observed without change.

Before this cédula reached him, Viceroy Matías de Gálvez, responding to that of 1782, asserted baldly that this cédula had been obtained by the "vices of obreption and supreption," the first by concealing knowledge of the ban of 1770 and the second by falsely claiming that the old style was still in force. Calling attention to the laws of Spain and the Indies,[25] the Council of the Indies said that for a romance surgeon it was sufficient to have five years' apprenticeship in a hospital or under some approved surgeon in order to submit himself to the protomedicato for examination. It then recommended that the king endorse such apprenticeship for romance surgeons and allow the professor of surgery in the Hospital de Jesús Nazareno to continue to certify those who had served internships under him. No one had to take the courses in the new School of Surgery in the Indian Hospital against his will. On the other hand, the council advised those who aspired to become Latin surgeons to take the courses in the new School of Surgery, something that would stimulate them to study their science more fundamentally. And, what was more natural than that there should be a distinction between the "mere *romancistas*" and these?[26] Clearly irritated, the king sharply ordered that the ban of Viceroy de Croix be followed on the terms "proposed by the protomedicato," despite the course advocated by the Council of the Indies.[27] After all, Viceroy Matías de Gálvez was the brother of José de Gálvez, the progressive, honorable, efficient, and sometimes arbitrary Minister of the Indies.

Prerequisites for Training in the School of Surgery

With the establishment of schools of surgery in America, the prerequisites for surgical education tended more and more to qualify graduates as Latin surgeons. Students did not normally come to the school with a bachelor's degree in medicine, but once they graduated they were not romance surgeons either. Between the authorization of the School of Surgery in Mexico in 1768 and the publication of the requirements governing matriculation in 1807, the prerequisites were fully elaborated. Between fifteen and twenty-one years old, the applicant must have no bodily defect and have Latin upon which the professors would examine him privately. Thereafter, the student must produce proof of his blood purity from the attorney of his town, certificates of baptism not only for himself but also for his parents and grandparents, both paternal and maternal, and another of *vita et moribus,* signed by his parish priest and the aldermen of his town. In addition, the student had to have a formal promise from a person of property agreeing to maintain him respectably and provide books and instruments. On the negative side, no student might take up with or study in a barbershop, which, "far from giving him useful instruction," would lead him into vicious habits out of keeping with the honor and respect due to the faculty he was entering. The regent of the royal audiencia and presiding judge of the Indian Hospital ruled that any student meeting these stipulations might "matriculate and take courses in the Academy."[28]

That these men, when they graduated, were not university-trained Latin surgeons disturbed them less and less, and finally not at all. The surgeons from the new surgical colleges in Spain regarded themselves as the best trained and most up-to-date. In fact, the graduates they trained in these new schools not only despised the romance surgeon but also acquired a growing contempt for the conventional doctor with his stereotyped language, conduct, and procedure. This passing of judgment upon the physicians by the surgeons turned the scale of judgment upside down. It was this feeling, reinforced by their Spanish spokesmen, that led the surgeons to fight so bitterly to certify their graduates instead of sending them through the royal protomedicato, where they merely had a representative.

Military and Naval Surgeons

In a government so centralized as that of the Spanish empire the total separation from private practice of army and navy surgeons, who yearned to combine their official posts with private practice in the civil population of the cities where they were stationed, or even where they put into port, was hardly expected and rarely achieved. Every regiment had its surgeon and, certainly in more important cases, his assistant, but individual ships needed their surgeons as well. The government was often so hard-pressed to find men for these posts that it often ended up with those who, if their credentials had been scrutinized carefully for a coveted post, were not legally qualified to practice. Besides, almost to a man, those all but impressed into this service expected some kind of official reward—exemption from some legal requirement to practice, promotion to consultant (*consultor*), or the right to awe the local people with some embroidered and fancily sashed uniform prescribed for his peers in Spain. Not the least of these latter gratifications was the freedom to operate without the intervention of the royal protomedicato, which was always loath to recognize any limitations on its powers.

In the early eighteenth century the crown usually appointed surgeons for the garrison regiments and other military posts in America, but when he thought fit the viceroy of New Spain appointed a surgeon and an assistant for the three companies of the palace guard in Mexico City and ordered the treasury officials to pay them a salary of ninety-three pesos a month. In those days of scarcity of money, moribund economy, and inefficient collection of taxes, the treasury passed the problem on to the Council of the Indies, which remitted the weighty matter to the king.[29] It should not surprise a student of Spanish imperial history in the second half of this same century that the king himself named these surgeons and ordered their salaries paid. In 1787 the Spanish government advised the viceroy of New Spain that it was sending the Spanish surgeon

José Morales to the Department of San Blas with his wife and two small children at the expense of the royal treasury in Mexico and had plans to send three more surgeons.[30] Surgeons in these ports retired as soon as they could at one-third of their salary, and unless they were unlike their kind turned to a practice where they could charge fees.[31] Vicente Ferrer, surgeon of a regiment of dragoons in Mexico City, for example, wanted to retire at full salary with "honor of consultant of the army."[32] No such request, however, except when based upon rigid custom, could hope for success. As honor and precedence were sought after as ardently as was money, the crown, which was notoriously tight with pesos, was also sparing with honors—except in return for money.

A fair example is Félix Cortés y Baro, surgeon of the First Battalion of the Infantry Garrison Regiment in Cartagena de Indias, who decided not only to slip into the practice of surgery but also to reinforce his boldness with the imposing and colorful uniform prescribed by the new ordinances of the colleges of surgery in Spain. Even after Cortés showed the governor a copy of these regulations, Cortés was ordered not to wear such dress. The governor, undoubtedly irritated that anyone outside the palace should assume so elevated a privilege, took his cue from the protomédico of Cartagena. When he discovered that Cortés had never presented his title, the protomédico ordered him to stop practicing. Little wonder that Cortés had refused, for as he explained it his formal title from the College of Barcelona had been lost in the course of the voyage. With an oversight that seems almost deliberate, the crown "condescended" to Cortés's petition and revalidated the title, not mentioning whether it asked the College of Barcelona to confirm the original and saying nothing about wearing the gold-braided uniform. The royal order also allowed surgeons to renew lost certificates, a move calculated to encourage a copious supply of medical intruders.[33]

How to handle these intrusions into the medical corps of the armed service, however, was still more complicated. For one thing, it was never quite clear in America whether the frequent reorganization of medical government in Spain had any bearing in America. Spanish armies, operating in America during the wars of independence, were thus caught up in uncertainty over medical policies. In Spain, for example, the royal protomedicato petitioned the government to abolish the posts of protomédico and chief pharmacist (*boticario mayor*) of the army and subject the military surgeon general to the civil protomedicato. Having already exempted all naval hospitals, vessels, and fleets from the authority of the protomedicato, in 1812 the Cortes again refused to allow the tribunal control over physicians, surgeons, and pharmacists in the army.[34] Ferdinand VII upheld this ruling two years later, but required army and navy doctors, surgeons, and apothecaries to have licenses from committees of their respective faculties, which had supplanted the general proto-medicato in Spain in 1811. These army physicians, surgeons, and apothe-caries, however, had to observe the pharmacopoeia prescribed by the civil authorities and cooperate with them in epidemics. If they practiced their professions illegally, they fell under the authority of the civil juntas. As an indication of how little bearing these changes of medical regulations in Spain had upon America when there was so much demand for army surgeons, Viceroy Calleja pigeonholed this one by turning it over to his auditor de guerra for an opinion.[35] Later, between 1827 and 1833, long after Spain's mainland empire was independent, the mother country did abolish the posts of army protomédico and surgeon general.[36]

The extraordinary tenderness with which the Spanish government treated those it recruited for service in American military and naval in-stallations shows that a mere commission in either service was not enough to attract licensed doctors and surgeons. Even surgeons who had gradu-ated from the College of Surgery at Cádiz and had taken courses in medicine there, though allowed to practice medicine also when they were aboard ship or otherwise isolated in the service, were really not eligible to practice ashore in America when they left the service, whether by ruse or with license.

Domingo Rusi, for example, surgeon first class in the royal navy, upon retirement from the service in 1760 went about making arrange-ments to practice both medicine and surgery in Mexico. Though he re-quested confirmation as chief surgeon of the Indian Hospital in 1761, he was still begging for the post in 1765.[37] Then, in the midst of this wait, he sought superannuation without salary but with all the privileges and exemptions his service entitled him "to practice freely the faculties of medicine and surgery,"[38] as "he had been doing in the navy." The crown adviser, however, immediately said that he could not practice medicine: he did not have the bachelor's degree from a university, and he had not passed examination by the royal protomedicato. In fact, Diego Porcel, the man rendering the opinion, questioned whether or not Rusi, or for that matter any surgeon superannuated from the navy, had the right to practice even surgery without taking the examination by the protomedi-cato.[39] When Commandante General Juan de Villalba named Rusi, who must have been a persuasive talker, as chief surgeon of the army,[40] the king refused to confirm the appointment on the ground that the creation of such a post was unnecessary.[41] Despite all these rebuffs, can anyone doubt that Rusi at least practiced medicine, as General Villalba tacitly admitted in an oblique reference that Rusi enjoyed "general acceptance and credit" in "that capital." In Cartagena de Indias, the surgeon Juan

Borrell, fiscal of the protomedicato, began as a surgeon in the royal navy and seemingly enjoyed every post at the disposal of the civil and ecclesiastical authorities there.[42]

Though the man with questionable credentials often looked for excuses to slip into practice at some populous center, it was far harder to induce the qualified man to come to America when there was little chance of side gain. In order to get Francisco Sánchez Martín to accept the post as surgeon at the port of Omoa in Guatemala, where he would care for the troops and the prisoners working on the fortifications, the crown offered a whole battery of extraordinary inducements. Though only 720 pesos a year, the salary was equal to that of the best-paid university professors in America. From the president of the Casa de Contratación he reserved two months' salary for expenses incidental to the voyage to Guatemala; he enjoyed half-salary from January 1, 1778, though his commission was dated January 18; and from the day he set sail he drew full salary without any levy upon it. The king also paid his family's passage and stipulated the same for his return, adding that, in case of his death, his wife and nephew might return at crown expense, while the widow, as a pension, might draw one-third of her husband's salary for life. To crown it all, Francisco might use the uniform of surgeon of the Spanish army and enjoy the honors attached to such posts.[43] Only those long acquainted with the inveterate penury of the Spanish crown can fully understand how much these concessions betray.

Spanish Colleges of Surgery and Surgical Reforms

In Spain the middle of the eighteenth century saw the development of a new concern for surgery that was bound to be reflected in America. In 1748 the establishment of the College of Surgery in the Naval Hospital in Cádiz (Hospital de Marina de Cádiz) was itself a reflection of the mounting concern of Spaniards, not only with the tragedies—reported and unreported—wrought by the host of romancistas among the people, but also with the very welfare of men in the armed services. When in 1748 the king authorized this college, it was to teach fundamental surgery to surgeons going aboard war and merchant vessels.

This "seminary or college," even with limited financial support, though perhaps impressive by the standards of that day, hardly seems adequate now. The royal order setting up the college obliged the Casa de Contratación to establish an enrollment of sixty students and provide a dormitory, corresponding refectory, and a salon for lectures and clinical observation of surgeons at work. The decree also called for a library, cabinets for instruments, and storage of "machines" needed in operations.

Hard-pressed as the Spanish government always was for money, it nevertheless stuck by its paternalistic responsibilities. Each student would receive a daily ration—elaborately stated, down to the very ounce—at the expense of the royal exchequer. Unless some relative could be found to sign a written agreement to provide clothing, that too would come at government expense. After three years in the college, these men would join others in actual practice for their internships.

The qualifications expected of these men still reflected the standards of the previous three centuries. Whereas the candidate for the study of medicine had to come armed with a bachelor's degree, the entering student in surgery at Cádiz had only to be able "to read, write, and count," but he had to provide proof of his blood purity and show that his father was not engaged in "any vile trade" and that his own behavior and attitudes were good.

The teaching arrangements of these men, though limited, were specific enough. Four masters and an "anatomical demonstrator," all under the supervision of the chief surgeon of the navy, took charge of instructing the interns. In order that these men not remain in ignorance of the composition of medicines, the "apothecary inspector of medicines," when he was about to make up a batch, had the obligation to notify the chief surgeon so that he could order all the surgery students to attend, hear the explanation of the samples used, the manner of dispensation, the dose, and the virtues of each. This surgical training would end in three years, and perhaps before, because annual examinations were staged to help the chief surgeon weed out the unpromising. Because the purpose was to put trained surgeons aboard ships, students might not linger more than six years, "because it is not suitable that they abide eternally" in Cádiz.[44]

Horrible examples and graphic pleas continued to plague the Spanish empire, however. Over twenty years after the founding of the college at Cádiz in 1748, while the protomedicato in Spain remained indifferent and even hostile, the struggle to establish a new college for Latin surgeons in Madrid forced the use of horror stories to discredit untrained or unlicensed romancistas and phlebotomists. And a good example was at hand. In 1765 in the town of Martín Muñoz de las Posadas, Eugenio Lázaro, a romance surgeon, putting a butcher's block on the bed and using a common cold chisel, had cut off not only the arm but also the life of the woman Josepha Redondo. As a preliminary to this delicate operation, he had seized the hand—burned while the woman was in epileptic seizure—and so twisted it that she "was left with one hand and the artificer with three." Family connections, when the case broke, protected this romancista from prosecution.[45]

What rankled and what got results was not the death of the woman but the disgrace to the nation. A crown fiscal stated bluntly that it was "unbelievable that in a civilized country the neglect of public health should be so pitiful and concern about it so slight. . . ." The case of Josepha Redondo demonstrated not only the pitiful ignorance of the surgeons but also "the indifference of the protomedicato, where the surgeons of the kingdom are examined," despite the "multitude of the maimed seen in the streets everywhere." At the same time, the damning opinion went on, there were chairs in some Spanish universities teaching surgery from Guido de Chauliac, "a work written in France in the time of St. Louis, some six centuries ago."[46] A better case of backwardness could be made for Spain in 1771, but, then, reforms are never made by proving them unnecessary, and this awakening led to a rapid increase in the number of Spanish surgical colleges. After the college of Cádiz (1748) came those of Barcelona (1764) and Madrid (1787), followed so rapidly by others that there were five before the end of the century and seven by 1818.[47] The zeal for overcoming the decadence that marked Spanish surgery at midcentury, despite the turmoil of the time, had achieved more than this concrete result: Spanish surgeons were moving into other countries to check upon and profit by any advances they found. Even when entrance requirements went beyond those projected for Cádiz and required courses in physics and other sciences, for example, students could not at first be found who could present them; Spanish preparatory schools had to have time to adjust to the new demands being made upon them. Despite what was at first a marked disappointment in enrollment, the influence of the colleges was felt throughout the empire.

At the very time that Spaniards were pressing to create a third college of surgery in Madrid, government officials in America felt obliged to expose the desperate situation there. In Guatemala the interim president of the royal audiencia, Juan González Bustillo, setting out the "notable lack" of surgeons in that kingdom, calmly stated that there was only one surgeon there, and that, because of frequent illnesses, he was unable to respond most of the time.[48] If there was only one in Guatemala City, the rest of the country was bound to be served by intruders or not at all. The president, in fact, had been obliged to suspend the French surgeon of the corps of dragoons for incompetence. That he was a foreigner could be forgotten.

To meet a crying need of this kind, two all-but-impossible things were necessary: to find the surgeons and to find the means to pay them without drawing upon the royal exchequer. In the whole Spanish world there was no place to turn, except to the colleges of Cádiz and Barcelona.

And men from these places were scarce and altogether indisposed to undertake hazardous voyages when the pay was not forthcoming. Despite all its writhing, the municipal council of Guatemala could never find the means to pay the salaries of the two surgeons from Spain. Beyond a half-hearted suggestion for assessing private houses, a slight tax upon indigo, and another upon the commerce of Guatemala City, they simply were unable to produce a workable plan. When the councilmen proposed that after eight years the surgeons might safely be left to their own devices, including their private practice, the accountant's office in Madrid countered that it was necessary to provide for the surgeons not only for eight years but also for all their time in service.[49] So feeble a response to so legitimate a cry seems all but pusillanimous, yet it is absolutely typical of the plight of progress and reform everywhere in the Spanish empire in the eighteenth century when, otherwise, the conditions were right. From the town council to the Council of the Indies, the government recognized the need for official intervention and had centuries of precedent to bolster it, but an inflexible economy or, perhaps, an inflexible view of it made this step no more likely than any other. The ayuntamiento in Guatemala City could point to only three "graduates" in medicine—one bachelor; one licentiate, past seventy; and one doctor, the professor of prima of medicine, who was about to vacate his chair without a candidate for the post in sight—a sad ending to the first century of the University of San Carlos de Guatemala. Another thirty years had to elapse before the government reached another peak in its effort to educate and make surgeons available in the empire.

The Royal School of Surgery in Mexico

In Mexico, as in Spain, a fresh interest in surgery and anatomy heralded the new age. At midcentury Dr. José Dumont not only initiated studies of surgery and anatomy in the Royal Indian Hospital but also began practicing dissections there—apparently the first in the viceroyalty.[50] The use of the facilities in the hospital—where cadavers were at hand—for dissections to determine the nature of the epidemic ravaging the city in 1762,[51] though these strange exercises horrified the Indian patients, gave the dignity of tacit approval to the method. Then in 1764 Antonio de Arroyo, the alert and aggressive administrator of the hospital, made an overture to the viceroy, the Marqués de Cruillas (1761–66), for the legal representative of the institution and even the royal protomedicato endorsed this petition, the new viceroy, the Marqués de Croix, submitted establishment of an anatomical amphitheater in the hospital. When the a petition to the Council of the Indies for a chair of practical anatomy and a plan drawn up by the surgeon Bernardo Cortés.

In Spain it met with quick success. For one thing it found favor with Pedro Virgili, surgeon of the king's bedchamber, who did so much to promote the modernization of surgery and surgical education in Spain in the second half of the eighteenth century; he also had a nephew—beautifully qualified, it must be said—at the right age and stage for the Mexican post. When the protomedicato in Madrid lent its endorsement, the Council of the Indies approved.[52] The king then confirmed the names submitted by Pedro Virgili. For the post of "master professor" of surgery, at one thousand pesos a year, he chose Andrés Montañer y Virgili, naval surgeon first class, "young, robust, and of proved good conduct," who had completed a course in anatomy at Cádiz. For the dissector, who would assist and substitute for Montañer at five hundred pesos a year, he named Manuel Moreno, then actual rector of the College of Cádiz. Since this new school was "in imitation of those at Cádiz," he enclosed a copy of the statutes of the College of Barcelona and the cédula founding the institution at Cádiz.[53] In Mexico the assignment for the new surgeons required them to give a course in practical anatomy and another in surgical operations "at the coolest time of the year."

Spanish authorities had made the best choices—choices so good that one wonders how these young men expected to improve their lot by a dangerous move to New Spain. By the next year (1769), however, Montañer and Moreno were in Mexico, making the sensible argument that for their theoretical instruction to be most useful, they also needed to have charge of the cure of patients in the wards and to make their rounds while both teaching and treating. Here we have a clue to the alacrity with which these men had agreed to come over in the first place: extra salaries might be involved. With Domingo Rusi, chief surgeon of the Indian Hospital, however, they could find "not the slightest fault." Back in Madrid, then, the government decided to leave Rusi in his post with the vacuous hope that this new joint arrangement would be no obstacle to the work of the new School of Surgery.[54] In the end, though, it took only about two years to usher out the aging Rusi.

Unfortunately, someone in Madrid slipped egregiously; both Montañer and Moreno arrived without their official titles to organize a school that had no rules beyond a vague deference to the statutes of the colleges of Cádiz and Barcelona. The Council of the Indies ordered these documents sent,[55] but quite discreetly and long before these precious documents reached Mexico City the two recent arrivals from Spain had launched "anatomical demonstrations" in the Royal Indian Hospital,[56] as a hedge, no doubt, against possible maneuvers of those looking for technicalities upon which to block them. Mexico now had its first college of surgery.

Despite four years of training, students of the new school of surgery did not receive academic degrees upon graduation. They underwent annual examinations for four consecutive years and, instead of taking a first or a second, were classified by the professor of surgery as poor (*corto*), medium, good, and outstanding (*sobresaliente*). Then, armed with a certificate showing they had passed this examination and a statement testifying to their standing, the candidates might present themselves to the protomedicato for examination. In the case of a medical student from the University of Mexico, a pass by the royal protomedicato entitled the candidate to receive the university's degree of bachelor of medicine. The candidate in surgery, however, did not qualify for an academic degree. In the same way university students and graduates were normally exempt from military service, while those graduating from the School of Surgery were specifically liable for military service when called by the government that both founded and financed the institution. Between 1770 and 1803, a span of thirty-three years, 122 men, an average of almost four a year, graduated from the School of Surgery. The next ten years 1803 to 1813, however, saw seventy-nine new graduates, an average of almost eight a year with certificates in surgery.[57] The sharp increase noticeable in the number of men graduating in all faculties from universities between 1790 and 1810[58] was a coincidental factor of great importance in providing surgeons for the levies already being called up for the war now under way and destined to last eleven long years. Still, the increase left the country short of surgeons to serve all the towns and hapless villages without them.

The Surgeons Struggle for Independence from the Protomedicato

By the nineteenth century the deplorable state of surgery—always hand in hand with pharmacy as nearest to total neglect of all the major medical sciences—had fully come home to Spaniards everywhere. What had brought it home was the resentment of the legitimately licensed surgeons, who not only deplored the "ruin" of their art but also writhed under the fees exacted from them by the physicians on the royal protomedicato. A half-century after the modern surgeon had begun to look upon medicine as stifled in tradition, the low prestige implied in this practice had even more weight with these Spaniards, whose sense of "honor, prestige, and merits" had declined very little since the sixteenth century. Even more powerful was the hope that they might break off from medicine and collect the examination fees themselves. The official separation of medicine from surgery by a cédula of September 28, 1801, placing the two upon an absolutely equal footing—at least in print—gave them their opening.

Not until 1804, though, did the surgeons' view get serious consideration. Then, on a most tentative basis, the royal government submitted to the American viceroyalties a draft of proposals by the Governmental Committee on Surgery (Junta Gubernativa de Cirugía)[59] that would strip the royal protomedicato of all its power over surgery and deposit it neatly and firmly with the committee itself. Critical to this plan was the creation of subdelegates who would conduct the examinations of surgeons under the rules prevailing in the surgical colleges of Cádiz, Barcelona, and Madrid until such time as surgical colleges in America should be established. Those who passed, while waiting for their titles from the junta in Spain, would receive temporary licenses from the subdelegates. Even the authority to suppress the illicit practice of surgery would fall under the jurisdiction of these same subordinates, who would give the unlicensed surgeon two years to present himself to his examiners with a certificate from the town council that "he had practiced with honor and good name." The penalty proposed was fifty pesos for the first time, one hundred pesos for the second, and two hundred pesos and six years' exile to a distance of twenty leagues roundabout for the third.

In doubt about setting up the system peremptorily, the Council of the Indies consulted the viceroy in Mexico with the concrete suggestion that he organize a commission to report upon the whole business. Viceroy Iturrigaray took a step that was bound if not designed to stir up a lot of heat and therefore a lot of information. For reports he appealed to Dr. Antonio Serrano, professor of surgery in the School of Surgery at the Royal Indian Hospital, and Dr. Vicente Cervantes, the professor of botany in the Royal Botanical Garden.

Dr. Serrano thus fell into a beautiful opportunity to write a brief for taking surgery from under the jurisdiction of the royal protomedicato.[60] First of all, it struck him as worse than unjustified that the protomédicos—all physicians—should call in a romance surgeon when they were examining a candidate to practice surgery. Even more outrageous was that when a romance surgeon was called in, as a rule, he was one of those most recently examined and most likely to be a relative, friend, or fellow student of the candidate himself. How could such a prejudiced judge, when he had no training in theory and no practice to speak of, be responsible? But were there not in the city, he asked, daintily and silently pointing to himself, qualified and honored surgeons whom the protomedicato could appoint on a continuing basis and thus avoid mischief to the present system? But no, the protomedicato wanted neither him nor other authentic graduates, preferring a mercenary romancista who, with his fee of twenty reales, would go away happy and raise no troublesome questions. Serrano's plain view was that, as the protomédicos had no surgical training, they could and did not properly correct malpractice. Moreover, in America the sum of fifty-eight or sixty pesos deposited for an examination was divided by the protomedicato, whereas in Spain after the distribution of some small fees, the bulk of the deposit went to the crown. Thus, in Spain an examiner could not live on the twenty reales he collected from some hapless candidate, but he sought the posts for the honor. In turn, he might expect to be retained by bishops, town councils, and hospitals and to hold university chairs and other appointments.

Serrano pounded very hard at the "desolation" prevailing in obstetrics that could be remedied by subdelegates, but he knew that if the subdelegations were not self-financing, the impecunious crown would never authorize them. He knew also that the fees attached to surgery would never suffice for their support. In this case he insisted that the subdelegates, far from serving for pesos and reales, would gladly serve for the honor. Such appointment, he said, would make a man more honored and more authoritative than his colleagues. With this change, men with legitimate titles could make a go of it against the slander and competition of illegal practitioners and approach the state in Spain, where every little place had its man with a proper license. With so few properly trained men to license as in Spain, no great sum could be expected from fees.

The salvation in New Spain, therefore, lay in the development of the Royal School of Surgery. Though it was authorized in a royal cédula of March 16, 1768,[61] and had kept functioning as long as the Spanish regime lasted, Serrano felt in 1804 that "he would not be true to his position" if he did not come out with the sad truth about the institution. From the date of founding, for thirty-six long years, he said, the institution had remained exactly as it was when founded with just the one professor of surgery, who served as director, and a dissector, the substitute in the chair. Thus, for nearly four decades, though they realized the need to have more chairs in order to train surgeons "for so vast a kingdom," the professors did not venture to petition the crown to bring the number of these up to par with the schools of Barcelona and Cádiz.

In the spirit of hope Serrano supplied the crown with the names of ten surgeons for the posts of subdelegates in ten Mexican towns. He admitted that "not all are Latin surgeons," but he could have added that only two in his list held doctors' degrees. The outraged surgeon then concluded that all surgery should be separated from the protomedicato, not only because physicians were incompetent to judge in these fields but also because with the fees previously collected new chairs could be created for the School of Surgery to relieve the royal exchequer of the salaries paid the professor and chief anatomist there.

The quiet disregard of anatomy and surgery in the University of Mexico and of their high place in the School of Surgery at the Royal Indian Hospital was both natural and justified. From the beginning until 1750 the teaching of anatomy in the university was stale and perfunctory if not nonexistent. The work supposed to go on in the chair of anatomy either did not go on at all or was irregularly and imperfectly performed. In 1714, when the chair fell vacant, Viceroy Duque de Linares (1711–16) refused to appoint any of the candidates proposed in the list of three submitted by the university cloister, saying that there were far better candidates available. Indeed, all of those seeking the post, though listed as approved surgeons and algebrists, were distinctly of the bonesetter class and, unless it was in another faculty, without any university degrees at all. When, however, those he named refused the post, including, apparently, his favorite "registered foreigner" Vicente Rebec of his own household, he settled for the appointment of the Augustinian friar, Bernabé de Santa Cruz.[62] Neither the humble nature of the post nor the humiliation of the appointment detracted from the high formality of Santa Cruz's inauguration. After taking the oath to respect the calls of the rector and to defend the Immaculate Conception, in the presence of the rector and "many doctors" of the cloister, and after a skeleton had been brought in, he explained the parts of the body and their functions until the examiners were satisfied and "the rector rang the bell for him to stop." He was now officially "anatomical surgeon."

More than half a century later, however, so little had been accomplished in this chair that some professors began to murmur that there was no use to dissections of cadavers and that comparative anatomies executed upon the bodies of animals were preferable. In fact, compliance with the statutes was so negligent that the dissections, if they took place at all, were almost always done upon animals. This practice was not because the full cloister disapproved of cadaver dissection, as one might gather, but because of the negligence of the professor and the indifference of the other professors and of the students.

Thus, the coming of Montañer and Moreno, the inauguration of the new School of Surgery, and the building of an anatomical amphitheater for the new school were bound to challenge negligent practices in the university. In this way, late in 1773 in its report to the viceroy, the full cloister went on record favoring dissections of human cadavers as prescribed in the statutes. Still, the university had difficulty in obtaining cadavers, and the new school refused to allow the use of its amphitheater for the required three dissections a year on the days when a fit cadaver was available. The rector of the university accordingly entreated Viceroy Bucareli to order the School of Surgery to comply.[63] The university's corporate dignity soon became so deeply involved that the editor of the 1775 edition of the university statutes, when he came to Constitution 146 outlining the work of the chair of anatomy, truculently added a footnote saying that this statute remained in force regardless of the new anatomical amphitheater in the Royal Indian Hospital.[64] As it turned out, surgical training continued to center in this institution, as Serrano's report clearly showed, although it was still problematical whether surgeons trained at the Royal Indian Hospital could get from under the thumb of the protomedicato.

The Spanish Colleges of Surgery and Control of Surgery in the Indies

Though stimulated by the example of the college of Cádiz, surgical education in America did not generate vitality. The School of Surgery in the Royal Indian Hospital in Mexico City, while it certainly was more clinical than the work done by the chair of surgery in the Royal and Pontifical University, itself lapsed into routine hospital procedures and failed to draw surgery into a new day. In contrast to the good health of the college at Cádiz, this lack of vitality left room for the Spanish surgeons to make an effort to assume direction of their profession in America. In fact, in 1801 the Principal Governing Committee of the Colleges of Surgery (Junta Superior Gubernativa de los Colegios de Cirugía) in Spain made a direct overture to the king, depicting surgery in America in ruins, carried on by individuals without knowledge, science, and a license to practice. Therefore, to end the ruin and neglect and "to contain the excesses committed," the junta proposed that pending the establishment of surgical colleges in America like those in Spain, Spanish subdelegations supervise the economic aspects of surgery in America, manage its government, and conduct its examinations. What is more, the king was so gracious—or so unreflecting—as to consent on December 29, 1801, as long as the junta presented all nominations for subdelegates for royal approval.[65]

Such gentle, self-aggrandizing remedies, however, were far too late. Before the king's resolution creating subdelegations could be carried out, evidence piled up in Spain that more direct, even desperate answers were needed. When in 1803 the king called upon the junta to nominate capable surgeons for the garrison at Portobelo and for the Auxiliary Battalion of Santa Fe, and after posting these possible appointments in the royal colleges, the junta had to report back that it could not be expected that persons qualified in surgery would volunteer to leave their own country and endure the trouble, hardships, and danger to reach such remote places "without some apparent advantages." One apparent disadvantage was the small but fixed salaries attached to such posts. As proof, six months after the call for a surgeon for the presidio of Bacalar near Mérida was published in the royal colleges, only two candidates presented themselves, and only one of these met the legal requirements. In Tierra Firme the governor of Portobelo thought that a salary of fifty pesos a month might bring out the applicants, but the viceroy of Santa Fe demurred, holding that not even this sum would get applicants. The junta, therefore, proposed a sixty-peso monthly salary to bring men from Spain, since America had no candidates to offer. Because the petition for subdelegations in America, made by the junta in 1801, was still unresolved in 1803, the junta could do nothing more than lay before the crown the need for schools of surgery in the Indies, starting with the proposed subdelegations.[66]

Despite the urgency of this matter, two years after they had asked the Council of the Indies for its opinion the king's officers were still begging for a report. Meanwhile, in the rare cases where candidates qualified or said they qualified for examination, there was no one to examine them except in the seat of the protomedicatos. Since there was no such tribunal in Puerto Rico, Antonio Abad de la Rosa, an intern in the military hospital there, applied to the Junta Gubernativa in Spain to permit surgeons to examine him there instead of requiring an impossible trip back to Spain. In such cases, the junta was willing to appoint examiners, provided the practice met with the king's approval, at least until the creation of the subdelegations for America—something that had been hanging fire since 1801.[67] The accumulation of cases supporting the urgent petition of the viceroy of New Granada led the Ministry of Grace and Justice to remind the Council of the Indies that it should render the report requested in January 1802.[68] Then, after waiting another month, the Council of the Indies replied that before it could render the report requested concerning the establishment of subdelegations and chairs of surgery and pharmacy, it needed copies of the decree suppressing the protomedicato and establishing a new control body, the Facultad Reunida, together with its bylaws (Reglamentos).[69] The royal government, acting with what was in those days almost supersonic speed, supplied the Council of the Indies with the decrees that suppressed the protomedicato and in 1799 established a governing agency called the Facultad Reunida, but the delay was so great that the same packet carried still another decree reestablishing the protomedicato.[70] This sudden abolition and reestablishment of the protomedicato in Spain no doubt played its part in frustrating the efforts of the Junta Gubernativa in taking over examinations in surgery from the royal protomedicato in America and giving direct orders to its subdelegations in America.

Yet when it finally took the matter up late in 1803 the Council of the Indies left strong reason to believe that it hesitated out of jealousy of its own prerogatives. Its first condition was that the law of the Indies requiring the council to approve every cédula or order going into effect in America[71] apply in this case also. Likewise, the council thought that the requirement that candidates for examination in surgery in America deposit examination fees in Spain amounting to more than 166 pesos worked an unnecessary hardship. It therefore recommended that deposits be made in the Indies for remission to Spain.[72] While all this was going on, the candidate examined and approved could be practicing. Instead of recommending the immediate implementation of the plan of the junta, the council advised that all the documents, especially those for the proposed subdelegations, be transmitted to the viceroys, governors, and presidents of America who would set up a commission composed of the regent, an oidor, the civil sala fiscal, the senior alderman, the *síndico procurador,* and a member of the ecclesiastical cabildo. Such a commission would hear the protomedicato of the district and any other doctors whose learning and judgment justified it, and then make recommendations at the first moment possible,[73] a moment that was long in coming.

The surgeons' quest for independence from the protomedicato and the attempt by the Spanish colleges of surgery to take control of the American scene ultimately failed, as the whole issue got bogged down in claims and counterclaims, reports, and demands for additional information. In Lima, eight years after the effort of the Spanish Junta Gubernativa de Cirugía to take over the government of surgery in Mexico, the surgeon José Pastor de Larrinaga petitioned for a whole series of posts, honors, and privileges, among them chief surgeon of the garrison in Callao and the right to form his own Junta Gubernativa de Cirugía with other surgeons he should name, "bestowing upon them the honors of surgeons of the king's bedchamber." He then crowned his request by asking that this junta be entirely free from the protomedicato.[74] But all the aggressive surgeon got for his efforts was total rejection and the Regency's strong support for the protomedicato, evidence that there had been no change in government attitudes toward surgery. In fact, the Regency was far too busy with other matters to deal with reforms in surgery in the Indies, no matter how desperately they were needed.[75]

WHEN THE ETERNAL judges hold their final hearing to determine once and for all the crowning folly committed in the name of medicine upon the planet earth, they, surely, will have dropped everything else to wrinkle their brows over a file labeled "Bloodletting." So great a hold did this overused and debilitating practice have upon men that it was simply not called into question until long after that period when a rigamarole in medicine was often a more solid proof than a demonstration. Little wonder that Father Feijóo in 1726, with his tongue in his cheek, agreed with Pliny and Solinus that man learned this art from the hippopotamus, "an amphibious brute which, when he felt very bulky, by moving himself over the sharpest point of broken canes, let blood from the feet and legs, and afterwards closed the wounds with mud."[1] The implication is that Feijóo thinks this is a perfectly appropriate way to learn such a doctrine. As a delicate afterthought, he makes it clear that the doctors preferred to take their precedent "blind" from Galen rather than from a more visible hippopotamus.[2] Regardless of what animal they learned it from, phlebotomy was a medical profession to the Spaniards when they conquered the Indies, as it still was when they left them three-and-a-half centuries later. The records of hospitals in Spain during the early sixteenth century run over with entries showing payments to bloodletters,[3] and a decade after the wars of independence got under way, the protomedicato in Mexico was still dignifying these practitioners—at least upon occasion—with solemn examination.

Qualifications, Practice, and Licensing of Phlebotomists

In Spain the practice remained monotonous from one century to the next. Almost casually the hospital accounts run, "four bleedings that a barber made, 136 maravedís,"[4] "168 maravedís for pitch to cover the case holding the barber's grindstone,"[5] and "a half real each for four live leeches for a sick woman."[6] Sometimes hospitals put these men under contract to come "to attend and to cure. . . ."[7] For all these documents tell, the phlebotomist was no more examined than was "the live leech." Though Ferdinand and Isabella had set up a systematic board of examiners to test practitioners of all branches of medicine, the few miserable maravedís for each operation make it unreasonable to believe that the operator could go to Madrid or, unless he lived there, to some other capital for examination.

In the Indies there was also good precedent for bleeding. Father Toribio de Motolinía, the Franciscan chronicler, observed that the Indians of Mexico were practicing bleeding when the Spaniards got there. As in nearly everything where they needed an edge sharper than they could get from stone, these Indians used "Itzli," or obsidian when they were well-to-do. If poor, they bled themselves with the awl-like spikes of the maguey plant.[8] The preponderance of bleeding by the Indians, instead of having a medical purpose, was in fact an invocation of the gods.

So, if the would-be physician could materialize on the heels of the conquest and flourish without a license, how much more so could the humble phlebotomist! In fact, the great danger was not that he would bleed without a license but that he would branch into the practice of medicine without one. Pero López, the first municipal protomédico in Mexico, as one of his first acts forbade the barber Pedro Hernández to cure buboes, so often brought on by the conquerors' "woman's sickness," but the justices and aldermen of the municipal council—who saw and felt this suffering firsthand—immediately reversed him and allowed the barber "to treat for the said sickness" as long as they saw fit.[9]

The assumption implicit in these two actions was that phlebotomy, like physic itself, fell under the jurisdiction of the protomédico appointed by the municipal council—until the council itself, which did not hesitate to take a position in technical matters of medicine, decided to intervene. Just at the beginning of the last decade of the sixteenth century with the viceroy, the Marquis of Manrique, threatening to appoint an examiner for bloodletters, the town council of Mexico City appointed its own,[10] a practice it silently discontinued three years later. However, as the city had contracted for the services of apothecaries and a bonesetter, especially necessary in cases of charity,[11] it began in 1610 to appoint phlebotomists and went on doing so for sixteen years.[12] Despite this burst of activity, the phlebotomist attracted no special attention and was, in fact, overshadowed by the bonesetter, Marcos Falcón. There is no indication either that these bloodletters enjoyed any jurisdiction over others.

In Peru medical problems as closely paralleled those of Mexico as did the conquest itself. Barbers and apothecaries eventually came under municipal inspection,[13] but upon occasion the city commissioned physicians to "inspect barbers and surgeons to see by what titles they practiced."[14] That Hernán Pérez, barber to his excellency, was bold enough to inform the municipal council of Lima that "he had need of the house where Carlos Barreta lives" in order "to be near the viceroy, his excellency Don Martín Enríquez," is a good indication of the high respect in which the bloodletter was held.[15] Since this special respect continued, the poor viceroy had no chance to escape the bleeder's dirty lancet. Scattered among the seeming trivialities of his diary, Juan Antonio Suardo left a pathetic record of five years of intermittent bleedings of the viceroy, the Count of Chinchón. Once when the doctors ordered him bled, "it pleased our Lord that he should get better,"[16] but as they later did the same thing when his excellency was suffering from a "terian fever," he "had a bad night."[17] After continued bleedings, with Chinchón still sickly, the doctors ordered him bled a second time, though "he had not profited from the first one two days before." In October 1635, when the suffering man was indisposed, "running at the mouth," the doctors had him bled again, and on the following day they varied their impotence by ordering the pulling of a tooth.[18]

Phlebotomists were not expected to have academic training, and as their examinations were oral they could pass the tests without being able to read and write. Whereas the physician needed four years in the faculty of medicine of an accredited university to go before the protomedicato, the bloodletter, following Spanish law, qualified by serving three years as an apprentice in a hospital[19] and for four years under an "examined and approved" surgeon or phlebotomist.[20] Because of the continued sway that bloodletting held over doctors, university students, though they did not expect to practice phlebotomy, were still much preoccupied with the notion that the remedy "for excessive fullness of the blood vessels consists in the quick release of the blood."[21] These academic exercises, however, indicated only that training for the doctor himself still rested upon the old hypothesis, as it did in England until 1837, when William IV's doctors added this unnatural ailment to an assortment of natural ones that, combined, hastened his departure into the beyond.

What the phlebotomist actually did in the Spanish colonies, at least what he did legally, may be deduced from the kind of questions the protomédicos asked him when he took an examination. Naturally, a knowledge of veins and arteries was critical if the bloodletter was to avoid tragedy. Beyond this elementary knowledge he had to know how to bleed properly and to put on cupping glasses and leeches. That the examiners expected him to know how to open ulcers and boils and how to cope with accidents and unforeseen problems indicates that the law, as it was interpreted, did not confine him to the blood alone. Questions on the extraction of teeth, particularly molars, are clear indication that, in that age when a whole viceroyalty might not claim three dentists operating under the law, somebody had to perform the basic if not the refined functions of the professional.

The few surviving records of examination of phlebotomists indicate that the "art of the phlebotomist" was still in such high respect on the eve of the wars of independence that, beyond proof of legitimacy produced in a certificate of baptism, the candidate merely needed to present various documents showing that his parents, as "old Christians," were "freed of all bad race of Moors, Indians, and others." Once having passed the examination, he took the oath to defend the "pure and Immaculate Conception." Thereupon, in those days before photographs could serve the same purpose, the clerk drew up a license that gave so minute a description of the bearer, including not only his features but also the shortest scar, that no thief could pass this document off as his own upon any alert official.[22] When the phlebotomist had run this gauntlet, he paid a stiff fee of fifty-five pesos and began his variegated practice.[23]

Wherever the difficulties of enforcement were insurmountable, the ideal requirements of the law meant that the regulations fell into abeyance unless some reason for their enforcement moved those charged with the king's conscience—such as the farming out of taxes or the collection of fees for examinations. In Mexico City itself, where the protomedicato was at hand to test any bloodletters who could qualify, practitioners often preferred not to face that formidable body and part with precious pesos for fees when the prospect of beating out unlicensed competitors—called *rapistas*—was also very uncertain. In fact, in 1795 at the expiration of the term of the renowned viceroy, the second Count of Revilla Gigedo, one witness to the improvements made in the Plaza del Bolador testified that in the interior, a short distance from the fountain, there were four nooks of beautiful workmanship where "certain barbers who, because they are not examined, set themselves up [and] apply their skill to the poor who come to be bled or to have their beard cut."[24] When, as a result of the agitation begun in 1798, the viceroy decided to permit examination of phlebotomists by delegates of the protomedicato, he gave an opening for the protomedicato to make the same plea on behalf of apothecaries.[25] In the towns apothecaries, too, were often poor with no one to leave in their shops. The fiscal of the royal exchequer was of the strong opinion that druggists should not be exempted from examination but from the necessity of journeying to the capital, yet a recent cédula had earnestly repeated the requirement that candidates for medical licenses should appear in person before the protomedicato.[26] Though the schedule of charges fixed in 1801 for various types of gracias al sacar assumed that "physicians, apothecaries, and surgeons" might be examined without coming to Mexico City,[27] it might seem—to collect the fees—evidence begins to creep out that, in the language of one of them, betting on the cockfights was more profitable than practicing phlebotomy in Mexico City. No doubt, although the bloodletter appeared for examination far more often than he did in the provinces, the evidence is that even in the viceregal capital an efficient, not to mention a total, enforcement of the law was a remote prospect. The extreme youth and immaturity of candidates under the scrutiny of the protomedicato, despite some evidence to the contrary, reveals bloodletting as declining in prestige. The prosecution of one of these, fortunately for history a headstrong and gabby youth, tells more of medicine than could a whole volume of viceregal bans.

The San Ciprián Case

The case began one morning in May 1791 when a few petty shopkeepers and casual passersby on the Street of the Clock in Mexico City looked up to see a young man running from his house, closely pursued by another stripling—this one wearing a blue cape and a white hat, brandishing a sword, and shouting to one and sundry: "Grab him! Grab him!" No one who heard him doubted that he intended to run his man through if he came upon him. Just as he was about to overtake the fugitive, however, he chanced to shake off his resplendent white hat, and in the moment it took him to stop and pick it up, his prey outdistanced him enough to take refuge in a confectioner's shop. A priest who happened to be in the shop, though, calmed the irate Beau Brummell enough to permit the Marqués del Apartado, who happened to be passing, to take the terrified youth under his protection and proceed with him toward the viceregal palace.

The marquis could hardly have realized that he had stumbled into a case showing the waning jurisdiction of the royal protomedicato. Yet, such was the main issue in this strange and violent incident. Despite the canopies and velvet-draped tables of the royal protomedicato, an insolent eighteen-year-old phlebotomist had ventured to challenge its power. Such an insignificant incident, to the patent disgust of the crown attorney, led not to just one but two different preparatory legal cases—one drawn up by the clerk of the audiencia and another by the clerk of the protomedicato.[28] This time Spanish justice, perhaps because of the competition between the protomedicato and the king's own courts, was not slow to move. Though the excitement began in the morning about 10:30, the clerks began immediately to take down the testimony and had both cases ready by the next day. It nevertheless took a favorable ruling by the judge of the royal audiencia—put in charge of the case by the viceroy—to enable the royal protomedicato to assume unquestioned jurisdiction.[29]

The case arose from the refusal of Manuel de San Ciprián, the man in flight, to close down one of the two "barbershops" where, after due examination by the royal protomedicato, he had practiced the art of phlebotomy. As this double-shop operation was a violation of the royal regulations governing the profession, Dr. José Ignacio García Jove, president of the protomedicato, had warned San Ciprián several times that he must close either one shop or the other. Yet it was not only just this act of disobedience but also the intemperate and insolent bearing of the barber that landed him first in trouble and then in jail. He was young—just eighteen—and what he did not really appreciate was that Dr. García Jove was a proud, domineering, and unrelenting man who did not take kindly to the reports reaching his ears that the insolent young bleeder was burlesquing the whole royal protomedicato, saying that body did not allow him two shops because he did not bribe them. Now, no doubt at García Jove's request, José Carabantes, an agent of the court, had arrived without a written warrant, as the victim saw it, to throw the screen, a kind of barber's pole of those days, and any other insignias of the bleeder's trade into the street, and to burn them there. His assignment, the protomédicos later insisted though, was to take the offending property "on deposit" and lodge San Ciprián in the court jail.[30] Though Carabantes testified that he delivered his warrant—a verbal one from the royal protomedicato—with soft words, San Ciprián and his wife testified that his manner was overbearing, peremptory, and insulting. At any rate, the barber quibbled, saying that he had no need of the royal protomedicato, that that tribunal was persecuting him for mere want of a bribe of twenty-two pesos, and that he did not intend to comply. In fact, he said, he would consult the viceroy first. As the arresting officer instructed his bailiff to bring in a porter to seize if not to throw the screen taken into the street, San Ciprián declared to the officers—so they testified—that he would cut their guts out, surely a strange thing to threaten when he was reaching for a cudgel. Thereupon, the son of the court agent, Demetrio Carabantes, unsheathed his sword, and San Ciprián, grasping at last that he was not dealing in mere bragadoccio, took precipitately to his heels, leaving his pregnant sixteen-year-old wife to cope with his enemies. Taking off in pursuit, Demetrio thrust her aside so roughly that he left a great bruise on her left arm as he dashed out after the insulting barber.

So it was from this scene that the Marqués del Apartado had brought San Ciprián when, passing the court jail, Carabantes, showing a surprising lack of respect for the marquis, caught up, and roughly pushed the somewhat chastened San Ciprián into the jail as a prisoner. Vicente Elizalde, one of the jailers, refused to accept San Ciprián because the officers of the protomedicato did not have a written warrant. Besides, he said, there was no precedent for receiving and holding prisoners of the medical tribunal. In consequence, he ordered the prisoner freed. Elizalde insisted that the secretary of the protomedicato, not Carabantes, had the authority "to conduct" prisoners to him. When Carabantes went to talk to the secretary, by chance standing at the door of the audiencia, San Ciprián ducked out and ran into the viceregal palace, reaching the guard post of the company of halberdiers. Though they still wanted to drag him away to another jail if necessary, San Ciprián managed to reach the viceroy, who gave an order instructing the chief justice of the phlebotomist's district to hear the case. There San Ciprián signed a complaint with such precipitation that his signature looked either like that of a palsied old man or of a gross illiterate. A little later, however, when he signed his more deliberate declaration, his signature had gained much in steadiness. His wife was obliged to allow the notary to sign for her; she could not write.

The protomedicato's case had a far different color from that drawn up by San Ciprián and certainly put a different complexion on the scene in the Street of the Clock. So great was San Ciprián's contempt for the royal protomedicato, they said, that when the protomédicos arrived he seated himself and with a show of nonchalance declared that he would not comply. He had no need for the protomedicato; he could earn more playing the cockfights than he could practicing phlebotomy. Indeed, if the protomédicos would return his hundred pesos, he would gladly hand back his license. For want of twenty pesos for Dr. García Jove and some miserable small doubloons for Carabantes, he was in this mess. All the rest of the protomedicato were thieves and swindlers, too.

Eventually, on May 26, Judge Miguel de Irisarri, who was hearing the case, turned both files over to Viceroy Revilla Gigedo who, naturally, passed the matter on to Fiscal Alva for review. The "king's mouthpiece," patently hostile to the protomedicato, referred bluntly to the "invasion" of San Ciprián's house; Escribano Espinosa certified both the injury to San Ciprián's wife and that the phlebotomist's house was not a shop, for the screen there only served to divide the room. The viceroy followed the fiscal's advice to ask for the protomedicato's own version.[31]

The formal report of the protomedicato[32] shows where its tender spots really were. It could not believe that Carabantes had exceeded his authority in making the arrest, as it would feel obliged to do had it not had previous knowledge that San Ciprián was "an audacious, insolent, and daring youth." On the other hand, they recalled, on the occasion of the "fandango" that followed his examination San Ciprián had burlesqued the police, who put him in jail but did not draw up an indictment. Carabantes was an old, reliable employee whose testimony was supported by witnesses. Most of all, though, the protomedicato cringed at jailer Elizalde's assertion that there was no precedent for receiving the prisoners of the protomedicato in the court jail. To his charge, the tribunal succinctly replied, "false"; it had sent its prisoners to both the court and city jails.

Fiscal Alva, to whom the viceroy now turned, remarked that the protomedicato threw no light "on the point of jurisdiction," which had led to the two separate preparations of the case in the first place, but agreed that both files should be turned over to the audiencia, which, according to the agreement, would advise on the question of jurisdiction.[33] When the audiencia then decided that the case belonged to the protomedicato, the viceroy duly authorized that tribunal to proceed. Thereupon, on August 8, 1791, it had San Ciprián arrested and lodged in the court jail where it had wished to lodge him in the first place. The unalloyed joy of the royal protomedicato at this act creeps through the faded record of the proceedings that followed. Manuel San Ciprián's "preparatory declaration,"[34] taken by the tribunal the very next day, finds him in a humbler mood and casts him, in addition to the other roles he had mastered, in the role of liar. Now, no longer pretending that he did not have two shops, he merely contended that he was keeping the shop in the Street of the Clock, with Dr. García Jove's permission, for a brother who was in the army and unable to submit to examination and start practicing. Dr. García Jove, he said, had advised his mother to pay the twenty-two pesos on "account" toward the cost of his brother's examination. Though he admitted that his stated reason for closing the shop was that he had not deposited the money and that he did say he could earn more betting on the cockfights, he claimed that he did not charge the protomédicos with being thieves and swindlers.

On August 12 and 13 came the cross-examination. In the first place the protomédicos wanted to know if his testimony that he was not operating the shop did not conflict with three depositions in which he said that he had no need for the protomedicato, that its members were a bunch of thieves, and that if they would return his hundred pesos they might have his license. His response was pointed: the depositions were false. Likewise, he denied reaching for a cudgel. Holding the cross-examination open for other developments, the protomedicato gave up on the note that his deposition was contradictory. The court read into the record the declaration made by its arresting officers on May 10.

Though the files offer no evidence on the final punishment meted out, they do show that San Ciprián did not languish forever in jail, as one is half-prepared to see him do. On August 16, 1791, the tribunal accepted a bond offered by Juan Beléndez and the next day permitted the release of the prisoner. In January 1792 the case was still pending, but by that time the poor whelp had already had punishment enough to match his offense and evidently remained at large.

More than a glimmering of the collapse of the independent "guild" jurisdiction of the protomedicato, which became so apparent in another case later in the decade, can be seen in that of San Ciprián. Once Dr. García Jove had slaked his thirst for vengeance on the petty offender, other judges of the tribunal were allowed to take over and even treat the harried youth kindly. Nothing short of a trembling fear for its jurisdiction and prerogatives could have led the protomedicato to start the preparation of a case against San Ciprián without waiting for an invitation from Irisarri, the judge to whom the viceroy assigned the case. In fact, the precipitation was so great that on mere rumor the protomédicos sent their countering documents to the wrong judge. In the end, there was little new in the viceroy's determining jurisdiction in the case, yet his referring the suit to the audiencia, when he could have relied upon his routine legal advisers, indicated that he understood the delicate balance involved. Evidently this dominant man, who accomplished wonders by dint of work and weight of personality, did not feel any particular jealousy of the exclusive jurisdiction of the specialized court. In fact, it was intervention from Madrid that soon wrested much of this independence from the protomedicato everywhere in America.

Licensing and Examinations: Other Problems

Recognition that phlebotomy was a poor man's trade and that its receipts and emoluments were insufficient to induce any sane man to journey all the way to Mexico City to submit to examination came very late—at the end of the eighteenth century. As happened in so many other fields of Spanish government in America during this half-century, the authorities began to see that it was better to be a little more efficient if a little less right. In 1798, for example, the intendant of Puebla, patently irritated with the indiscriminate mix of trimming the beard with bleeding the customer, told the Viceroy Miguel José de Azanza that it was the practice in his city that no one be allowed to have a shop without passing examination by the protomedicato. He thought the regulations of the tribunal both sound and just. He would be the first to enforce those regulations to prevent barbers from "sticking their noses in" to become phlebotomists and tooth-pullers without any proof of their expertise or of their having passed examination, proof such as the signboard that all should have at the doors of their shops. He therefore endorsed complete separation of pure and simple barbering from bloodletting. He did not think that shaving a man should require the barber to submit to an examination by the protomedicato. Only the man performing the actual bleeding operations had any such need.[35] The protomedicato thereupon informed the viceroy that neither the tribunal nor its delegates outside the city had ever exempted those who bled from examination and that the simple haircutting barber had always been independent of the protomedicato. If, however, the ordinary barber should exceed his privileges and begin pulling teeth, it became the business of that body. The protomédicos informed the viceroy that a curtain (*cortina*) and a hanging basin were the proper signs for a mere barber. If, they said, the bloodletters at the same time exhibited their traditional lattice (*celosia*) and signboard (*tarjeta*), the distinction between mere haircutters and shavers on the one hand and licensed phlebotomists on the other would be quite sufficient.[36]

This solution was not acceptable to the fiscal who now made a cynical and more nearly correct analysis. Barbers and bleeders in separate shops could still be confused. Because of "the attractiveness of gain," many would surely operate on the sly without shops. To ferret out and punish all these violators, he thought fanciful. He accordingly recommended to the viceroy that no change be made and urged the continuance of the laws of Castile and of the Indies[37] that barbers without distinction be examined and approved by the royal protomedicato. Because those who had had public shops were the ones who practiced bleeding, a sweep of these should catch the offenders.[38] Taking his assessor's advice,[39] the viceroy then published a ban throughout the towns and cities of the viceroyalty that barbers might do their work without examination by the protomedicato, if they distinguished their shops with a screen and a hanging basin, and if they did not bleed, use the leech or cup, pull teeth, or practice any other of this type of operation. Otherwise, the inspector of the royal protomedicato should start proceedings against them.[40]

Though the bloodletter outside the city was most often neglected, the protomedicato could become petulant when an unlicensed phlebotomist presumed to set up shop in the seat of the viceroyalty where it functioned. In 1693 Protomédico Félix Vela del Castillo fined the notary clerk of the protomedicato for not executing orders to close shops in Mexico City where the operators had not been examined. Having illegally closed shops on his own authority, Vela del Castillo found his order reversed by the president of the protomedicato. Charging that Vela del Castillo was persecuting him for not closing the shops again in defiance of the president of the protomedicato, the secretary successfully appealed to the viceroy for relief.[41] This squabble does indicate that in the seventeenth century where the protomédicos stood to collect fees, they did show a kind of self-centered zeal in prosecuting phlebotomists operating illegally in Mexico City. In these cases, although nobody puts it in words, the aroma of bribery can be distinctly smelled.

If one assumes that some of the barbers throughout the viceroyalty were qualified phlebotomists willing to submit to examination, they could not do so because of the great costs of the trip to the capital and the neglect of their shops during a long absence.[42] The delegates of the protomedicato outside Mexico City, who reported this situation to their superiors, stood to gain by allowing these men to be examined in their respective districts. The protomédicos then passed the petition to the viceroy with a recommendation that phlebotomists be allowed examination in their own territories. Though they added that the fees be adjusted "in accordance with the ban of June 24, 1795," they admitted that they did not know what the increase should be.[43] The regular fee in New Spain was stiff; it had been fifty-five pesos since 1759 and in 1813 went up to seventy-five pesos,[44] though in 1791 phlebotomist Manuel San Ciprián, the utterly unrestrained lad, protested that if the protomédicos would return his hundred pesos they might have his license in return. The royal treasury recommended the application of the schedule of gracias al sacar[45] and suggested that at twenty to forty leagues from Mexico City the extra cost should be five pesos; at forty to seventy leagues, seven pesos, four reales; beyond seventy leagues, ten pesos.[46] Though the ministers of the Tribunal de Cuentas suggested moderating the fees set out by the royal treasury, Viceroy Iturrigaray issued two printed bans, one permitting examination of phlebotomists in their own territories[47] and the other putting that schedule in force.[48]

One way of escaping this close governmental supervision, especially for those "barbers" who attended the natives too poor to live inside the city but clustered in its environs, was to set up shop "beyond the walls." Run by mixed-bloods referred to as *chinos* by officials,[49] these shops so greatly increased in number that at the beginning of 1636 the viceroy, the Marquis of Cadereyta (1635–40), gave strict orders that no more than twelve of these with government licenses should be allowed to operate. Fourteen years later another viceroy reiterated this decree and reinforced it with a threat to proceed against violators as stipulated in the original document.[50]

The bloodletter who did not wish to run from the city, however, could hide himself among the stalls of the great squares. When the attorney for the second Count of Revilla Gigedo called upon the protomédicos and other prominent doctors to testify on the subject of the count's struggle to clean up the city, one of them, Bachelor Juan Bermúdez de Castro, said plainly that many unexamined phlebotomists had their shops in the Plaza del Bolador where the poor people came to be bled and have their beards cut.[51] They were thus protected both by custom and by the disorder and squalor that repelled inspectors and offered a refuge for criminals.

The unlicensed bloodletter, clandestinely practicing where there was no one else to help the people, sometimes in all modesty appealed to the royal protomedicato for a license to practice openly. His method was the same as that invoked everywhere: to prove by the testimony of those he had helped or cured that the public would suffer if he were not licensed. That he would have to prove by all this generous and unimpeachable testimony that he had established a reputation by violating the law gave nobody pause. An Indian cacique from Otumba, Juan Cárdenas de Espinosa, descended from the conqueror Antonio de Luna, brought a successful appeal before the royal protomedicato to examine and license him as a phlebotomist on the basis of his reputation[52]—all this four years after the opening of the nineteenth century. The whole countryside rushed in to support him. The subdelegate Manuel Ignacio Gómez, a strong advocate of Cárdenas de Espinosa, presented a witness, Visencio Antonio, severely gored in the scrotum by a bull. Antonio testified that after his wife had called Cárdenas de Espinosa, that "surgeon" pushed back in the testicle that was torn out and dangling, sewed up the wound, watched over the patient for a while, and soon had him completely well.[53] After establishing that the applicant was "free of all bad race,"[54] the protomedicato exempted him from the required internship, examined and licensed him, but imposed one inevitable condition upon him: that he "show charity to the poor."[55]

This case, however, was not typical. The suits and appeals in cases against "mere bleeders" who quietly slipped into the practice of surgery were "almost interminable." To relieve the governors, the protomedicato, and the audiencia, the king issued a cédula in 1799 transferring jurisdiction to ordinary magistrates provided these had the offenders at their disposition. The drastic scale of punishment is an index to the frequency and growing seriousness of the offense. For the first offense those guilty would pay a fifty-peso fine, the costs of the action, and exile to a point beyond twenty leagues. For the second, the magistrate doubled the fine and fixed the same exile, while the offender guilty a third time got a fine of five hundred pesos and ten years in prison. That the denouncer got one-third of the fine brought greed to the support of the law.[56]

If it proved both uneconomic and impossible to get phlebotomists and surgeons to come up to the capitals of viceroyalties to be examined by the royal protomedicato after their apprenticeship, what happened where there was no protomedicato and no examiner? At the beginning of the seventeenth century a man in such a place actually had to face the prospect of going all the way to Spain to be examined. Juan Pérez, for example, had lived for fifteen years in Havana and served the four years' apprenticeship required by the ordinances, but when he sought to go back to "those kingdoms" for examination and licensing, "the convents, inhabitants, and people in the presidios of this city" would not hear of it. Among them, although unlicensed, he had recorded a host of important cures and enjoyed the grateful "acceptance" of the city. He therefore petitioned the king to allow "any physician to be found in this city, together with those who should come in the fleets or galleons," to examine him as surgeon and phlebotomist and license him in case they found him "able and sufficient . . . as was done with Julius Caesar. . . ." In case the petitioner's story was found to be true, the king authorized the doctors and surgeons of the fleet guarding the Indies to examine the applicant and, if called for, to license him.[57] How little imagination is required to see that practitioners of so lowly an office as that of phlebotomist, less successful than Pérez, would never bother the king to get a license!

Naturally, in case of a medical practice so deep-seated as bloodletting, not just the civilians but the military were its victims. In 1767 at the time of the expulsion of the Jesuits from America, Juan Almeida, a licensed bloodletter from Mérida de Yucatán, made an appeal that tells something of the prestige of his art in his time. He had served in the Spanish army when it proceeded against the rebels of Quiste and become an intern (*practicante*) in the Hospital Real de San Juan de Dios de Montesclaros of Veracruz, "attending, bleeding, and doing the rest of the operations" that came up among the sick soldiers. For these reasons and because the Tribunal del Protobarberato of Madrid had passed and licensed him, he asked the king to make him phlebotomist of the Real y Militar Hospital de Nuestra Señora de Loreto in Veracruz.[58] That Almeida tacitly admits that he had no license when he went to serve as phlebotomist in the army and in the military hospital in Veracruz shows how, in instance after instance, unlicensed men who established themselves as doctors and surgeons in the army and navy, once accepted by the public, remained in America to practice in great dignity—sometimes as protomédicos—and in the rare instances when some rival challenged them refused in silent hauteur to discuss examination.

The Spaniards in America recognized that bleeding left many "crippled and invalid," but this disastrous result they attributed not to the unsoundness of the practice but to the barber's lack of expertise, which was, no doubt, also true. Of two victims called to the attention of the municipal council in Mexico City at one session in 1776, one was injured by a bleeding and the other by "some caustics." Hence, the proto-medicato could respond only with measures calling for "examined barbers" to exhibit a lattice window painted green and those only shaving and cutting hair to show a white one.[59]

Pricking a tendon or slitting a vein could be fatal. And how many persons died from infections following the use of unsterilized not to mention dirty knives and lancets! This complaint against the inexpertness of the phlebotomist continued as long as the practice of bleeding itself. In 1813, when Mariano Bermúdez tried to resign as *"regidor constitucional"* of Quito, Dr. Pedro Jiménez assisted him with a deposition[60] to show that "Presbyter" Antonio Bernal prescribed "too abundant" bleedings that, in his opinion, caused the alderman to lose his sight. Bermúdez, however, admitted that he had pneumonia and "hemorrhoidal effusions," which, after exercise, wracked his insides and gave him convulsions "in the parts most necessary." Not even an excuse such as this, in a part of the world where avoiding this particular civic duty was hard to accomplish, proved sufficient; Bermúdez had to go on in his post.[61]

The curious mixture of the yen to collect fees and the need to suppress the illicit practice of phlebotomy thus crops up in every century. Having seen eight years of armed rebellion come and go in Mexico City, the increasingly bold Dr. José Ignacio García Jove issued an order to begin an investigation of the barber, José María Orijuela. The barber claimed that, though he had no license, he had bled only one person, and that person upon the orders of the surgeon Mariano Alarcón, whose apprentice he was. When not only the surgeon but also the patient bore out this testimony, García Jove turned over the papers to Oidor Felipe Martínez de Aragón, then serving his turn as judge of the protomedicato, for sentencing. Taking a reasonable yet firm position, Martínez warned Orijuela that if he repeated the offense the full weight of the law would fall upon him; the bailiff would carry him off to jail with no more authority than "this document."[62] The phlebotomists in Peru felt the same need to submit to examination, but there is no more evidence there than in Mexico that the wars of independence, under way for eight years, had lessened the respect for the practice of bleeding.[63]

Yet the government did not suddenly ban bloodletting as a result of some even more sudden awakening of science or some disaster to a patient. Instead, that art fell into a state of decay at the end of the Galenic period, and having no justification to match the importance given to it ever since the hippopotamus suggested the practice, it did not rise again. Where it was possible to prepare for examination by apprenticeship, bloodletting declined because the phlebotomists neither made money nor respected their own profession. Like midwives, they simply drifted along, rarely submitting to any kind of official test. The lower in the scale of dignity, prestige, and remuneration a medical profession fell, the less likely was the practitioner to hold a license. To them, the examination was a mere pretext of the protomedicato to exact fees. Surgery, on the other hand, gained in importance for two reasons. (1) Since 1770 in New Spain, the government in Spain and in Mexico City had modernized and dignified the subject in the viceroyalty by creating a college of surgery and by requiring the presence of a surgeon on the examining committee. (2) The civil war that in the long run became the wars of independence, moreover, greatly increased the demand for surgeons in the field and in the cities and towns where troops were billeted.

The reign of Charles III was the best time in history for the government to put an end to bloodletting. Had it not ventured, among other steps, to set up a board to stop the rehashing of inanities in universities, to purify style by eliminating "weary pomposity" and "tired rhetoric," and put some limit upon argument as a method of learning?[64] Why could it not do the same in the case of bloodletting? The answer is that the government in Spain, not being an omniscient physician, no more had a way of being certain than it did, for example, in England. Of all professionals, doctors were the most bound to appear certain of what they were doing—both to give reassurance to their patients and, if Spanish satirists are to be believed, to maintain their lofty importance. But what difference does the doctors' refusal to admit their uncertainty make when "their perpetual contradictions make it perfectly patent to us"? The only route for the layman to take to gain some certainty, and nearly the only one chosen by doctors, was to read the "medical authors," where they might learn, for instance, whether the astrological signs were the same for both poles. For the same sickness, some said bleed; others said do not. If some illustrious medical writers, even before the time of the astute Feijóo, "not only condemned bloodletting as useless but also as harmful, did it not follow that bleeding is always damaging"? Feijóo thought that, except for some "accidents" in which bleeding appeared to help the patient, there was not even any "seeming" support for this "barbarism." But, alas, as some patients die and some live, "he who favors the remedy applied attributes recovery to the remedy if the patient lives, and death to the insuperable force of the illness if he dies. He who is against the remedy, attributes death to the remedy and recovery to the robustness of nature. . . ." What else but robustness could it mean, Feijóo implies, if the "Leopold Academy," thinking to bolster bloodletting, reported an instance of a nun who recovered from a quotidian fever after "having had about ten pounds of blood taken from her veins in the space of two months"? Even in such remarkable escapes "from the violence of the doctors" as this, the patients were often left so weak that they soon succumbed, if not to some other infirmity, to the dragging on of the old one.[65] Yet, nearly a century later, as many phlebotomists as physicians presented themselves in Mexico for examination and licensing.[66]

WHEN SOME KNIGHTED English physician wryly observed that modesty had killed more people than war, he referred, no doubt, to the Anglo-Saxon habit of indefinite postponement of acts of elimination while waiting, sometimes in vain, for absolute privacy. He must have known also that modesty, because it obstructed the development of obstetrics, took its unfathomable toll in childbirth. The obvious result of such coyness was to turn attendance upon childbirth over to women in an age when the female was nearly everywhere shut off from even such education as men might get. Since a midwife had to be either an "honorable widow" or a married woman bringing a certificate of consent from her husband, she was frequently a curandera and nearly always poor, ignorant, and superstitious. The more educated men passed obstetrics by because, when noticed at all, the subject was connected with surgery, itself spurned by university men who allowed most of its practitioners to present themselves for examination without a certificate of blood purity.

A byproduct of this outlook was that the weight of government was rarely if ever felt in obstetrics. Where the government was paternal and ever-present, this fault tells a great deal. The royal protomedicato did not very often bother, or have occasion to bother, with something so far down the professional scale as midwives. In consequence, there were no regulations for their guidance or for their punishment—this in a system where too many professions and trades had their elaborate and rigid "statutes." In the American countryside the ignorant Indian and mulatto midwives very soon did feel the hand of authority, but it was that of the Inquisition. Here, however, the charge was that the poor women crossed the boundary of science—or, rather, theology—into superstition and witchcraft.

Spanish Models

At a high point of development at the time of the conquest, Spanish institutions proved most durable in America, but midwifery in Spain had not developed in accord with the wishes of Ferdinand and Isabella. In contrast, the records of Spanish hospitals reveal the calm, institutionalized acceptance of practices that persist without change and show no improvement for a full century. Those who came to deliver the poor, unfortunate women in the beds of these institutions were themselves women. And the main point of the records is the amount paid these midwives, ranging from two to four reales, or, from a quarter to half a dollar, or piece of eight.[1] Anyone inclined to exalt humankind should remember that the services of a goat that nursed the infants in the hospital for a week was worth two reales.[2] Thus, lacking government regulation, so conventional in nearly everything else, the care of mothers and the delivery of children remained unchanged in that long period from Ferdinand and Isabella to the middle of the eighteenth century.

In 1751 Eugenio Muñoz lamented that "for more than two centuries midwives in the kingdoms of Castile have gone without examination, approval, or title," except for the hereditary custom by which the practice passed from mother to daughter. Indeed, the forward-looking Catholic Kings, Ferdinand and Isabella, following "ancient practice," required in their "fundamental ordinances" that midwives submit to examination. The protomédicos took advantage of the law to examine and "fee" unqualified persons and to levy penalties right and left upon those "unexamined." So great was their zeal, if not their greed, that they illegally examined across the "five-league" circuit surrounding Madrid. These "excesses" led Philip II in 1567 to confine the official examination to physicians, surgeons, and druggists.[3] Though the protomédicos might, upon the insistence of the applicant, issue a certificate to a midwife, they explained at the same time that they were not permitted by law to subject her to an examination.[4]

If considered normal for two centuries, the results can well be imagined, but at long last in 1750 the royal protomedicato of Madrid set afoot a motion to examine and license midwives. That tribunal told a tragic tale of heartrending happenings "at court and in other principal towns and cities in Castile. . . ." There, "strong young women with every expectation of happy and natural deliveries," "died at the last moment" on account of the incompetence and "want of conscientiousness" on the part of "the women called midwives [*parteras*]" and some men who, in order to earn a living, have taken up the "occupation of assisting in childbirth." Moreover, this "universal damage" had been caused by the long suspension of the examination of midwives by the royal protomedicato. A suspension sound in the time of Philip II, the protomedicato insisted, constituted an intolerable abuse in 1750. To the royal protomedicato it was unthinkable that these ignorant, often unscrupulous midwives—male and female—should make declarations admissible in ecclesiastical and royal courts in "cases of the greatest importance, matrimonial as well as hereditary successions, and estates entailed under terms of primogeniture." The protomedicato therefore proposed that all those delivering infants be examined by a person satisfactory to it and appointed by it.

The schedule of fees for these examinations, submitted at the request of the Council of Castile, is strong proof that abusive exaction of fees had caused their suspension over a century and a half before. Though the schedule provided for the payment of one hundred reales for examinations in Madrid, no fees might be collected for examinations outside the court jurisdiction, especially in Valencia, which had its own system. Moreover, the crown required the protomedicato to forgo fees "in needy cases," because some persons of "notorious sufficiency" had eluded examination in the capital and in some other cities for want of money. With these stipulations, the government entrusted the examinations to the protomedicato, requiring it to appoint examiners to conduct the tests beyond the established five leagues around Madrid and to formulate "prudent rules" for their conduct. Most critical of all, in some respects, was the related charge to the protomedicato to draw up instructions for the guidance of midwives.[5] An indication that the profession of midwife was to acquire dignity lies in the requirement that the applicant present a proof of blood purity, a birth certificate, testimony of "good conduct and customs," and, inevitably, a deposit of 128 pesos to cover fees and other expenses.[6]

In Valencia, where the custom of requiring midwives to take examinations had survived "from very remote times," the right to conduct the examinations in 1677 fell to the "Medical College," which retained the privilege until 1736 when the "colleges" of medicine and surgery in Valencia were incorporated with those of Castile. Thus, in 1750 the many licensed midwives in Valencia could not be reexamined unless they voluntarily appeared for that purpose. Because this royal cédula did not prescribe formal instruction for midwives, American historians, bent on saddling the Spaniards with the responsibility for the backward state of obstetrics in the New World, have assumed that the protomédicos of Spain felt no concern.

This position is false, as anyone can see who takes the trouble to read the work of Dr. Antonio Medina, prepared at the request of the Spanish protomedicato.[7] Medina felt that the towns and magistrates should see that midwives were trained. Delivering the young, he thought, was the peculiar function of women, but he made it plain that in the case of a difficult delivery "a good surgeon" was necessary. Even the surgeon-obstetrician should keep his "decorum and respectability" and enter only those cases the midwife could not cope with. To see that women were prepared for the examination, Medina directed his *Cartilla* to "women who could read and write," hoping to overcome their natural "aversion to study." Only in this way could men hope to avoid subjecting their women to the mercy of ignorant people "without skill and without practice." Since the Council of Castile required an examination on "knowledge of everything pertaining to the art" (theory) and in "the execution of methods, rules, and doctrines" (practice), those who did not pass in both theory and practical skills might not practice. It was to meet this requirement that Dr. Medina prepared his instructions—something closely resembling the little booklets issued in the twentieth century.[8]

Dr. Medina's list of qualifications for those who should become midwives is an instructive index to the standards of his day. First, the woman should be literate and young enough to spare some preliminary years for theory and practice, because if she should go into the profession when already old, she would be past the proper time to learn, with her "understanding and senses already weak" and "her bodily strength insufficient." On the other hand, very "young girls and maidens" should be barred except when they wanted to serve as apprentices to a qualified midwife or surgeon. Though the candidate should be in "robust health" and strong enough for the tasks necessary, her hand should not be horny or deformed, especially with bent fingers. There were, too, features of character as well as of body that should be sought. The midwife should be "vigilant and careful" and not so self-confident as to fail to call for expert help if needed. She should also be merciful enough to go to the aid of the poor as quickly as to that of the rich. Such a person would be "kindly, patient, cheerful, modest," and not disposed to intemperance—especially in taking wine. Last of all, she had to know how to keep faith and be silent to avoid the dishonor of giving away secrets.[9]

Medina regarded certain anatomical knowledge essential to the midwife. Thus, a "distinct knowledge" of the bones of the pelvic area and the "lower parts called genitals" were especially essential to a midwife. Her information on bones, moreover, should come not merely from books but through demonstrations staged by a master anatomist upon a skeleton. The instructions, using the question-and-answer method, gave a description of these bones: five vertebrae, the sacrum, coccyx, pelvis, and innominate bone. It is a comfort to observe that she also had to know the womb, the orifice of the uterus, mons veneris, frenulum clitoridis, vulva, clitoris, urethra, nymphas, and hymen. As elementary as were these data in obstetrics as a science, they were also critical in cases involving "doubtful virginity, rape, or impotence." In fact, exact knowledge was so critical that Medina advised the midwife to consult a "learned physician" before presenting any written legal depositions on these subjects to judges.[10] Indeed, notarized testimony on "doubtful virginity" by a woman who did not know what the hymen was might just be embarrassing.

Questions that impinged upon theology and popular belief as well as upon medicine intruded themselves initially. The first of these theological problems—at least for the midwife—was what to do in case a woman "illicitly pregnant" should ask the midwife to help with an abortion to avoid scandal and dishonor or for any other "grave cause." The antiphonal response: it is not licit to give her advice or means that could point toward an abortion. In proof, the "highest pontiffs" as well as secular judges had judged this offense a capital one. It also made no difference whether the "creature" had reached the "animate" stage, for from the first instant of conception it had had the "potentiality" of possessing a "rational soul." It therefore devolved upon the poor midwife to dissuade the unhappy but pregnant woman "in fear of God and justice" from having an abortion. Then, after learning what the fetus, the membrane, the amniotic fluid ("licor"), the umbilical cord, and the placenta were, the midwife learned the time necessary "for the fetus to enjoy a rational soul." That occurred, the *Cartilla* answered her, when the embryo became "so organized" as "to exercise its vital functions"— something that occurred sooner in some than in others. Because the contrary was "vulgarly believed," she also learned that the embryo in the uterus "neither breathes, excretes, nor weeps . . . ," why the umbilical cord was so long, and the symptoms of pregnancy. When pregnancy was indicated by these symptoms, the midwife was to counsel her patient to avoid frequent intercourse in order to prevent miscarriage, not to take unusually vigorous exercise, to take off all corset stays or anything else causing pressure or putting weight upon the belly, to keep serene, and to call the doctor in the case of anything unusual—advice that has stood up pretty well for the last two centuries.

At every turn it is apparent that the midwife did more than merely deliver babies. The royal protomedicato, for example, expected her to distinguish a true from a false conception. Dr. Medina's instructions told her that "the elevation of the womb" in a false pregnancy was "the same in all parts"; in a true pregnancy, milk appears after the third month and not at all in the false, which had "no regular movement." Besides, among other inconveniences in a normal conception, there was greater difficulty in urinating. In the same way the task of determining whether an infant in the womb was dead or alive fell to the midwife. Indications of a stillbirth were the following: the fetus "fell like a stone to the other side" when the mother leaned over; and the woman had a bad color, suffered "sicknesses," and emitted a bad smell from the mouth and from the "moisture" of the vagina. Thus, when the midwife observed these signs, her next step was to call the doctor and surgeon.[11]

Dr. Medina also expected the midwife to understand the basic elements of delivery such as the position of the parturient—"some prefer to give birth standing up"—and what to do after the child was born. In a dangerous case, however, the midwife had no legal right to give medicines—only to call the physician.[12]

Obstetrics and Midwifery

No branch of medicine suffered more between the fall of Tenochtitlán in 1521 and the fall of Mexico City in 1821 than did that of midwifery. The surgeon Antonio Serrano, in reporting to the viceroy on surgery in 1805,[13] offers plentiful proof that the more advanced medical men in Mexico knew full well that, except for the seats of the major towns, the towns of New Spain had neither good nor bad practitioners—only a "plague of curanderos, destroyers of humanity." Even in Mexico City, complained Serrano, women, without any knowledge at all of the "art of midwifery," so vital to the state, by a "desolating routine, acquired from mother, sister, or relative," do great damage to humanity that, "in these days, horrify the true protectors and lovers of humanity."

Serrano had no compunctions in putting this fault at the feet of the government. The country had no trained midwives, he said, because there was not a single chair of obstetrics in the whole kingdom. He might have added that, in his own preliminary statement, he had not mentioned midwives—male or female—as among those "received" for examination of the royal protomedicato. Outside Mexico City, not only in the countryside but also in many towns, there were no practitioners. The reason was, he asserted categorically, there were too few of these for such a vast kingdom. There were, of course, a few in the capital, both Europeans and "sons of this country," who "finding themselves mired in the greatest misery" go from one place to another when told of some populous place without a doctor. Besides, the swarm of intrusos and curanderos put them in such a bad light with their wild prognostics that they drove the true practitioners out of their professions. Still, Serrano was sanguine enough to suggest that the establishment of the surgical subdelegations, proposed in the cédula of that year, meant that the men who had been driven away by quacks could be legally commissioned by the subdelegates in the various intendencies and presidencies and attack the charlatans judicially.

There was contagion in Serrano's feeling of distress, and the viceroy of Peru was as ready as the viceroy of Mexico to grasp and endorse any straw thrown into the wind by the specialists themselves—as his strong, quick sanction of the cesarean shows. In Lima José Manuel Valdés, writing a series of articles under the pseudonym of Joseph Erasistrato Suadel, characterized the midwives of Lima as "without principles and rules" and as fit only "to take the infant" upon delivery and "cut the umbilical cord."[14] Then, in a couple of essays unmatched for classical allusion and pomposity, he gave a set of rules for pregnant women[15] that neatly balance the harm and the good they might do. He advocated fresh air, a good diet so frugally taken as to curb the appetite and keep down undue rise in weight, and the avoidance of strong, "piquant" drinks so "popular among the common people." He knew enough to warn that suppositories, injections, and emetics were "vicious and frequently mortal."

Unfortunately, he reflected the tone of eighteenth-century European books on obstetrics, most of which had been published more than a half century when Valdés gave his grandiose advice in 1791. Despite much good information, Valdés, as was natural in 1791, elaborated on the utility of bleeding pregnant women. The theory was that as the blood usually lost in the menstrual flow, no longer having a free outlet, was detained in the vessels and loaded the membranes of the uterus, the nerves became irritable, and the whole system was thrown out of order, producing vomiting, etc. For these reasons, because nine of ten miscarriages occurred in the third month, bleeding was indicated not only then but at any other time miscarriage was threatened.[16] Even after the third month, headache, sleeplessness, hard breathing, flushing, and the "full pulse" should be relieved by bleeding.[17] Valdés perhaps reflected his European education when he recommended putting the parturient on a bed or, as was conventional among the well-to-do in the colonies, upon an obstetrical chair.

Lack of Training and Schools for Midwives

Historians of obstetrics in the Spanish empire denounce colonial medicine, at least by innuendo, for the low place accorded obstetrics—as if the art was practiced by ignorant midwives solely because, so intimately related to the genitalia, it was beneath the dignity if not the notice of the pompous man of science.[18] This, however, is an appraisal by modern man using his own standards, not those of the epoch he is writing about. In the eighteenth century, for example, the view was that in normal deliveries the work could be performed by persons trained in a limited way to take care of limited contingencies. Between the midwife and the Latin doctor, therefore, the profession of obstetrics as a specialty on a par with medicine did not develop. For one thing, the surgeons opposed the examination of male candidates for the role of midwives on the ground that obstetrics was a part of surgery upon which surgeons were examined. No one ever contended that the surgeon and physician were too good ever to intervene. They appreciated the importance of hygiene but did not understand how filth operated to produce disease. A midwife with a good anesthetic sense was as likely to be correct on this point as the physician. There was, in fact, much insistence on cleanliness, because, for one thing, when the true causes of disease could not be perceived, the blame was often put upon filth and litter or their "miasmic exhalations." Spanish doctors also recognized that there were not enough men with medical degrees to see to every birth occurring in the whole kingdom.

In fact, the state of American life, more than the law, explains the lack of training for midwives. The law required the midwives to have four years with a licensed master. That obstetrics did not become a separate teaching field in the colonial university, however, does not mean that the subject was not taught in the chairs that did exist. What happened was simply that the protomedicatos throughout America had no means and perhaps no inclination to harass the poor women who were helping other women to deliver their offspring. Indeed, few of them could pay appreciable fees, anyway. The formalities of the apprenticeship were thus overlooked, and in 1813 in Mexico the outstanding surgeon Dr. Antonio Serrano testified that the protomedicato did not subject those delivering babies to any kind of examination.[19] The profession then, as in Spain, was all but hereditary, passing from mother to daughter.

In Chile Dr. José Antonio Ríos ransacked the record in 1796 for the laws that required their examination and concluded that the protomedicato in America had both the right and the obligation to conduct it,[20] especially in Chile, where mulatto women, "without God, . . . without law," and without being able to read, practiced everywhere. He felt that intelligent, literate women of Santiago de Chile would not touch the occupation "when everything persuades them that this is a low-grade, disgraceful profession. . . ." So great was their arrogance, in fact, "that one who is perhaps barely white is already the kinswoman of countesses and marchionesses." In Chile, Dr. Ríos lamented, the protomedicato came too late to improve the situation. Though these female practitioners did not have the approval of the protomedicato, they could not obtain it because they could not read the "primers" issued for their instruction. As in all of these cases of a gross deficiency in both numbers and education, Dr. Ríos came up with a sensible but, as he admitted, a hopeless plan. He proposed the selection of two able women, presumably literate and white, to be given thorough obstetrical training. These two, in turn, would establish a school to instruct all the other midwives who would then be subjected to examination by the royal protomedicato. Licenses would be issued to those who passed, and those without the proper certificate would be prosecuted. The stumbling block, as he saw it, was finding two literate and acceptable women to form a school, because he was certain they would not wish to associate with the "rustic" mulatto midwives.[21] The case closely resembles that of Lima where, at the same time, the entrance of mulattoes into surgery and medicine had all but driven the whites out.

Such schools were all but impossible. In Lima, José Manuel Valdés said bluntly in 1791, it was a pity that in a city of that size there was "not a single woman capable to teach obstetrics to those who wish to follow in her footsteps."[22] When such a woman—Paulina Benita Cadeau de Fessell—did appear and got her school under way (1826), Peruvian independence was five years old. Paz Soldán remarks that such a foundation ran nearly a century behind similar institutions in Europe.[23] This lag was not exceptional and, given the isolation of America by the frequent wars between 1739 and 1824, not particularly discreditable.

Standards of Obstetrics and Midwifery

Before the arrival of the current school of medical historians a generation ago, writers in Hispanic America wrote very much as if the foibles—even the horrors—of previous centuries in medicine were owing somehow to a backwardness altogether unnecessary. A quick check of the status of medicine in other parts of the world will reveal that this assumption is only slightly true. Though no responsible scholar will deny that, by absolute standards, the medical picture was bad—even deplorable—he will have to say at the same time that the Spanish colonials were as aware of their situation and deplored it as much as anybody else. It is the contemporary criticisms that writers have resorted to in order to establish the worst, yet it was precisely when there were few or no criticisms that the situation was at its worst. When complaints rose, hope mounted also.

The last three quarters of the eighteenth century witnessed a crescendo of jeremiads about medicine in Spain and in the empire. In Spain itself, Feijóo wrote the first of a long series of pieces aimed at the ridiculous dogmas of medicine.[24] And when Mexicans, for example, got around to deploring the terrible state of the medical professions, they wasted their first breath on the blighted—the "abandoned"—faculties of pharmacy and surgery, which theoretically included obstetrics. The medical graduate of the University of Mexico in 1772 knew as well as those of today that the obstetricians were, even in the capital, nearly always "most ignorant little old women," whose authority rested, first of all, upon their having given birth themselves. So, midwives, like medical practitioners in general, got their bad names and "perhaps the maledictions of the people" because the quacks among them edged the others aside. Dedicating his work to Viceroy Bucareli, José Ignacio Bartolache thought that "graduated" and licensed doctors did not do much to wait upon women in childbirth. To end all of this trust placed in "false doctors," he recommended proceeding with all the rigor of the laws, "so prudently made," to eradicate these adventurers. To this end, he thought Feijóo's famous essay[25] on medicine should be written on the walls of physicians' houses.

For the miseries of childbearing the women themselves were at fault, but, then, little was done to sharpen their critical faculties. These "secular ladies" gave themselves in their pregnancies and deliveries to the care of midwives, "whose handiwork had nothing to do with licenses." So, women who disliked a medicine prescribed by a learned physician would not hesitate to take "the most absurd and crazy brews, so long as this is by the order and at the hand of the midwife." Moreover, they suffered her to manipulate them to "put the creature in its place," and take a mysterious bath, with the same old woman presiding over the ceremony. To Bartolache, such an "expert" was only fit to "receive the child and change the clothes [diapers] of the parturient."[26]

By the beginning of the next century these plaints had become pitiful enough, for the men as well as the women suffered in ever-recurring tragedies. For one, Dr. José Miguel Guridi Alcócer, in the vanguard of modernization in the University of Mexico, played a role as priest and confessor of the privileged classes in Mexico City, where he observed some strange conduct, and left, albeit unwittingly, striking commentary on the pathos of obstetrics. Quirós Rodiles takes from the priest's *Memorias* a pathetic account of the delivery of "the little countess of the Presa de Jalpa." At her feet squatted the midwife and—a most unusual thing— to one side a surgeon stood on call while the priest, Guridi, waited at the door to enter and baptize the infant the moment it was born. The mother, throwing herself back in the obstetrical chair of that epoch, when the baby had been "hung" for a long time (the expression used by the priest, "suspended" [*colgado*] points to a breech birth, for it is hard to imagine how the child could be "hung" with only the head protruding) kept asking whether it was alive. When the midwife and surgeon reassured her, she plaintively asked why it did not cry. The infant was finally born dead, and before the mother could expel the aftermath, the priest, who was reading the "convulsions and movements" better than the surgeon and midwife, gave her absolution when he saw a sudden change in "her beautiful colors changing to yellow." With that, said the priest, "all of my blood went to my feet." The learned churchman blamed the surgeon and midwife because "they did not recognize gangrene introduced into the womb," but not even he suspected the hemorrhage that must have struck the tragic "little countess." This, nevertheless, was an aristocratic delivery; for most mothers in New Spain there was neither surgeon nor "chair"—this latter undoubtedly a blessing.[27]

Despite the eloquent helplessness, despite the incisive reporting of the distinguished Guridi y Alcócer, a feeling of revolt was beginning to emerge among laymen. The government could do nothing until the professionals knew what to do and made it known. In 1806 a man widowed unnecessarily, he thought, "from one morning to the next" threw himself against such fate in the columns of the *Diario de México*. On the other hand, of course, the technique of speaking through another man, whom the readers could not get at, was typical of the coy reform editors of his day. The case was that when his wife was about to deliver, he sent for the midwife who, "after some flattering words [*chiqueos*] and impertinences," finally sauntered in. Her measures applied, among them a brew "she poured in," the childbirth "went awry and the infant and the mother lost their lives together." And, supporting the suspicion that "the widower" was a mere foil for the worried editor, the *Diario* insisted that women, even those taken for learned, thought that to have a happy delivery they should submit to the ridiculous operations "that midwives do in the womb," which consisted of "pressings" and other "impertinent jigglings" to put "the infant in its place."[28]

Here was ground for philosophy. The widower reflected that because of a squeamish conception of modesty, his wife resisted his wish that a surgeon attend her. Now that he had time to reflect, he wrote, "With my whole heart I curse" my weakness and the custom so generally accepted that makes us avail ourselves of some barbarous women with no more schooling than that they themselves have given birth. If such events were an everyday occurrence in the viceregal capital, he felt the situation in the backcountry was bound to be even more tragic. The bereaved widower thought, since such cruel and unkind cuts struck at "our very happiness and lives," they should not be taken as fate. He could not understand why if there were studies, examinations, inspectors, and proctors for barbers, shoemakers, and tailors, "there were neither schools, examinations, nor precautions for so delicate . . . an art as that of helping a woman give birth."[29]

The imagination, if the historians would permit it, could be trusted to picture the horrors of launching life a century and a half ago. Yet the documents, scattered though they be, are as graphic as the most active imagination. The Mexican doctor, Juan Manuel Venegas, whom the protomedicato honored as "the protomédico of the countryside," in the case of a dead infant in the womb recommended the application of clysters, "a chicken cut open down the back," a mule's sweatpad cooked in urine, and infusions of feathergrass and leaves of senna, before giving the crowning drink of horse manure dissolved in wine to speed up the delivery.[30] And Fernández Lizardi in his *Periquilo sarniento* (México, 1816) had a most ignorant midwife "clawing" out a fetus with "talons of silver" and with other "infernal" instruments and so lacerating "the passage" that "the skill of no surgeon could stanch" the bleeding that promptly killed the mother.[31]

Cesarean Births

Just as Medina's instructions, authorized by the protomedicato of Madrid, emphasized theological problems, so too did this element take precedence in America in the second half of the eighteenth century. The great revival of interest in the cesarean operation, by then all but forgotten, sprang more from the accidental raising of a theological question than it did from the protomedicato. When in Mexico in 1772 the Franciscan José Manuel Rodríguez published a translation[32] of the Italian edition of Father Cangiamila's *Embryologia sacra*[33] he unwittingly raised a hue and cry that lasted a quarter of a century. It began when Viceroy Antonio María de Bucareli immediately issued an edict putting his full weight behind the operation. Also when an episcopal edict followed soon after, it suggested that the viceroy and Archbishop Alonso Núñez de Haro were working in close concert.[34]

What kind of arguments could have been convincing enough to get such quick action and keep the discussion alive in America for so long? Father Rodríguez, aglow with pleasure at the approval accorded his work by the proprietary professor of theology in the University of Mexico, roundly endorsed Cangiamila's theological arguments as "solid, secure, and sound." The "law, from the first age of Rome," had made it an ordinary criminal offense not to take out the fetus before burying the mother—a law not merely just but Christian. In fact, survival of these fetuses would increase the number of the faithful.

The design of the book was to overcome the scruples of priests to authorize someone to do the operation or actually to do it themselves. In the first place the rule against the practice of surgery by priests was not valid when the "soul and body" of the child was at stake. Of this error even an archbishop, "otherwise learned and zealous," could be guilty, for on one occasion when a curate implored his archbishop to let him make the incision because there was no time to get a surgeon, the archbishop forbade it, threatening him with "irregularity" and saying "that soul was lost"[35] when the "law of charity" demands that the "spiritual" be respected over the bodily. If the obligation to baptize, as many theologians insisted, required a priest to baptize a dying child in heathen country at the risk of his life, how much more logical to allow the cesarean for the same purpose?

Other taboos kept the cesarean from taking immediate hold. For one thing, was it a mortal sin for a male midwife to perform a cesarean when nobody else was available and when the mother and, naturally, the fetus would otherwise die? To sustain that it was no sin to do it—he had recourse to the example of a priest who found a woman by the roadside in such difficult childbirth that both she and the fetus were in danger of death. The priest heeded the pathetic plea of the woman and assisted her to a safe delivery, saving both mother and child. Still basing himself upon Gobat, Rodríguez concluded that the priest, especially if he were the parish priest, should do whatever he had to do. This conclusion established, the priest should keep a knife or razor handy so that the midwife, "or somebody else with the courage," could perform the operation when there was no surgeon.[36] Rather "than send the soul to limbo, he should himself make the incision. . . ."

Of course, there were bound to be many questions frightened people standing around a dying woman could not answer, and these Rodríguez sought to satisfy in advance. First of all, he insisted, the ecclesiastical authorities should compel "the expert" to perform the operation after the death of the woman without allowing the husband and relatives to interfere. That the operation had never before been performed in a country, moreover, should never be accepted as an excuse for not doing it the first time.[37] Nor should the operator take anybody's word that the fetus was dead, since it is not necessarily dead when it does not move. Thus, a person who impeded a cesarean or neglected to perform it might become a criminal. As a precaution, the priest, when about to administer the viaticum to some married woman, "will delicately inquire if she is pregnant." In the case of a single woman, perhaps trying "to conceal some carnal sin," the case was all the more urgent. Upon her confession, the priest should oblige her to entrust her case to some agency outside the confessional since the salvation of the soul of the issue took precedence over everything else. After making certain tests with cotton, wool, and candle to determine whether the parturient was breathing, the operator should introduce a tube through the mouth to let out the "vaporous gases," enough in themselves to kill the fetus. Moreover, since fetuses had been known to live twenty-three or twenty-four hours after the death of the mother without the aid of the tube, the operation should be performed regardless of the lapse of time. Then, if the operator put her hand on the head and the *arteria magna* was observed to pulsate, the fetus should be baptized.[38] At the same time, even if it should appear to be a monster, the weight of the evidence was against the supposition that the fetus was "not of the human species" and without a "rational soul" since in Genesis God commanded even the trees to reproduce their own kind. The fetus should therefore be baptized conditionally.[39] A "monster" in the eighteenth century was thus not, for example, merely a bifurcated human being but possibly the offspring of a brute fertilized by a man, or a woman fertilized by a male beast.

Moreover, according to Rodríguez, it was the duty of the parish priest to see to it that there was a person instructed in the cesarean, midwives in particular. Though a midwife intimate with a family might, more than others, be expected to help conceal a birth, Rodríguez argued at the same time that a woman with the family's confidence would "excite less horror" in the husband and relatives than a strange man and be "more decorous and suitable" for both the deceased woman and the surgeon.

Since the authorities had to assume that the person performing the cesarean operation had never seen one before, they gave minute instructions on the most obvious points. For this reason Rodríguez published a series of "corollaries," beginning with "precautions to prevent the death of the fetus." The first step was to tie off the umbilical cord four fingers from the belly of the infant and cut it off one finger beyond the string, cauterize the cut with a lighted candle, and clean the nose of any "filth" to permit breathing. Then a little liquid might be introduced into the mouth and the infant swaddled in cloth. The second corollary contained instructions on procedures in the operation such as place and type of incision, in which learned medical terms gave way to popular ones. As always, the writer remembered to sound that delicate note of modesty. It would, for instance, be "very fitting" if the two people to take up the dead woman should be women. As the last corollary, the operator got directions on how to treat the wound in the woman should she, by chance, be discovered to be alive "oppressed by some hysterical passion." Somehow it seems very Spanish that the stitches should be made in the "leather dresser's" style and that the thread should be "guitar strings."[40]

A practice so sound theologically and so quickly endorsed by the viceroy and archbishop was still not destined for immediate and universal acceptance. In fact, the next sign of the problem after the publication of the viceregal ban in 1772 was still another set of instructions for midwives lifted from Cangiamila, translated into Castilian, and published in 1775.[41] Twelve years later, when the protomedicato in Mexico did venture before the public, it was in the form of a notice from the president of the tribunal, Dr. García Jove, that washing and baptizing the "fleshy substance" in miscarriages was in error, as this pouch was merely a cover for the body, which, of course, should be baptized.[42] Thus, even the president of the royal protomedicato showed himself more concerned with baptism at childbirth than with, say, the physical problem of the cesarean. Some signs of reviving concern appeared when in 1793 Viceroy Revilla Gigedo gave the royal protomedicato orders, under threat of the direst penalties, that surgeons and midwives should go immediately to the aid of a parturient directly upon being called. Since Viceroy Bucareli in 1777 had made the same threat to physicians who did not respond when called, now, after sixteen years, the professional dignity of midwives and surgeons was recognized; they came under the same disagreeable orders as the physicians.[43]

The viceregal ban of 1772 calling for the cesarean everywhere had no direct, immediate effect, and twenty-three years elapsed before any sure evidence of the performance of the operation appeared. Then the *Gazeta de México* began to report a series of this operation in extremis. In 1795 Frigida Ruiz, five months pregnant, died in Chiautla, and a cesarean produced a live girl infant who, after baptism, lived only a short time,[44] as was to be expected. Three years later came the report of a similar incident—this time from Mission San Antonio de Oquitea, Sonora. When the Indian woman María Antonia Zapatito died after "five or six months" of pregnancy, Friar Ramón López succeeded in baptizing the unborn infant—a matter of preoccupation, as great to judge by the tenor of all reports, as was the simple requirement of keeping the infant alive. The missionary, however, did not do the operation himself; he turned it over to a midwife and a sergeant, who cut open the right side of the belly with a "barber's razor," and the midwife extracted the placenta "in the short time of two minutes" and baptized it.[45] This same pair soon performed a second operation on a certain Ignacia Martínez. The next case at faraway Mission Santa Clara in New California was even more curious. There, the operators were not pioneering medical men either, but two friars, José Viader and José Viñals, in desperate straits, yet mindful of plain civil and canonical injunctions. With no knowledge of anatomy, no books, and only "an obscure report on the manner of doing" the operation, but "eager to unite this unborn child eternally to God," these two men took the infant from an Indian girl, a neophyte, already pregnant eight months. The child, though starved on account of the spotted fever (*tabardillo*) from which its mother died, did live seven hours. To editors in Mexico City this example proved two points: that the participation of these two men did not produce the slightest outrage "to the most scrupulous propriety . . . ," and that in the future such unborn infants need not "be the victims of irresolution and fear."[46] Then, in 1800 the *Gazeta de México* reported that severe rains had collapsed some adobe houses in León, Guanajuato, "between ten and eleven at night" that "suffocated" four people, among them, María Barboza, a pregnant woman. The account does not make it clear whether she died immediately or not, but when the parish priest came, sixteen hours later, at two o'clock the next day to bury her, he ordered two "practical physicians" to perform the required operation. These two, "with the greatest dexterity," took out a live child. As had all the rest, it died soon after baptism. The reporter rejoiced that the unborn had thus escaped "eternal unhappiness."[47]

Unfortunately, Mexico remained on the brink of the old barbarism in obstetrics while at the same time it appeared to skirt modernism too. As early as August 11, 1784, Juan de Puertas, "chief surgeon of the Royal Hospital of San Carlos and surgeon of the royal navy, second class," performed an operation on the *symphesis pubis,* separating the bones of the lower anterior abdomen of Juana Gertrudis Hernández, a woman twenty-two years old, taking out "a well developed" but dead girl child of nine months. Within thirty-two days the mother was well and the incisions perfectly healed. In this way after eight years an operation developed in Paris and first performed there in 1777 reached America.[48] The absolute lack of precedent, no doubt, delayed the operation until the fetus was dead—a circumstance that did not tend to encourage drastic steps. For a long time in the future, as well as in the long past, both mother and child went on dying.

Such an issue cannot be called skirting modernism unless placed in opposition to a case that occurred under the noses of the royal protomedicato not a decade before. In 1776 María Bernadino de la Rosa, a woman of thirty-four, married sixteen years and already the mother of eight children, began to have symptoms that made her seek medical advice. When the "established doctor" arrived, he treated her as a consumptive and prescribed an enema because of "the dryness of her bowels." Then, without suspecting to that moment that their mistress was pregnant, the domestics noticed that the enema was forcing out her entrails, which they tried to push back. But lo! what they saw as a *"prolapsus"* was the foot of the first of five infants about to descend upon them. The husband, who made the discovery, forthwith called in a midwife who assisted in the delivery of the rest of the quintuplets. As was natural in an age obsessed with monsters and other extraordinary events of nature, the president of the protomedicato, Dr. José Maximiliano Rosales de Velasco, took time to inquire into the particulars and report them as "curiosities" to the viceroy. Astonishing as the story was, Dr. Rosales could not resist the urge to cap it: he knew the grandsons of two women in Seville who had given birth to seven infants at one confinement. So eager was he, however, to regale the viceroy with details that he let out, quite incidentally, that the Mexican woman was very fat indeed—the only type with any prospect of concealing a quintuple pregnancy.[49]

These frontier cesareans tell more than they seem to. Surely women in difficult labor died in Mexico City—or even Lima—as well as in Chiautla or San Antonio de Oquitea. Why, then, did the *Gazeta de México* report no operations by the surgeons of the capital? Opening up a woman from "a powerful house," even if she was dead, was no matter to be undertaken lightly, but there is no report of such an operation upon even the humblest servant girl. Could it be that an operation upon a dead woman would scare off a whole gamut of superstitious patients? It is likewise strange that surgeons from Europe, such as Dr. Antonio Serrano at the School of Surgery, who had certainly read Feijóo's "Discourse" on obstetrics, would have known that women doctors, as early as 1723, had saved not only the fetus but also the mother by performing the cesarean. If a soldier on the frontier with no training could surgically extract a live infant from a dead mother, why could not the most highly trained surgeon in Mexico City not try to save both? The answer is not clear.

Rodríguez's little book on cesarean operations led other friars here and there in the empire to undertake the preparation of a similar tract. In Guatemala the Franciscan Pedro Mariano Iturbide, after his work was sanctioned by the government in 1787, published an abridgment of this work and of Cangiamila's tract, upon which in the end they were all based.[50] Iturbide had come to the subject by the conventional but oblique route of the obligation to baptize fetuses—both those aborted and those left unborn because of the death of the mother. Domingo Juarros goes so far as to say that experience had shown the usefulness of this little treatise, because, though it hardly covered two sheets, many people with it alone "had successfully performed the cesarean operation."[51] If Juarros was right, the Guatemalans were singularly alert and bold; and, as we have already seen, the *Gazeta* in Mexico was boasting of similar feats on the frontiers of New Spain two decades later.

The tradition of publishing works in imitation of Cangiamila was continued in Peru by the friar Francisco González Laguna, who had far more than merely religious preoccupations. Laguna collaborated with the famous botanists, Hipólito Ruiz and Joseph Dombey,[52] experimenting for them in El Jardín de la Buena Muerte, becoming a member of the Amantes del País, and publishing in the *Mercurio peruano* under the pseudonym of Thimeo.[53] He was, then, not merely a friar or a monk, preoccupied with the otherworldly problem of baptizing fetuses, but a true member of the new scientific vigor now so distinctly felt throughout the Spanish empire. Laguna's work endorsing the cesarean operation in 1781[54] shows, once again, that the Spanish government in the Indies, far from thwarting scientific progress, all but enforced it. Viceroy Agustín de Jáuregui, too, was eager to endorse the new humanity and immediately published a ban requiring surgeons "in certain cases" to perform the cesarean.[55] In fact, the proclamation came with martial formality. The public crier, Joaquín Cubillas, accompanied by a picket of bugle-blowing troops, published the proclamation according to the "usage of war." Yet there was no impatience with the theological preoccupation, for the first point of the document was "the eternal felicity of infants shut up in the wombs of their mothers" and unable to receive "the holy sacrament of baptism" for want of the cesarean.

Jáuregui's justification for this firm step pulls the curtains back on the plight of obstetrics in the eighteenth century. He deplored the neglect of the "cause of unborn infants." Indirectly, he charged that the parents, relatives, and even "surgeons, barbers, and obstetricians" resisted the cesarean with the argument that the "locked-up" child was not alive and excused themselves with other "frivolous and malicious pretexts. . . ." At the same time, he lamented, such practitioners could and did administer abortives and, if they got results, they threw the fetuses away without even examining them and, of course, without "procuring them spiritual life" and without attempting to start their breathing even when this could have been accomplished. In the swollen official language of the day, this was an "offense against religion, humanity, and the state."

Such was the basis upon which the viceroy issued his order, bolstering it with particulars to perform the cesarean that was published not only in Lima but also throughout the whole viceroyalty. He accordingly notified bishops to have the priests cooperate. As soon as they got word that a pregnant woman was on the verge of death, or it was feared that she might soon be, public officials all over Peru were ordered to throw the weight of the government behind the cesarean operation, with everything in readiness, and a surgeon or barber summoned, or wanting these, "any person" able to perform the operation. Then, after "some intelligent person" had examined the mother and declared her dead, the operation proceeded. As soon as it saw the light of day, of course, the infant received baptism. The emphasis in the viceregal ban, however, was upon keeping the "creature" alive.

The presence of the civil power, though, was still required. The king's officers, in fact, had instructions to proceed, without admitting any excuse, against all those who either obstructed the operation or even those who failed to give notice in time. If the case was flagrant and plain enough, they gave due notice to the viceregal government, heard the evidence, drew up charges, and prepared the case against the offender as guilty "of a grave crime." One thousand pesos was the minimum fine for failure to prosecute.

Many chapters of Laguna's book illustrate the state of obstetrics with even more pointedness than the viceroy's unequivocal and hard-hitting proclamation. Though high in his praise for Cangiamila, Laguna gave realistic and fresh advice on difficult childbirths. On the basis of "thirty-six years' practice," he flatly denied the dictum "Vinslou and Bruhier" that "putrefaction was the only sure sign of death." On the contrary, there were three other "principal and unfailing signs" that death had occurred: (1) a "pallid, yellow, and leaden countenance," (2) stiffness and inflexibility of the muscles and inability to close the eyes without special effort, and (3) the lassitude and mistiness of the eyes when the cornea loses its transparency and the light becomes entirely "obfuscated."[56]

Laguna was specific enough to show the state of knowledge on the cesarean. Like Rodríguez, he recommended a long incision rather than a cross, as easier to repair in case the mother was not dead. Unless some swelling indicated the fetus was more to the right, the cut should be "slightly above the navel and four fingers to the side, down to the upper part of the empeyne." How primitive to Laguna was the "science" of obstetrics can be seen in his detailed advice on cutting through the peritoneum, "the white cloth-like parchment that covers the intestines." For example, the author counseled his operator not to cut the bladder, "taking it for the uterus," as "the urine will render the operation more difficult." No wonder he felt it necessary to remind "the surgeon" that pregnancies are not always in the uterus, but sometimes in the "abdomen, falopian tubes, and in the ovary." How necessary it was to be able to proceed expeditiously he illustrated with the case of a two-headed child, born in 1709, when the proper prelate waited four days before making a reply to an urgent overture. In fact, Laguna did not even say what became of the "monster." Thus, the high place given to baptism is illustrated by Laguna's devoting considerable space to "baptism by injection."[57] Since destroying a fetus soon after conception was a sin, Laguna was bound to notice that "voluntary abortions" were owing to the lack of foundling hospitals—"an insult to nature, religion, and country."

Three decades after Alfonso Josef Rodríguez published his little book in Mexico, there were only a few scattered cases of the cesarean—cases that had more relation to the saving of souls than to the saving of lives, but back in Spain complaints kept coming in. Finally, one of these got action. The government in Madrid decided to "require" the performance of the cesarean operation "in the dominions of the Indies and Philippine Islands." First, however, the king called upon the College of Surgery of San Carlos to draw up instructions for the operation, which had to presuppose the possibility of an operation where there was no person trained or licensed to do anything surgical. A committee of professors (*junta de catedráticos*) submitted its draft, the protocirujano approved it,[58] and the Council of the Indies sent the document with a covering cédula to the Indies.[59]

The procedures were much the same as those set up by Viceroy Bucareli in 1772. These required the attendant to report an apparent death immediately to the parish priest, who was then to summon the surgeon, should there be one to summon. Because there had always been a great resistance to medical calls at night in the towns of the Spanish empire, the cédula specifically stated that the priest and surgeon should "go at once, day or night, to the house of the deceased." After making sure that the woman was dead and in the absence of a surgeon, the priest simply named the person who, in his judgment, was best qualified to carry out the operation according to the "Instruction" supplied by the crown. Moreover, he might not consent to the burial of such a pregnant woman "regardless of what class she might be from" and regardless of how long she had been dead before the operation. Should the family insist upon immediate interment, he might call in the civil authorities to enforce the regulations.

In the actual performance of the operation, the instructions[60] were adapted to the circumstances of the countryside. After applying hydroxide (*alcali volatili*) to the mouth, nose, and eyes, the operator stuck a pin under the fingernail to make sure the woman was dead. He then examined the mother, cut through the abdominal wall between the pyramidal muscles, and opened the pouch around the "creature" with "care." Presupposing an amateur operation, the instructions were specific when the woman was in the latter months of pregnancy and the womb in the middle of the belly, "rising nearly to the breast." What the "surgeon" would need would be a convex cutting scalpel and "another ending in a button." Failing these, as was bound to be the case, a razor or a penknife would "be the only instruments needed." Placing the body on a bed or some other place a little to the side "without uncovering more than necessary," the operator would "compress the abdomen moderately," make a light marking cut a little less than six inches in length, and proceed through the skin, by the muscles, and into the peritoneum. In order to avoid cutting or damaging the bowels, intestines, or stomach, however, the operator should start with a slight opening—about two inches—and, introducing two fingers, should raise the wall and enlarge the opening by using a scalpel with a button or razor.

The incision, of course, would need to be on the side of the abdomen raised the most where "the infant presents itself," and it should be "transversal two fingers from the edge of the lowest ribs and four fingers from the front toward the spine." After this step, the same thing followed in the womb, "which is a great pouch like flesh. . . ." Then, following the opening of the membrane, which, "like a cloth also in the form of a pouch," immediately enclosed the creature in the womb. Meanwhile, the operators should absorb the blood with a fine sponge of cloth. If, at this point, the infant showed no signs of life, the operator might not remove it "before it was baptized conditionally." If, however, it was alive and robust, it should "be taken out by the feet, which takes less effort," and be immediately "baptized by sprinkling water on the head." Once the enveloping membrane was out, the operators should tie the cord two fingers from the navel and cut it off two fingers more above the ligature. The next step was to take out the placenta, "and if this should have adhered, it should be unfolded with great care, and lightly detached with the fingers, the nails cut, or better, with the side of the hand." Since sewing back the opening was "repugnant," a towel, moderately adjusted, from back to front, would have to suffice.

The notes to this piece are instructive in many ways because one has to return to the eternal question of baptism. Thus, in the case of a bad delivery, the placenta should be most carefully opened and when the creature appears, "even though it should be but a grain of barley, if it moves at all, it will be baptized; and if it does not, this will also be done conditionally." The surgeons at the San Carlos College of Surgery also thought of other complications such as "a hernia or a rupture, and a very low uterus, or the placenta over the point of the incision." Since such contingencies required a surgeon, they very appropriately regretted that all such brief instructions, prepared to be understood by those who had no professional knowledge, would "like these, always be defective."

Innovation in Childbirth Techniques: Dr. Narciso Esparragosa

The campaign to perform the cesarean upon a pregnant mother unable to give birth as soon as she died so that the saving water of baptism could reach the fetus before it too died had one unforeseen but saving grace: all those writing pamphlets to advocate and explain the cesarean took the occasion to comment upon the horrors of childbirth in America—plain indication that the best informed in the empire fully understood how backward was obstetrics. In Guatemala the energetic and highly original Dr. Narciso Esparragosa,[61] horrified at the havoc wrought by "mangling iron forceps," began work in a most peculiar way on an "elastic forceps [*asa elástica*]" for taking infants sealed up ("nailed up" was the graphic untranslatable Spanish expression) in their mothers' wombs.

Cloth fillets, to which the harried doctor had had resort from ancient times, became useless and unmanageable from moisture. Esparragosa therefore devised an elastic "loop" that he personally wove of whale bristles, something soft that would still resist moisture. This loop he proposed to insert under the chin with a cross band over the brow. Raising the hips of the parturient to allow the fetus to recede momentarily, he inserted the loop under the chin and the cross band over the brow. This done, he applied traction in rhythm with the woman's natural labor pains by pulling the rings at the two ends of the loop with his right hand while at the same time he flexed the head of the fetus with the other. In this way "the infant was delivered without decapitation, without lacerating or crushing the skull, and, supposedly, without tearing the neck muscles in the case of a breech delivery, and without 'offense' to the mother."[62]

In botanical research, paleontology, or anything that required gathering and classifying, the Spanish government in the eighteenth century was alert and competent, but it had so little experience with pure experimentation, unless it was with mining, that it rarely promoted a scientific experiment until some individual came along begging the government for help. Then it was willing enough to recognize and, when it could, reward the merits so acquired. For his innovation in Guatemala, Esparragosa gave the facts of his obstetrical loop to the *Gazeta de Guatemala,* which, in keeping with its innovative and "useful-knowledge" slant, called attention to the illustrative plate about to appear in print.[63] Moreover, in a most disinterested and totally scientific spirit, he strove to put his invention to the critical test and all but begged doctors and "practitioners" in Guatemala to call him at any time day or night when they had an obstetrical case threatening mother and infant. In the same spirit of largesse, in the year 1798 he published a pamphlet at his own expense describing the device and giving instructions for its use.[64] In its own way, after the fact, the Spanish government recognized this contrivance as a "service" of Dr. Esparragosa, one of those enviable accumulations upon which the Spanish government based its honors and preferments. Thus, the captain general of the Kingdom of Guatemala advised his government that "conceding" the "uniform of a physician of

320 THE ROYAL PROTOMEDICATO

the King's Bedchamber" to Esparragosa would do much to relieve the low esteem in which the public held "surgery," of which obstetrics was then considered a part. At the same time it would stimulate "studious youth" to follow his example, especially if he were allowed to wear this uniform to cloister meetings of the university in place of the conventional "heel-length" dress. The king not only conceded him this right, but after imposing consultation with the College of San Carlos, the new surgical college in Madrid, ordered the cloister of the University of San Carlos not to hinder the honored man from wearing his suit of honor in the cloister meetings,[65] which brought together all the professors and holders of higher degrees in the city and five leagues round about. Nevertheless, back in Madrid, the faculty of the College of San Carlos meeting in weekly session to discuss, approve, or disapprove scientific papers and innovations, quietly decided that Esparragosa's whale-bristle forceps were not "useful."[66] Yet the little pamphlet carried enough professional weight to lead to its republication in Barcelona eighteen years later, bolstered this time by the promise to publish some of the many testimonials from doctors to the "excellence" of the little tract.

Dr. Esparragosa also gave a series of five lectures, "not counting," as Mariano Padilla says, "a work on obstetrics,"[67] something that does not appear along with the manuscript lectures in the National Library of Guatemala. From all of this, one must deduce that he even had resort to education in his efforts to relieve a state of obstetrics already recognized by the professionals as deplorable.

Superstition and Obstetrics

In obstetrics, developments took place that, in retrospect, seem extravagant. There is, though, little difficulty in accounting for them. Obstetrics was in the hands of women who could not read and write, and the superstitious rites they were bound to introduce were condoned by the women of the most aristocratic families. In fact, it would be hard, if not impossible, to find a mulatto midwife who did not resort to some kind of magic. Since the civil authorities took no note of what was going on, it is only when these women "assumed the power of God," or ran into black magic by "making a pact with the devil," that the Inquisition assumed jurisdiction, and, here and there, preserved their records for posterity. It was more or less a matter of chance when such a sorceress was dubbed a midwife, for these people, who issued their own license to practice, were free-ranging indeed.

One poor woman has enjoyed a celebrity beyond others of her kind for no other reason, it seems, than because the index of the archives of the Inquisition in Mexico lists her file (1648) as that of "midwife." This woman, Ana de Vega of Puebla, who included obstetrics in the range of her general practice, only did what others did—in thousands of recorded instances. Her battery of fraudulent tricks was very normal, though, likely enough, she believed in some of them herself. She used redwood, flatulency—windiness—and against "hexing" and love potions she resorted to the head of a scorpion. To bring up the phlegm, she tried wild cinnamon (*bolitas*), an Indian remedy. Since horsehair was always to be found near or on the person of a sorceress, Ana de Vega made haste to explain that her collection of the hair was for her husband "to make halters for beasts." Though she had driven three devils—one with a big tail and two with little ones—from a woman with oil of coconut and Indian palm, she "did not know the devil or have any pact with him." How little the judges believed her may be deduced from the sentence. With a symbolic rope around her neck, a green candle in her hand, and mock crown with writing on it upon her head, "with the insignia of witchcraft, in conjuration of Levi," she was ready for the rest of her sentence: 200 lashes and perpetual banishment from Puebla.[68]

In obstetrics, except for that vague thing called "pact with the demon," white magic differed little from the black. Juan Bautista Chirino, a native of Mexico, stated in 1752 that in the case of a difficult labor, in order to produce immediate birth, one had only to enter the room with a turkey heart. At the exact moment of delivery, however, it was necessary to withdraw—turkey heart and all—otherwise the woman would go on with the delivery until she had delivered her entrails also.[69] There is, though, something exceptional in this case; the denunciation was made by an educated man.

In the main, denunciations were first made by rivals of no more elevated culture than the witch herself and passed on to the curate or friar, who sometimes passed them on to the Inquisition. This step, however, was no light one, for the Inquisition required that denunciations not spring from malice and that all charges be legally established, something that most of the clerics involved were not up to. Technically, too, the Inquisition did not have cognizance in cases involving the offenses of Indians. True, most of these charges sent up to the tribunal in Mexico City were against whites, mulattoes, and mestizos, but in the mass of trifling cases nobody was particularly interested in who had jurisdiction.

Secret Births

The shame that attached to legitimate birth was stretched to tragic length when the mother was single or, occasionally, when the husband had been away for appreciably more than nine months. Perhaps for this reason sympathetic concern for the problems of maternity came last among the many charitable undertakings of the Spaniards in America. Hospitals for Indians and orphanages for half-breed children appeared before the conquest was over, yet it was not until 1806 that a maternity house was founded for women who, if they could not give birth in secrecy, were forced to the brink of infanticide.[70] Thus, Viceroy José Iturrigaray, who was to see the war of independence break around him, authorized the taking of a small part of the endowment left by "the Indian philanthropist," Captain Fernando Zúñiga, for a "Department of Concealed and Secret Deliveries."

One Mexican medical historian uses the preamble of the *Ordinances* of Zúñiga's institute to describe the circumstances of founding. Even those sympathetic with their dilemma thought primarily "of the fear, shame, or desperation which possesses unchaste and weak-of-will women after they have stained their reputation, the honor of their marriages, or the distinguished class of their families compels them to bury themselves in oblivion or embrace the most cruel, bloody, and horrible measures against themselves and against the fruit of their own wombs. . . . Thus, the unfortunate women who should have been the surest protection of their children by the use of the powerful abortives, gave birth in the most secret of places, attended by vile persons who published their infamy everywhere. . . ." Religion, nature, and public piety cried out together to "protest against such execrable evils." Dr. Quirós Rodiles deduces from this preamble that the morality of the "privileged classes," for whom this house of "concealed" births was founded, was not "enviable." When the parturient arrived, the "surgeon" covered her face so that no one could recognize her. The midwife, called at the very last moment, took an "oath of secrecy," as did the parturient's confidant, and a chaplain who was called in case of danger. Even in the moment of birth, the suffering woman, if she wished, kept her face covered. In case the surgeon found it necessary to prescribe medicine, only the confidant could uncover the face to administer the medicine. (Physicians and surgeons "intervening" at such moments were also under oath to divulge nothing.) Unless the mother wished to take the infant or send it to some place of her choosing, it went automatically to the orphanage (Casa de Expósitos). Even death itself was not enough to uncover the identity of the parturient. The chaplain, posted close by, entered at the last moment to administer the last rites and the nurse notified a deputy to arrange a burial by the Junta de Caridad. The burial went forward at night in the greatest secrecy, the face still covered to hide it from the pallbearers. When the deputy made the last record and listed the effects of the deceased, he used no name. Even the historian is denied the sight of her face—the sure test of secrecy.[71]

Attempts at Reform and Change

The response to all these lamentations on the state of obstetrics, untrained midwives, secret births, and prevailing superstition was slow. As late as 1793, when the professors of the University of Mexico were pressing for an increase in the funds for raising the salaries of their chairs, the need for reform in the regulation of midwifery came up repeatedly. When called upon to render a report, the royal protomedicato volunteered that "it is certain that among the rudest artisans there is no idiocy like that of our midwives."[72] The surgeon and "master of anatomy" Miguel Moreno y Peña remarked that the "swollen crowd of women who have introduced themselves into this city" practice at the expense of the lives of both the mothers and the fetuses. When the municipality authorized him to examine midwives, he responded by asking for the endorsement of the royal protomedicato, which had jurisdiction in the examination of midwives. In addition, he made it clear that examination was futile unless only those examined and licensed were allowed to practice.[73] The protomedicato, as he no doubt foresaw, summarily rejected the request of this "suppliant."[74] The city attorney, on the other hand, was so impressed with the need for improving the quality and regulation of midwifery that he proposed—"when this war is over"—opening and financing the school of obstetrics that the city "has considered so many times."[75] The attorney general also proposed that means should be found to finance the school proposed by the syndic.[76] This solution—and on this note the file abruptly ends—was little better than a veto, though the agitation did have the virtue of putting new stress upon obstetrics in the chairs of surgery in the city.[77]

In America, chronic financial stringency had prevented any effective response to this plainly recognized need until the colonial period was over. While Antonio Medina was preparing his instructions for midwives in mid-eighteenth-century Spain, the king ordered the protomedicato to put the licenses of midwives, as well as those of physicians and surgeons, on first-class stamped paper.[78] However, practically nothing has survived to indicate that the regulation of midwifery in America under the Spaniards ever reached the point of effective licensing. The scattered records of the royal protomedicato in Mexico—the most complete of any in America—while revealing annual examination and licensing in branches of medicine as low as that of phlebotomy, turn up only two cases of licensing midwives: in 1816, Angela María Leite petitioning from Puebla to be examined in her own city by an agent of the protomedicato,[79] and in 1818, María Francisca Ignacia Sánchez undergoing examination by delegation in the same city.[80] That same year these two women were listed among those getting their titles in the medical professions.[81] There is no indication that any other midwife in Mexico or any other city received a license.[82] Indeed, in 1830, nine years after independence, there were only two recognized midwives in the whole Federal District of Mexico.[83]

D ESCRIPTIONS OF THE practice of medicine leave the contemporary observer with a distorted view of Spanish colonial medical
education. The fault could lie with the observer, however, because one should not judge medicine of the sixteenth and seventeenth
centuries by the standards of the twentieth. But if such judgments are
made, an observer might also ask whether the English, either in London
or in America, had a system of medical education for their colonies any
more adequate than that of the Spaniards. In fact, by European cultural
and institutional standards, one might say that the Spanish more closely
approximated European models than did the English. They at least had
their model universities and their system of medical chairs at hand.

Chairs of Medicine in Spanish American Universities

After 1617 Spanish universities approved for conferring medical degrees
had to have at least three chairs of medicine. Thus, since getting even one
chair of medicine in an American university was difficult, only here and
there did American institutions fully qualify under Spanish law to train
and graduate bachelors, licentiates, and doctors of medicine. The custom,
however, sometimes with the support of a royal cédula, was flexible
enough to allow the graduation of candidates prepared by only a single
chair.[1]

The pace of establishing new chairs in the Indies was exceedingly
slow. The University of Mexico, the first major university in the Spanish
empire, took twenty-seven years to secure its first chair of medicine, forty-
eight to secure the second, and seventy to gain the legal minimum quota
of three. The stumbling block, as in the case of nearly every forward
step in the history of the Royal and Pontifical University, was viceregal
finance. In 1575, when the rector consulted the full cloister, that body
could think of no way to pay for a chair of medicine except by suppressing the chair of rhetoric and using the salary thus saved to pay a professor of medicine. In a city all but destitute of doctors, the only notable

demurrer, as a cynic might observe, came from the professor of rhetoric himself; he thought something more suitable and important should first be provided for Master Diego de Frías, the holder of the chair.[2] Two years later the university made its request.

This chair of medicine, however, came into being by action of the royal audiencia, not the viceroy. Upon the urgent petition of the rector of the university in 1578, the Audiencia of Mexico ruled that the chair be created with a salary of 150 pesos oro de minas to be paid exactly as were the other professorial salaries. The university then posted the oposición, the traditional trial-lecture competition for the chair, but as only one contestant appeared for this ordeal, it could not be staged. After some uncertainty, Dr. Juan de la Fuente, the solitary opositor, took formal possession of the chair on June 21, 1578. In 1582 at the end of the four-year tenure of this winner of the temporal chair, on the grounds that he was well deserving (bienmérito), the rector and cloister appointed de la Fuente for a second term without holding an oposición, in curious violation of Spanish university law. Three months later, however, they made the chair proprietary. If they had reversed the order, making the chair proprietary and then appointing a professor without an oposición, the full shock of what they had done could have provoked sharp dissatisfaction. Their strategy was well planned, for Dr. de la Fuente was held in such high esteem that he was appointed medical inspector protomédico of Mexico City at least eleven times between 1563 and 1591.[3] In this way the university and the city council, long before the royal cédula of 1646 required it, had instituted the practice of appointing the holder of the chair of medicine as the protomédico of the city.

At the very end of the sixteenth century the University of Mexico was at last able to establish a second chair of vespers (vísperas) of medicine because the king had just released three thousand pesos annually to the university from the revenue of the convoy tax (avería) and duty imposed at Veracruz. Among the chairs erected as a result of this rare largess was a "temporal" chair of vespers of medicine carrying an annual salary of three hundred pesos. After the oposición was gazetted in 1598, four men, each on a separate day, discoursed in Latin upon an aphorism of Hippocrates while the sand trickled down in the hourglass. Dr. Juan de Placencia, in competition with such celebrated figures as Dr. Juan de Cárdenas,[4] won by a plurality of one vote among the forty cast by members of the full cloister, who then served as judges, and took possession on January 7, 1599.

The application to New Spain of the cédula of 1617 requiring a faculty of three members in medicine to certify doctors resulted in the creation of the third chair of medicine in the University of Mexico. In

1620 the fiscal of the protomedicato, Dr. Francisco de Urieta, asked for this document and formally requested that the University of Mexico follow its stipulations. The result was that in 1620 a "third pragmatic" came into force in Mexico. As a result, at the beginning of 1621 Dr. Cristóbal Hidalgo Vendábal offered to teach the chair of medicine free of charge at a fixed hour, solely in order to help the university provide able physicians to be a credit to it. The rector accepted, and the viceroy of New Spain confirmed the appointment.

A chair of surgery and anatomy was virtually forced upon the University of Mexico. Put in force by the royal protomedicato and the university in 1620, the pragmatic of 1617 stipulated that no bachelor might graduate in medicine except in one of the three approved universities in the Peninsula, or, at least, in a university having no fewer than three chairs of medicine—prima, vísperas, and surgery and anatomy. In the fall of 1621, after suggesting that all degrees conferred in the University of Mexico that had no chair of surgery and anatomy would now be null and void, Dr. Rodrigo Muñoz offered to serve in the chair without salary or stipend of any kind. When the rector requested Dr. Muñoz to produce his certificates of examination, approval, and degrees, he retorted indignantly that a man graduated from the University of Mexico in medicine had no need to present such documents. To any man accustomed to evasions in matters of nonexistent medical diplomas, this is only the legal way of saying that he possessed no such papers. His justification was that he had studied surgery and medicine in the course of his medical education, that he held the degrees of bachelor and licentiate, and that he had served the chair of prima of medicine to the great profit and advantage of his students. His greatest claim to legitimacy, he asserted, was his person and skill—something not recognized in surgeons, who in dangerous cases were required by law to attend their patients in company with a physician. When the protomédico, Dr. Jerónimo de Herrera, and the professors of medicine in the University of Mexico refused to answer Dr. Muñoz's complaint, he demanded that they be held in contempt and that their claims be dropped by default. Dr. Cristóbal Hidalgo Vendábal, the professor of method *medendi,* did respond, but when he did so it was to offer to teach surgery and anatomy in his chair free of charge, thus fulfilling the requirement of the pragmatic of 1617 that the third chair deal with these subjects. Either because he suspected Muñoz's credentials or because he disliked his aggressive personality, the rector of the university accepted Dr. Vendábal's offer and ordered him to teach surgery in the chair of method.

The appearance of medical chairs in the University of San Marcos de Lima was no less instructive than in the University of Mexico. In fact, it was not until 1634, eighty-three years after a major university was authorized in Peru and some fifty-eight years after it began to function, that any medical chairs at all appeared, whereas the prima chairs in all other major faculties came into being with the university itself in 1576.[5] In the same way, all these chairs—theology, law, and sacred canons—carried annual salaries of slightly over 1,300 pesos except theology, which paid 1,390 pesos, 6 reales. The professor of prima of medicine, in contrast, got only 600 pesos, paid from the income produced by the monopoly on corrosive sublimate (mercuric chloride). After 1687, when the income from the mercury monopoly ended, the salary went up to 780 pesos, 2 reales, of which 300 was paid by the university with the rest from the income of vacant bishoprics. There was also a corresponding discrepancy between the salaries of vísperas and those of other major faculties.[6] The third chair of medicine, founded in 1690 at San Marcos, enjoyed neither endowment nor salary, while the professor of anatomy, finally endorsed in 1711, had a salary of 312 pesos, 4 reales drawn from the doubtful and variable fees and fines of the royal protomedicato.[7]

In reality, according to the pragmatic of 1617, about one in eight of the colonial universities ever qualified during the colonial period to give medical degrees. Mexico and San Marcos de Lima eventually met the standards, and the constitutions of the University of Havana, endorsed by the king in 1634, also provided for a medical faculty of prima, vísperas, and surgery. Universities in Guatemala, Quito, Caracas,[8] Bogotá,[9] Santiago de Chile, and Guadalajara had chairs of medicine, but these, with two or three exceptions, came at the very end of the eighteenth century and hardly had time to organize before the wars of independence were upon them. Besides, these universities had only a single chair, not the three required by the Spanish reforms of 1588, 1593, and 1617. In a situation so distressing with so few licensed doctors practicing, however, the king and everybody else could hardly blink at the conferring of a medical degree upon any candidate responsibly presented by anybody. But, after all, if a standard any more severe than this were applied to the English mainland colonies, hardly a school would have qualified before the American Revolution. Thus, the Council of the Indies endorsed seventeen medical chairs in America, eleven of them concentrated in three universities.

Though three chairs were the standard requirement for medical degrees, petitioners, sometimes in a mood nearing despair, continued to beg for even a single one. In 1682 the generous rector of the University of Mexico, for example, transmitted to the crown an urgent call for a chair of law and another of medicine in the College of Santo Tomás in the Philippines, where they were already teaching "the rudiments of

Latin and the faculties of philosophy and theology." If not granted, the islands would be all but stripped of their rights for want of lawyers and without relief from disease and epidemics for lack of doctors. Coming to the University of Mexico was too forbidding for Philippine students, because besides the prohibitive cost the voyage took at least seven months. Spaniards in the Philippines wanted exactly the same "preeminences and privileges" as other universities, with the right to confer both bachelor's and higher degrees and with suitable income for these two chairs. After all, had not the king established these chairs in Guatemala to the "considerable" benefit of that kingdom?

The best the king could do in this instance, however, was highly tentative. First he asked the viceroy to take into account the impending report of the Audiencia of Manila on the method the islands proposed for financing the chairs. If then, after a thorough discussion with the Audiencia of Mexico the viceroy still favored the proposition, he might proceed to set up these two chairs in the form proposed by the rector of the University of Mexico.[10] It was a forlorn prospect; even the government of the Philippines required an annual subvention from the viceroyalty of Mexico that had already gone on for seventy-six years and was destined to go on for 122 more.[11]

Both the foundation and the operation of chairs of medicine in the remoter regions of the empire were seriously handicapped by the trifling and sometimes nonexistent salaries. The establishment of a chair of medicine in the College of San Fernando in Quito in the early 1690s,[12] fortunately, rested squarely upon an endowment of 6,000 pesos, which yielded a salary of 300 pesos, an arrangement endorsed by the king in 1693.[13] But since such funds were often put at *censo*—deposited in trust with the crown on condition that it pay a fixed annual interest—these small endowments fell heir to the vicissitudes of a poor government almost constantly at war. Though this was infinitely better than leaving these endowments for private misinvestment,[14] the interest rates were subject to change—and sometimes downward—at the whim of the government.

Private arrangements for the financing of medical chairs could also slip. Because of the distances as well as the difficulties and dangers of travel both over land and along the coast to the universities of Guatemala and Mexico, a chair of medicine in the city of León de Nicaragua was vital, for the city was without even a bachelor of medicine. In the early nineteenth century in recognition of this dire need, the bishop of Nicaragua, Josef de la Huerta Casó, personally financed chairs from the income of his miter in the seminary in various subjects, including surgery and medicine. When he died, however, these chairs ceased. The Audiencia of

Guatemala and the Cortes of Cádiz could only hope that the new bishop would follow the example of the old.[15] Here, then, was an institution with an income of only 1,500 pesos aspiring to become a university in a place where one was sorely needed.

Even the chairs founded in the eighteenth century suffered and sometimes floundered because they carried no salaries. Dr. Lorenzo Campins y Ballester, the founder of medical education in Venezuela, actually assumed the chair of medicine in 1763[16] with the promise to teach faithfully in it for six years free of charge. At the expiration, whoever then held the chair might draw one hundred pesos a year from money invested at censo.[17]

In Havana none of the chairs at the University of San Jerónimo carried income when that institution was launched in 1733. The statutes of the institution provided only that the holder of a chair, who should duly qualify after serving for six years, might be given a doctor's degree absolutely without fees.[18] The sponsors of such an institution hoped that regular financing could be provided after this lapse of time. Yet more than thirty years after the founding of the University of Havana, doctors in major faculties were so busy with their government posts or with their lucrative practices that only the youngest and least prepared of all the possible candidates could afford to take the professorships. Aside from getting a doctor's hood, they might pick up occasional fees from those graduating with advanced degrees, but this was of little help, for sometimes years passed without a candidate, and then when he did appear, what he paid in fees had to be prorated among a multitude of eager doctors.

The selection of professors by the trial-lecture system, which was extraordinarily persistent, often resulted in bitter controversy and sometimes in riots. Because doctors of medicine were scarce and because they were all from the same university faculty during what Mexican medical historians used to call "the metaphysical period," contention was rarer among them than among the doctors of theology, who tended to split into schools. The cloister of the University of San Marcos de Lima, in fact, at one stage in 1631 thought fit to fill vacancies in theology without any competition in order to avoid "great riots"[19] that experience had taught them to expect. In Mexico, though the prestige of holding a medical chair was considerable, the transition from one professor to the next went smoothly by the eighteenth century.[20]

But there was one element in the filling of chairs that seriously weakened the effectiveness of colonial university education. Temporal chairs, in which the holder had to enter into competition with his rivals every four years to keep his chair, carried both less salary and less prestige. The proprietary professor, who held his chair for life, by a practice called *jubilación* could step aside after twenty years and have a substitute take over his teaching duties,[21] while the proprietor continued to enjoy all but a fraction of his salary. What is more, since there was no sliding scale up to the proprietary chair—the best in the system—a young man graduating as a doctor of medicine at age twenty-one could immediately contend for any chair falling vacant. If he won a proprietary chair at age twenty-five, he might retire at forty-five and therefore draw his salary for forty years more. For replacement of these early retirees, the salary of the substitute was insignificant and the prestige increasingly thin—as was likely to be the instruction. Only two or three universities, however, were old enough and sufficiently staffed for this handicap to come into play. The rest, in the main, were creations of the eighteenth century, in which the founder of medical instruction held on out of sheer zeal, sometimes to the very eve of independence. But during this epoch medical students were exceedingly scarce both because of the disdain felt in the best families for medicine as a profession and because of the refusal to let castes into the universities. In the less important audiencias, such as the Presidency of Quito, higher studies in medicine hardly took hold at all. As late as 1800 medical instruction had to be terminated in that capital for the good reason that no students appeared to be taught. With the realization that the curanderos were carrying the day and reenforced by the demise of the chair of medicine, Dr. Bernardo Delgado, no doubt by virtue of his being professor in the chair without students, became the first royal protomédico in the presidency in 1800.[22] Thus, it is doubtful whether even a handful of medical degrees were conferred in Quito during the 110 years between 1690 and 1800.

Requirements and Degrees

The medical degree and the legal requirements for the practice of medicine remained stable from the sixteenth to the nineteenth century. During all that time any man with a bachelor's degree in medicine from a university approved by the royal government might then begin practice. To reach this stage, however, he had to spend eight years in a university—four earning the bachelor's degree in arts and four in the study of medicine. Then, with a certificate from an established physician that he had interned two years with him,[23] the candidate might present himself to the royal protomedicato for examination. If he passed, he received both his bachelor's degree and his license to practice.[24] Since his bachelor's degree in arts consumed what, in current American terms, would be the high school years, he entered professional school at approximately the time the modern student enters college. Thus, he could get his professional degree at the age the modern student graduates from a college of arts and sciences and be fully qualified to practice.

Two more medical degrees—the licentiate and the doctorate—were possible. Of these only the licentiate involved the additional work that might indicate greater learning, but even this degree did not involve any more classes or laboratory work—only the reading and the memory required to perform the "acts" and stand the examinations, some such as the funeral night (*noche fúnebre*) by tradition both long and savage. The doctor's degree, however, though it involved some light performances, was like a modern honorary degree, conferred merely to collect money—this time in the form of entertainment and fees—and sometimes was conferred upon a candidate only a few days after the licentiate.[25] Thus, a *doctor* of medicine always held three degrees, any one of which was sufficient academic qualification to practice.

Normally, medical students pursued a course of study prescribed in the constitutions of the university and confirmed by edict of the king. For the most part, teachers drew their materials for medical instruction and learning from Hippocrates, Galen, and at the very most Avicenna. In Mexico, nevertheless, after Palafox's reforms of 1642, the selection of medical books by the rector and a committee of professors[26] made it possible to adapt instruction to new and even the latest doctrines and discoveries. The points selected for the examination, while they long came from Hippocrates,[27] could be used like a musical theme around which to play variations from the latest authorities.

But this was not always the case. In 1803 Dr. Felipe Tamariz in Caracas complained that Dr. Lorenzo Campins, who founded the single chair of medicine in the late eighteenth century, during his entire professorship had his students write out, recite from memory, and explain three paragraphs from a manuscript that had neither author nor title— an exercise that took the entire hour. His successor, Dr. Francisco Medina, then adopted this method without the slightest variation. Tamariz observed charitably that this system enabled the student at most to get some idea of "this or that disease," but did not enable him to acquire any idea of the fundamentals of medicine or profit by the experiments being made every day in an experimental faculty. Accordingly, he preened himself because he resorted to the *Medicina práctica* of Dr. William Cullen, which he implemented by a course in surgery. Cullen's work, he noted, was peculiarly adapted to the Caracas climate, despite the fact it had been adopted widely as a text throughout Europe. With this innovation his students had at least some chance to understand a whole range of diseases, not just those that happened to be embraced in some anonymous copy-book.[28]

Actually toward the end of the eighteenth century, it made little difference how or what students were taught because so few matriculated in medical facilities. In the decade before the general outbreak of the wars of independence in 1810, a medical career remained so unattractive and the opportunities to pursue it with dignity so few that only a tiny number of students elected it. In Bogotá only fourteen students, with a few auditors, chose to enter the first class of medicine opened in 1802, the first since 1774. Only ten of these reached the third year, and as the course required eight years for one man and his assistant to finish, the students who finished their prerequisites in 1803 had to wait out the eight years to start a new course. Thus, the years a man had to spend getting a medical education had to be counted in multiples of eight—a forbidding prospect.[29] In Caracas at almost exactly the same time Dr. Felipe Tamariz reported that he had fifteen students, but these did not register at any set date. They simply dropped in at any time of the year they chose—a telling index to the informality of medical education in 1803, the best time for medicine in the history of the audiencia.[30] That Hipólito Unánue had only fourteen students when he opened his modern College of Medicine and Surgery of San Fernando in Lima is still another example of how few students were electing medicine as a career even in the best of circumstances.

Promotion of Medical Research and Learning

What then was taught by these august chairs of medicine, and what was the stance of the government? Taken all together, the policy of the Spanish government in America was one not of mere sufferance but of actual encouragement of the circulation of medical literature. Of course, medical books as well as books of all other kinds were subject to the scrutiny of both the government and the inquisitorial censors. In the course of the two centuries and a half before the wars of independence, however, the greatest handicap to the spread of medical literature was the high price of books. Dr. José Ferrer Espejo, a medical student before independence, told his own student, the Mexican medical historian, Francisco A. Flores, that it was very difficult to get books shipped from abroad and that, when these arrived, the prices were "exaggerated."[31] In those times an excellent way to realize money was to sell even outmoded, or, as they then said contemptuously, "rancid" books. Still doctors did manage to accumulate medical libraries that included not only the classic texts but also the most recent publications in medicine and surgery from every important country in Western Europe.

As the nineteenth century approached, medical works were more and more contemporary. Once established as classics, medical books like Gray's *Anatomy* today tended to hold popularity a long time, if not indefinitely. After the long domination of Galen and Hippocrates, this rule still held good, but to an ever-decreasing degree. Medical theses defended in Mexico in 1771 gave evidence of familiarity with the works of Lorenzo Bellini (1643–1704), Friedrich Hoffman, the "immortal" Boerhaave, the "ingenuous" Johannes de Gorter, and the everlasting Hippocrates.[32] In Guatemala the library of Dr. Manuel Dávalos y Porras, who died soon after the defense of his thesis, contained not only an extraordinary variety of medical works from Spain, France, Great Britain, and Holland, but also other scientific works including at least one on chemistry.[33] A quarter of a century later, when Dr. Narciso Esparragosa y Gallardo was preparing his surgical course, his students were drawing upon and defending European works on surgery, many of which had not been off the press more than a decade. In view of the time consumed in ordering and shipping books, this showed exceptional alertness.[34]

The repeated use of some of these works, especially that of the great Hermann Boerhaave, who emphasized modern discoveries, should put an end to the debate about whether the Spaniards, especially in America, were aware of the circulation of the blood before the second half of the eighteenth century. Wherever Boerhaave was known, so was the circulation of the blood. Besides, does it seem likely that a Spanish work, the *Institutiones medicae* of Andrés Piquer, published in Madrid in 1762, should be adopted as a text at Montpellier[35] if it overlooked so important a matter as Harvey's famous discovery? In fact, if neither the Inquisition nor the Spanish government barred Leibnitz, Bacon, and Newton, why should it bar Harvey's work on the circulation of the blood? But the dissemination of great discoveries was everywhere, even in continental Europe, gradual and exceedingly slow. John Milton opposed the views of Copernicus in the seventeenth century, and John Wesley was still firing away at them in the eighteenth. The gradual acceptance of the discovery of the circulation of the blood in the Spanish world, given the all but continuous warfare between Spain and England, was in no special way different from the gradual acceptance of other discoveries in other countries.

It should be an axiom of those versed in Spanish culture that the state of one branch of learning is an index to the state of progress in all the others. Given a fair picture of the development, say, of philosophy at an unspecified time during the eighteenth century, the expert cannot only fix the period but also outline the progress of science, medicine, or even literary style. In fact, as time passed, the conventional image of a government repressing learning and individuals struggling to be free of such restraints, if anything, should be turned on its head. By 1770 the crown had authorized "royal censors," not just to protect or promote regalism but to rule out "weary sycophancy" and to encourage pure straightforward language.[36] In time, the king turned to these censors to promote change and enforce greater liberty of learning and expression in America.

Jerónimo Feijóo, who was adroit enough to have done so if he wished, did not blame the Spanish government for any shortcomings he professed to see in Spain. Rather, he bemoaned the failure of the public to appreciate the achievements of a scientist during the learned man's lifetime. He therefore regarded it as a miracle that when that "most subtle Englishman," Isaac Newton, had "changed everything," the scientists of his country immediately accepted his discoveries and became his disciples and followers. Other scientists, however, might wait for public approval until they died or passed the point where they cared.[37] This is not to say that this universal failing of mankind meant that Spanish institutions always closed the door upon scientific discoveries. Copernicus, for example, met with a remarkably favorable reception. With the approval of the government, professors and students defended the Copernican system in Salamanca.[38]

The current of denigration that was running against Spain, especially at those times when Spaniards themselves suspected there was some ground for it (as in the case of botany and surgery), could be not just provocative but profitable. The Spaniards, after spectacular innovations in botanical research during the sixteenth century, now returned in the eighteenth to make another effort that spread over and reached the Western Hemisphere. Spaniards had begun to realize too that their surgery was static and that much was needed to keep it from falling indefinitely behind. When they quickly founded the first three of a series of surgical colleges, their emphasis was upon the armed services, where international rivalry was most concrete.

From such movements clinical medicine began to emerge, and in Spain and America it was the scientific investigator who did most to establish clinical medicine. In Spain Andrés Piquer, with his wide-ranging interest in physics and his prolific production of books, promoted clinical study. In America in Lima the Peruvian-born scientist, Hipólito Unánue, fell in with the drift of the times when in 1792 he announced the establishment of clinical lectures in the Anatomical Amphitheater. Stimulated by the example of the University of Halle in Germany, he tried to raise clinical medicine to the dignity it required. Both students and professors were observers at the Thursday clinics. In Mexico a movement started in 1796 culminated in the creation of a chair of clinical medicine in the Hospital of San Andrés in 1805. Candidates preparing for examination might count the time observing the holder of this chair as a part of their internship,[39] an innovation welcomed by the University of Mexico. In part out of respect to Dr. Luis Montaña, the holder of the chair, the cloister ruled that students as well as those interning might also attend these sessions.[40]

On another front wherever the creation of the protomedicato was the result of the efforts of an individual physician, the event was soon followed either by a great reinvigoration of medical training designed to close the gap between standards in Spanish cities and those in America or by a branching out into medical research and experimentation. This stage was also paralleled, as in Guatemala, by a shift from Latin to Castilian as the language of instruction, the language of publication, and the language in which to defend theses.[41] In 1798, for example, Luis Franco and Mariano Antonio de Larrave, two students of Dr. Narciso Esparragosa, in theses printed in Castilian, offered, among other things, to set out the surgical method for handling ulcers by making sutures and for treating wounds to the head, breast, abdomen, and tendons. Franco and Larrave offered to solve these problems through the doctrines of the "most accredited authors," especially those published by the royal academies of surgery and medicine in Paris.[42]

Doctors who had both training and certification were necessary for research. That there should be men to attend the sick, much less to conduct research, was hardly possible. In the old universities, such as those of Mexico and Lima, the brilliant professor was more likely—at least until the time of Unánue—to spend his time in a multiplicity of academic acts designed to show off his virtuosity rather more than to set out a new course or to conduct experiments. Even in the nineteenth century in Mexico, the medical historian Francisco Flores, when he sought to touch the high spots in the careers of outstanding doctors, emphasized their "defense of conclusions." Even Dr. José Ignacio Bartolache, who observed comets and experimented with iron pills (*pastillas marciales*), won high praise for a "brilliant" performance in these acts.

The Protomedicato and Promotion of Medical Research

As it stabilized in Mexico and Peru, the protomedicato was not concerned primarily, or even in considerable part, with the promotion of research.

Routine tasks of the tribunals absorbed the time protomédicos could spare from their teaching and private practice. Carrying on research was not one of these tasks, and even if it had been, the protomedicato had no budget to meet the inevitable expenses. Yet whenever there was a ripple of scientific activity, the investigator and the protomédico tended to become one. For one thing, regular payment of money for research was not conventional, not even in the eighteenth century. Appointing a man protomédico was therefore merely one way to compensate him for doing unprecedented work. In 1570 Francisco Hernández, physician of the king's bedchamber, became protomédico in Mexico without any intention of consuming his time in the suppression of illicit medical practice; his aim was field research in natural history, especially in the medicinal properties of Mexican plants.

In the same way two hundred years later the eminence of José Celestino Mutis as a scientist and his prominence as the director of the botanical expedition in New Granada made it difficult but not impossible for him to avoid becoming professor of medicine and protomédico also, because the two went together. In the same way Hipólito Unánue, the very year after he published his famous *Clima de Lima,* became protomédico in the City of Kings, but he never published another book. In contrast to Mutis, Unánue could accept the office, for the powers of the protomedicato were in keeping with his aims. He was a conscientious and persistent observer, but he had other professional purposes that burned as brightly as the scientific: he wished, first of all, to suppress the curanderos. To avoid the jurisdiction of the protomedicato, these "curers" were so bold as to come out into the open in Lima under the leadership of the charlatan, José Larrinaga, falsely to assert the "independence" of surgery and pharmacy. Larrinaga's chances of remaining an associate judge (*conjuez*) of the protomedicato would have been better had he not trapped himself in a laughable squabble with the protomédico in which he maintained that a woman on a plantation some distance away had given birth to a pigeon.[43]

Thus, the office of protomédico and medical research, though expressly connected in the title given Francisco Hernández in 1570, did not go together. The ideal of combining the two was never precisely lost, but there is scarcely an instance in which one function did not give way to the other. It was not just the absorbing police function of his office that kept the protomédico from becoming a scientific investigator; the medical doctor came into the office of protomédico by virtue of winning the prima professorship of medicine, a responsibility that confined him to the university almost exclusively.

Promotion of Research: A Case Study of José de Flores

The career of the scientist Dr. José de Flores offers the clearest illustration of the incompatibility of research and the more routine duties of the protomédico. When named first protomédico of Guatemala in 1793, Dr. Flores had behind him a formidable record. He won the doctor's degree in medicine at a time when there were not enough qualified doctors in the kingdom to examine him. When the king called upon authorities in Guatemala for the remission of medicinal plants, the captain general turned to Dr. Flores, considered the leading botanist in the kingdom. In an era when professors in Mexico and Peru were heralding the opening of anatomical amphitheaters, Flores, for want of cadavers, fashioned perfectly natural looking skeletons and other anatomical figures of wax "with such art that they did not lack the slightest thing that went to make up the harmonious composition of such a prodigious mechanism." In fact, they were so articulated that the student could see each part in its proper place with the same color and shape as in the human body. Working in isolation from his colleagues in Europe, Flores later claimed that he had produced figures that could be taken apart and reassembled to suit the convenience of the instructor or student. What is more significant, they may well have antedated the more perfectly executed ones of the Abbé Félix Fontana, which have been credited with being the first.[44] Not content with this accomplishment, Flores also brought to the faculty of medicine "a considerable collection of machines, instruments, and books," with no other purpose, so his associates reported, than the advancement of medicine in Guatemala.

Thus when Flores drew up a memorial to the king in 1793 soliciting the post of first protomédico in Guatemala, he tapped a veritable well of support. Joaquín Viejobueno, assistant consultant in surgery of the royal armies and chief surgeon of the infantry regiment in Guatemala City; the president and regent of the royal audiencia; the town council; and the former and actual prior of the Hospital de San Juan de Dios, who had witnessed Flores's success with smallpox inoculation in 1780, all joined in an endorsement of the petition. The university, however, refused its support. Flores had insisted that those coming up for the bachelor's degree in medicine could not be properly examined and legally qualified.[45]

Interestingly, in his petition Flores did not mention his earlier promotion of meatballs made from the newts (*lagartijas*) of Lake Amatitlán as a cure for cancer, syphilis, and leprosy, an episode that tells a good deal about medical research and innovation in the Spanish empire. His pamphlet published in 1781[46] had set off a wave of interest in Mexico and an investigation by a number of individuals and governmental institutions, including the protomedicato and the town council of Mexico City. One of the protomedicato's choices to make its recommendation on the new cure was Bachelor Juan Manuel Venegas, citing the English physiologist John T. Needham, who had observed that these particular newts had a split tongue, while others also had a split penis, and "that in sexual congress both partners so twisted together that they look like a single body with two heads." It was believed analysis of these aquatic salamanders had produced both oil and volatile salts. Oil from the newts was useful in destroying spots and ringworm of the face and, rubbed on the head, helped make the hair grow. When rubbed on warts, newt blood made them disappear. Powders made from lagartijas, when applied to the roots of teeth, made them easier to extract. Newt excrement was useful for spasmodic ophthalmia.

But so much for Needham in London, Venegas had his own ideas. He deduced that since the broth made from the newts turned green when left sitting, especially when this fact was combined with the "nausea, vomiting, and slaver" of the patient, corrosive poisons were present. Either these newts were not for internal use, or, he conjectured, Dr. Flores's lagartijas were a distinct species, or the skink had been mistaken for a newt. Since he had heard no report of cure from lagartijas, he recommended that the newt found at Ayotla at the source of Lake Chalco be brought to Mexico for analysis and experiment because a report indicated that this specific had been used successfully in combating syphilis. And thus he left the matter, no doubt to the joy of the protomédicos in Mexico City, grateful to him for leaving the problem open and them uncommitted.[47]

At this point the town council reported on its investigation. Its medical commissioners administered the newts to eight lepers, and after examining the eight patients reached a curiously unanimous conclusion. Six of the eight should be sent back to the hospital as incurable. Two had shown some progress and should continue treatment with the newts, although some investigators recommended their use combined with mercury.[48]

A case against Flores's new meatballs was more plainly stated by Andrés Montañer y Virgili. Appointed to the board of inquiry by the protomedicato, he was the chief surgeon of the Royal Indian Hospital and the nephew of Pedro Virgili, one of the great spokesmen of Spanish surgery in that epoch of reform and the founder of the colleges of surgery at Cádiz and Madrid. Montañer agreed that the six lepers dismissed were incurable and capable of communicating the disease, but that the newts might retard the progress of the disease in the other two. He would not, however, testify that these two had enjoyed any amelioration;

he had not seen them before the treatment. He did observe, though, that this kind of remission was common to the disease without the use of lagartijas. At any rate, there could be no certainty of a total cure short of a year. Besides, as reports of untoward consequences had come in from other places and since there was no solid evidence of therapeutic value in the administration of newts to lepers, he thought the continuation of the experiment useless and inadvisable. He added the observation that he could see no ground for believing that in the treatment of cancer and syphilis the use of lagartijas had any value at all.[49]

This negative view prompted an optimistic rebuttal by Antonio Velázquez de León, the chief surgeon of the Hospital Real de Amor de Dios, whose observations were prolix—an indication of uncertainty in all cases. The greater the ardor for the new remedy, the greater the classical allusion and the more elaborate the verbal dress. The motive for endowing the poor newt with great medicinal virtue was so great to Velázquez de León that he presented extensive reports on the treatment of syphilis with these lagartijas. A man with his testicles afflicted with syphilitic ulcers had so thoroughly yielded to treatment that twelve doses produced such a perfect cure that only a small scar remained as a reminder of the disease. In another experiment with seventeen patients suffering from syphilis, Velázquez de León had to admit that the twelve treated with mercury recovered faster, but he still held out hope for a cure or improvement in the five treated with newts, though he felt some terror because he was not sure his lagartijas had the same virtue as those used by Dr. Flores.[50] After weaving in and out of the subject for page on end, Dr. Francisco Rada professed to detect some improvement and in the end reached the safe conclusion that whatever helps should be continued.[51]

In the end, though, Dr. Flores himself probably believed he had been carried away by his new cure—probably superstitious in origin—that lagartijas were a specific for so many of the direst maladies. His hope, surely, was sustained by occurrences and symptoms during treatment that had nothing to do with lagartijas. And, of course, where there is so much hope in an experiment, something to sustain it is likely to be found. Not even the Mexicans, who had more facilities for such chemical analysis as was then possible, were successful either in proving or disproving the claims of the Guatemalan scientist.

Support for the idea, because it promised so much, built up in rushing crescendo and died down in diminuendo. The insistence of those reporting officially that at least a year was needed to make sure of the results of testing did more to end the use of lagartijas than could have any vehement statement against the practice. They vaguely sensed that they did not know what they were talking about and were reluctant to risk their reputations on any clear, decisive opinions. That the proto-médicos held aloof is no sign of special illumination, for their reserve was one of protocol; they simply could not accept a place second to that of the city council in a medical matter. Though he had created an international hubbub with his pamphlet, Dr. Flores himself, in 1793, eleven years after its publication, passed it over in silence when drawing up the list of those "merits and services" upon which he based his hope of appointment as first protomédico.

Under the Spanish system, despite the lagartijas episode, a swelling wave of accomplishment and appreciation like the one Flores was riding was the ideal basis for a significant royal favor. Yet Flores had enjoyed no rewards. In Guatemala medicine was "looked down upon with disdain," and in towns with the greatest population with no qualified doctors, those without licenses and unable to explain the elements of medicine "made bold to practice it to the grave detriment of humanity." The upshot was that, because the captain general and the royal audiencia felt that the circumstances in Guatemala did not permit the immediate establishment of a classic, full tribunal of the protomedicato, the king appointed Flores first protomédico, with all the honors, privileges, and powers attached to an actual tribunal.[52] The next year, on March 10, 1794, the king authorized the full tribunal.[53]

To Flores, appointment as first protomédico of Guatemala was a block to his personal and scientific ambitions. Though obliged to remain in Guatemala City by the terms of his title, in such quick order did Flores work that the very next year, 1794, the king honored him with the title of Physician of the King's Bedchamber, which carried with it the coveted treatment of *señoría*[54] and allowed him 1,200 pesos expense monies annually, charged to the funds generated by communities of Indians,[55] to enable him to go to Europe "to improve his own lights" and to carry out scientific work. By the time this document had reached Guatemala, all arrangements made, and the impatient doctor embarked for Spain, some two years had elapsed.

Once in Europe, Flores immediately launched into the travels that in his utopian hope and expansiveness were "to improve his lights." He scurried from one scientist to another in Germany, Holland, and France, only to hasten on to Madrid where he moved almost frenetically, only to hurry off on another jaunt that carried him not only to other Spanish cities but also took him anew through France, Switzerland, and Italy, where, in 1798, he visited the Abbé Félix Fontana, who was perfecting his sectional wax anatomical pieces.[56] By the end of two years, however, the exaggerated confidence that Flores reposed in European scientists had begun to wane; it was almost a disappointment to find himself, a mere American, generally up with if not sometimes ahead of them.

In this mood he began his experiments in the refraction and reflection of light that was to dominate him for many years and to run, intermittently, with all his other projects until age and lack of financing stilled his restless energy. The problem was that when lenses were substituted for reflecting glass in telescopes, as they had to be in order to increase the power of these instruments, the result was the long, troublesome chromatic aberration—a rainbow-like halo around the images because, when refracted, each colored ray in the spectrum had a distinct focus. By the use of a mercury-coated concave and a convex mirror and a very thick *"lentilla de agua,"* Flores produced an instrument that he said corrected the chromatic aberration as well as did the flintglass lens. After working until 1801—sixteen months in his own room and using his own money—he succeeded in getting his telescopes examined and approved by Juan de Peñalver, the director of the Royal Museum of Machines (*Real Gabinete de Máquinas*) in Madrid.[57]

In the range of his interests Flores could move without a tremor from the development of an achromatic telescope to the preservation of meat in a fresh state. That he had reached Europe only by taking passage on a neutral American ship, and certainly after hardships at sea, did not lessen his curiosity about the great historic plague of ocean travel—scurvy. By the end of the eighteenth century, however, seamen even if they had never heard of vitamins understood the role of fresh food, especially fresh vegetables and citrus fruits, but they did not have the technology to keep these foods fresh long enough to prevent scurvy. Exuberant, extremely curious, and always feeling himself on the verge of a breakthrough, Flores was just the man to turn to that grave problem.

So sure was he that he had the solution that he put his own life in jeopardy to prove it. He had observed that when the king called for specimens and artifacts from America to exhibit in the Museum of Natural History, organic substances came in brandy, the most convenient form of alcohol. It was this example that Flores proposed to follow in the shipping of meat and fish. Though he had begun to develop this idea two or three years after reaching Madrid, he was able to subject it to the trial of a sea voyage only in 1809. In that year, carefully immersing his meat in brandy according to his formula, he set out upon a voyage to England that did more than test his idea. In the shipwreck that followed, Flores himself survived, but later managed to recover his precious barrel of meat, but with the bunghole open and the preserving liquid gone—quite enough to suggest that seamen as well as the sea had had a part in the episode. He was satisfied enough, however, to insist that his method had survived this trial by ordeal. If he published his results, they have not been discovered, but Flores's demonstration was convincing enough for the government to commend him on his discovery that "promises so much for humanity and the nation."[58] Not satisfied with a limited experiment, Flores extended his method to include keeping fish fresh with a solution of brandy diluted in water.[59]

Flores's absorption in building a steamboat in Spain—though it was launched a decade after that of Robert Fulton—is, even more than his other scientific plans, shrouded in an obscurity that not even the zeal and industry of his very competent biographer could completely lift aside. Flores was working on this preoccupation as early as 1804, and a decade later, at the request of the Secretary of State, presented his model to the Junta de Marina. The launching of the Spanish steamship *Rey Fernando* in 1817, despite the lack of concrete proof, could very well have sprung from the industry of José Flores or from the irritation that his persistence could have provoked.[60]

Having to depend upon the fiscal responsibility of Guatemala, Flores was bound to suffer eventually. Spain had been so constantly at war in the eighteenth century, and particularly since taking up the old fight against England in 1779, that the economy of Guatemala had collapsed. Owners of indigo plantations that had once brought 18,000 to 20,000 pesos found themselves gladly accepting 1,000.[61] Smallpox, not the rapacity of the Spaniards, said Dr. Flores, had wrought such havoc as to leave tigers and serpents in possession of the desolate villages.[62] As if smallpox were not enough, swarms of locusts laid bare the lands of prostrate Indian communities. Clamor from the president and Audiencia of Guatemala ultimately arose to spare the kingdom the burden of perennial stipends to an absent scientist, particularly funds from Indian communities. In 1810, therefore, the Audiencia of Guatemala declared that Flores's pension of 2,000 pesos was an unbearable burden upon the Indian communities and that this outlay to the absentee doctor—now abroad for more than twelve years—was the one farthest afield from the original purpose of the fund.[63]

When the audiencia asked the Council of Regency to suspend the salaries of Dr. Flores in case he did not return to Guatemala, the Council of the Indies acceded. Then, on November 8, 1812, the Secretary of the Exchequer with what appeared to be great precipitation suspended the 2,000 pesos allowed Flores. There followed a veritable barrage on the offices of the Regency exchequer, whose secretary, José de Limonta, in turn, bombarded other offices.[64] Following a resolution of the Cortes on June 28, 1813, the Regency issued an order continuing payment of the original grant of 1,200 pesos, not from Indian communities but from the treasuries of Guatemala, although it suspended payment of the additional grant of 800 pesos made to him in 1801 when he won authorization to carry forward his work in the Royal Glass Factory at San Ildefonso. But there was a rider attached: he must return to Guatemala within one year or have his appointments terminated and payment of his salaries discontinued.[65]

Flores's economic plight, though it waxed and waned, steadily deteriorated. In mid-July 1813 he was still not getting the 800 pesos annual stipend. Soon after his return in 1814, however, the king, for some mysterious reason—perhaps the sheer pleasure of undoing what had been done in his absence—reversed the Cortes and Regency and ordered Flores paid all suspended salaries. Such a sweep of the pen, though, did not necessarily sweep down the bureaucracy. It was 1819 before Flores's attorney got any back payments at all, and then only one-half, about 5,000 pesos. He was still making the futile rounds of waiting rooms for the rest when the declaration of independence in Guatemala—September 15, 1821—left him destitute in Madrid. The annual pension of 12,000 reales, which it took him nearly three years to secure, finally arrived a little over three months before his death in 1824.[66]

Flores's exponents in the last quarter of a century have been able to establish to their satisfaction that the Guatemalan savant is entitled to priority in a whole battery of critical advances in science, but priority born "to blush unseen and waste its fragrance on the desert air" is not enough. When Flores visited the Abbé Fontana in 1798, the abbé was then working on his sectional wax anatomical pieces, which Flores was rigidly honest enough to admit were more finished than his. The implication generally left is that, as Flores asserted later, his anatomical pieces antedated those of Fontana. Is there satisfactory evidence, though, that at the time of this interview the abbé had just started on the sectional figures? Moreover, Flores's work, except for the advantages it offered in vitalizing the teaching of medicine in Guatemala, had no effect at all upon the world of science during the time when it might have been both original and helpful. By Flores's time, however, as the superstitious awe of cadavers slackened or collapsed, wax figures remained little more than curiosities anyway. In the same way Flores was a pioneer among Spanish men of science in planning and advocating the application of hydraulic force to the propulsion of ships. There is proof positive that he drew plans and made models of a steamboat, but only conjecture to support the idea that the first Spanish ship propelled by steam was the result of this work. Here again, even if the claim is correct, his only distinction lies in his preceding some other Europeans, and it took the world until 1960 to learn, and tentatively at that, what his role had been. In contrast, Robert Fulton, who, like Flores, came after other pioneers, carried through and made a practical success of the steamboat in 1807, ten years before the launching of the first one in Spain, which may have owed its creation to Flores. The failure of Flores to force his refinements through to triumph and to herald them in the scientific world of his day was unfortunate.

Medical Training and Learning: A Case Study of José Hipólito Unánue

In Lima the career of José Hipólito Unánue, the father of modern Peruvian medicine, illustrates first a medical precursor, then a precursor of independence, and finally a geographer and literateur. Fortunately, nice discriminations need not be made here about where the great anatomist and educator must first be viewed, but his career in many respects shows where enlightened medical training and learning had progressed by the time of the wars of independence in Spanish America. Born in Arica on August 13, 1755, José Hipólito Unánue studied there as a youth and later was brought to Arequipa by Bishop Chacón y Aguado, who had recognized possibilities in the brilliant boy from Arica. The Catholic piety of his home and the domination of ecclesiastical influence when his preliminary studies were finished naturally gave the youthful Unánue an ecclesiastical bent in a society where arms and orders were the only two avenues open to men of his extraordinary stamp.

Fortunately, when coming to Lima in 1777 to continue his training, Unánue was placed in the residence of Friar Pedro Pavón, his maternal uncle. A professor of anatomy in the University of San Marcos from 1760 to 1766 and of method in 1765, Pavón enjoyed an enviable reputation.[67] Perhaps Pavón, a little older and apparently recognizing the incompatibility between his situation as a member of the Congregation of San Felipe Neri and his position as professor in San Marcos, actually insinuated the study of medicine into the boy's head. If he did so, it was a signal service to Peru, for Unánue selected what was then "the most difficult and least appreciated of the professions."[68] Directed by the distinguished mathematician and cosmographer Gabriel Moreno, Unánue doubtlessly maintained close ties of friendship with him in the restricted academic world of Lima, for Unánue's greatest and most mature scientific work[69] was dedicated with affectionate gratitude to Moreno.

It was at the side of Moreno in his observations in the Hospital of San Andrés and under the protection of the Landaburu family that Unánue became a doctor. Some time before 1788, most likely on January 9, 1786, after successfully passing by the bachelor's and licentiate's degree, Unánue got his degree as doctor of medicine.[70] (Apparently in 1784 or 1785 he had been officially made a medical practitioner by the medical tribunal.)[71] To the question, put in one of the literary exercises that spread the fame of a student, "Will medicine prove more useful and illustrious when accompanied by *belles-lettres* and the exact sciences?," Unánue was in a brilliant position to give a startling answer. Student and friend of Moreno and well versed in the classics of Spain, Greece, and Rome, he spoke with a knowledge that convinced and in a language that enchanted distinctions. This led to his selection as secretary of the enlightened group of Peruvian Lovers of the Country (*Amantes del País*).

After a famous oposición, Unánue came to occupy the chair of anatomy in the University of San Marcos on February 1, 1789. Although only thirty-four years of age, he was, after Moreno and Cosme Bueno, the first medical authority of the viceroyalty. Concerning this academic competition, in which one is tempted to place the beginning of modern medicine in Peru, the facts are only piecemeal, but in the contest for this chair were elements of both pathos and irony. One contender against Unánue was none other than Dr. Miguel Tafur, who might have been the first medical doctor of the realm, but Tafur, doubtless concurring in the opinion of his contemporaries that defeat at Unánue's hands involved no dishonor, maintained in his breast the warmest friendship for his rival and stood by his deathbed as Unánue's personal physician.[72]

Although there is no concrete evidence that the necessity of an anatomical amphitheater was urged as a prime requisite of medical instruction in Unánue's opposition for the chair of anatomy, such an assumption seems highly logical. In the pages of the *Mercurio peruano*,[73] which began publication in 1791, the advantages to be derived from such an institution were boldly set forth by Dr. José Manuel Valdés under the pen name of Erasistrato Suadel. Unánue certainly urged such ideas on the viceroy who perhaps became interested through an essay on typhus[74] to give a quick response. On November 21, 1792, the Anatomical Amphitheater in the Royal Hospital of San Andrés was inaugurated. On this occasion, which was the first of Unánue's three major medical achievements in Peru, he himself appropriately delivered his celebrated discourse on "The Decadence and Restoration of Peru." The eloquence and feeling of his oration, its graphic description of the deplorable state of medicine, the obligation that the tenets of public health imposed to improve the teaching of medicine, and the necessity of producing physicians capable of coping with diseases indicated that Unánue was fully aware of the epoch-making significance of the event.

While a medical college for Lima was also revolving in his mind and awaiting the opportune moment, he did his best to fill the need by makeshift measures. In lectures at the amphitheater he called to his side the most reputable talent of Lima, even enlisting the services of the mulatto José Manuel Dávalos, doctor in medicine from Montpellier, who had not fared as well among established doctors as his superior education merited.[75] Taking his model from the best medical establishments of Europe, especially the Institute at the University of Halle, Unánue regularly assembled all the doctors and students of medicine in the city to discuss medical matters. By August 20, 1795, these meetings had been held fifty-four times.

His Royal Amphitheater had a social significance as well as a pedagogical use. By the fourteenth and fifteenth article of his plan, he called not only for looking after the indigent diseased who appeared and dispensing medicines gratuitously if necessary, but also when the evidence warranted it, actually sending doctors to those unable to appear—a long stride forward in medical service. He also rendered advice on public health in the *Mercurio peruano,* advice that would not be considered anachronistic in a modern journal of hygiene.[76]

The Royal Amphitheater of Anatomy and the publication of the *Observations* were a first and a second landmark in Unánue's enviable medical career, but a third, setting up the San Fernando College of Medicine and Surgery, marked the zenith of this career. Although a plan for a medical college had probably long been formulating in his mind, the first indisputable evidence of the project bears the date November 29, 1807, when Unánue addressed a tenderly impassioned memorial to Viceroy José Fernando Abascal (1806–16) soliciting its foundation.[77] Exactly one month later Abascal directed a communication to the Brotherhood of Our Lady of Santa Ana disclosing his intention of erecting the college in their hospital building.

In his enthusiasm for the college Viceroy Abascal appealed to all the available agencies of the realm: the cabildo of Lima, bishops, intendants, protomedicato, the miners of Hualgayoc, every significant organized group. Responses were numerous, and money was provided from many quarters. Most unique in providing the finances of the school, however, were the proceeds of a bullfight given by Hipólito Landaburu, a patron of Unánue's, and also the income from Wednesday afternoon cockfights. These funds thus provided for a building that evidently took three years to build (1807–11).

Strangely, despite the great fervor in Peru for creation of the Royal College of Medicine and Surgery, it was inaugurated without any fanfare on October 1, 1811.[78] Without ceremony, students were assigned their rooms, and the holders of medical chairs at the university transferred to the new medical college. Why there was no formal installation ceremony is not clear. Normally an institution like this would be launched by a gala, spectacular university procession with the viceroy in solemn attendance, but the inauguration of the College of San Fernando took place so quietly that it not only came into existence without the proper respect that pomp alone could pay in the colonial epoch, but also its quiet, almost furtive beginnings have shrouded its early history in mystery.

Unánue developed a vital, enlightened faculty. In the new college Unánue himself was professor of anatomy, Dr. Miguel Tafur professor of methods of medicine, Dr. José Pezet substitute professor of anatomy, and Dr. José Vergara, substitute professor of vísperas of medicine. Unánue also created a chair of external clinics and entrusted it to the aged Dr. Pedro Belomo, physician of the naval base at Callao, surgical examiner of the board of medical examiners, and well known for his administration of smallpox vaccine. Belomo was succeeded by Félix Devoti, whose bachelor's thesis on smallpox presented in 1803 was considered a model of elegant Latin. Dr. José Gregorio Paredes, professor of mathematics in San Marcos, ultimately assumed that same chair in the newly formed medical college that initially had twelve students, ten Peruvians and two from the Río de la Plata.[79] Also achieving a record for brilliance in these early days were assistants to the regular faculty, among them José Falcón, Juan Antonio Fernández, Juan Miguel de la Gala, José María Galindo, and José María Pequeño.

Unánue's appetite for expansion and excellence in the training of medical practitioners was never sated. Soon after his college got under way, he added two more faculty members to handle the vaccine for smallpox and to teach its use. One of these, Dr. José Manuel Dávalos, was a mulatto. Also playing upon Abascal's penchant for promoting the college, Unánue petitioned the viceroy to help him get new chairs in chemistry, physics, medical institutions, botany, surgery, obstetrics, and pharmacy. In 1812 the viceroy responded with a personal gift of twelve thousand pesos and a decree joining the Royal Anatomical Amphitheater with the College of Medicine and Surgery of San Fernando. He also declared Unánue protomédico general of Peru and director of the new medical college.[80]

This flurry of activity that came with the creation of the medical college seemed to promise great improvement in medical education in Peru, but unfortunately the outbreak of the wars of independence and the disruption of government in Spain caused by the Napoleonic takeover slowed the pace of reform. Moreover, Unánue himself became involved in the political upheaval. In 1814 he journeyed to Spain to take a seat on the Cortes, but the return of Ferdinand VII and his rejection of the Constitution of 1812 frustrated that aim. Being in Spain, however, allowed Unánue to pursue the needs of his beloved medical college. On May 9, 1815, his persistent efforts led to a royal cédula confirming the foundation of the College of San Fernando, but more than that, the suppression of the chair of peripatetic philosophy at San Marcos and provision for two new ones in experimental physics and chemistry were seemingly other victories for Unánue.

But when this reform triumphed officially—when the cédula reached Lima—the viceroy could do little to implement it. The turbulent enthusiasm created by the declaration of independence in the Río de la Plata by the Congress of Tucumán on July 9, 1816, pushed medical reforms into the background. About the only result of the cédula was the agreement by the learned conclave of doctors who acknowledged it to begin certain sessions with a religious act, to hear Mass every day, and to take instruction in the catechism of Pauget every Thursday and Sunday night. Also a new chair of practical surgery was set up, but little else of import in medical training and research marked these years prior to Peruvian independence. For his part Unánue deserted his anatomical amphitheater and college to connive with José de San Martín and to enter the political realm, less compromising in its call upon men of public spirit than medicine. The Lima medical students, too, also scattered in response to the drum and fife of the recruiting sergeant or the oratory of a Bernardo de Monteagudo. Thus, the scientific work of Hipólito Unánue came to an end.

The late eighteenth and early nineteenth century in Spanish America seemed to presage a more modern, more enlightened age in the training of medical practitioners and in medical learning generally. For better training, the creation of a Royal College of Surgery in Mexico City, additions of new chairs to medical faculties, and Unánue's Royal Anatomical Amphitheater and Medical and Surgical College of San Fernando gave notice that a new age had arrived. In medical research Narciso Esparagossa's invention of the innovative elastic forceps of whale bristles, the ready acceptance and use of Edward Jenner's smallpox vaccine in Spanish America, the gradual rejection of the Galenic pharmacopoeia, and the scientific activities of José de Flores—despite his lagartijas— showed a new spirit of experimentation and change. Such advances, it appeared, would ultimately give a new prestige to the practice of medicine and take it out of the disreputable state in which it was mired. More and better-trained professors, tested and proven cures, and greater government support of the kind provided Unánue by Viceroy Abascal in Peru seemed to augur a new day.

But alas, two factors, one old and one new, restrained this rapid drive toward modernism. The first—lack of money—had always held back development of medicine, in fact cultural and intellectual life in general, and continued to do so. If Unánue had had his way and the Medical and Surgical College of San Fernando had been allocated monies to realize all his plans, it would have become one of the most advanced centers of medical learning in all America or Western Europe. Scarcity of funds, however, prevented him from realizing his plans. So too did the second factor: the coming of Napoleon Bonaparte to Spain. Not only did this create an upheaval in the Peninsula, but it also set off a constitutional crisis in Spanish overseas kingdoms that caused revolt and ultimate separation. In this milieu medical learning and training suffered the repercussions, sadly, in an age when medicine seemed to be casting off its traditional shackles.

A S UNDERSTOOD BY Spaniards and Spanish Americans in the eighteenth century, public health was somewhat different from the contemporary American perception of that same enterprise. In fact, public health for the eighteenth-century Spanish American meant the proper licensing of doctors, phlebotomists, surgeons, and pharmacists; the inspection of hospitals and apothecary shops; the control of false or dangerous medical information; suppression of fakes and quackery; and rendering justice in medical cases. The modern American, however, views public health as the enforcement of sanitation and drug standards, detection of disease, and preventive medicine generally, usually at no cost to the individual.

To some degree enlightened Spaniards and administrators in the Spanish Indies had the same view, and in fact, the protomedicato performed many of these public health functions. For enforcement of laws against promotion of false cures and for revealing new remedies to the waiting public, the protomedicato played an important role. In times of public crises, however, particularly when epidemics occurred, the protomedicato was on the fringes of efforts to remedy public health problems. Because they had both the authority and the money, viceregal or local officials were the ones to take action with the protomedicato providing advice and counsel.

Urban Sanitation in the Late Eighteenth
Century: Mexico City and Lima

In his impassioned panegyric defending Spain in the Indies, the Spanish author Salvador de Madariaga eloquently describes the elegance and richness of the cities of colonial Hispanic America. But more than that, he praises their cleanliness, particularly in contrast to their European counterparts. When compared to London at the end of the seventeenth century, for example, Mexico City was elegant and noble—and clean. St. James Square, he points out, was "a receptacle for all the offal and cinders, for all the dead cats and dead dogs of Westminster." Drainage was bad; streets abounded in potholes; and windows opening on to London streets were used to rid households of excrement, garbage, and refuse with little or no regard for the passersby below. By contrast Mexico City was a virtual paradise, "clean and well policed."[1]

This was hardly the case in the late eighteenth century. In 1789 when the Second Count of Revilla Gigedo became viceroy of New Spain, he encountered sanitary conditions that could best be described as stomach-wrenching.[2] Walking toward the Zócalo, the central square, and the Plaza del Bolador, where the decline in sanitation was particularly manifest, he observed the bodies of dead dogs, killed after curfew by the night watchmen, half-floating in the shallow, sluggish canals. Because they were cleaned only every two years, these canals were clogged with garbage and dung flushed into them from the street in the afternoon rain. On the banks of the canals men and women squatted facing each other, "doing their operations," at the same time conversing with unaffected ease and cordiality. His cicerone might nudge him to notice that the windows of houses were tightly closed to hold out "these rotten exhalations." And if one of these windows suddenly opened—shades of London a century earlier—the passerby had to step lively, unless he was prepared to get an odorous shower, whether gaily and deliberately or accidently and routinely tossed. The drainage ditch running down the middle of the street, graded down to the center for this purpose, was clogged with the manure and urine from animals and human beings alike. In low places rotten puddles, laden with essences that not even an insane chemist could have thought of, concealed their ultimate possibilities until, in the dry season, some colorful carriage with red wheels and liveried outriders dashed through them to stir up an "intolerable fetor." Here a sagging black lead pipe bringing water from the mountains to the "powerful houses" of the city, battered by the constant bouncing of carriages over the cobblestones above it, gave way to the soft bottom of Lake Tezcoco, broke, and mingled its contents with this pestilential ooze. Once at the square he could not safely cross it, except by concentrating on his footsteps alone. If he retreated toward the cathedral, he found that its atrium had become a latrine.

At the fountains he saw Indian women indiscriminately washing their heads along with their infants' diapers and swaddling clothes, and prostitutes taking such baths as they took at all. As the time to eat approached in the Plaza Mayor, the fountain became the receptacle for all the refuse of cookery as well as for the dead animals already thrown into it "by mischievous boys and others." Vending stalls, so long tolerated, pushed into the very entranceway of the royal audiencia and of the viceregal palace itself, as if these were some kind of warehouse for their stock. Here and there, bleeders escaped the vigilance of the royal proto-medicato by losing themselves among these vendors. Whoever ventured onto a balcony overlooking this bedlam, be he viceroy or royal oidor, there beheld "the lugubrious aspect of the gallows, silhouetted between the latrines and the fountain." As they waited for their masters, coach-men washed their vehicles in the patio of the palace itself while their animals spattered the paving stones with manure.

At night the square took on the aspect of an encampment of no-mads in hostile territory. Every abomination had its corresponding sound. The "continual shouting and hubbub of a thousand dissonant voices . . . , obscenities, curses, and blasphemies" struck the ears. Cows and oxen, ravenous with hunger, bawled, sometimes charged, and always threatened the visitor with impalement. Attracted by the prospect of food, dogs took up with the Indian families sleeping in their stalls and charged "like lions" upon anybody "not dressed like an Indian." Others showed by their furtive movements and incessant barking that "they acknowledged no master." These so much disturbed respectable people that, upon the viceroy's command, the police killed and piled them in corners to await the cart drivers who, after daylight, dumped them somewhere in the country. Under cover of darkness, men and women in the square "aban-doned themselves to the most complete acts of sensuality." In the Plaza del Bolador "a vicious brothel" faced the Royal and Pontifical University, where, by Salamancan precedent, it might reasonably expect customers. In the squares and especially along the unlighted streets, and in the very houses, stabbings and murders had gone on until, in a single outrage, ten members died at one time in the house of a Joaquín Dongo.

The horrible conditions that Revilla Gigedo observed led him to take immediate action. Two or three elements probably moved him. First, Mexico City badly needed cleaning up. Second, the viceroy himself was full of the preachments of the Enlightenment that dwelt upon use-ful knowledge and projects. Moreover, Revilla Gigedo was enough of a dandy to recoil with abhorrence at the frightful scenes, sounds, and smells that greeted him in the Zócalo of Mexico City. In fact, he was so given to taking baths that he signed his viceregal papers there. Also his cabinets and dressing tables of his toilet were stocked with an assortment of "soaps, brushes, clean uniforms fragrant with cedar and sandal, light colored trousers and discreet perfumes," which "smelled of health and good conscience."[3]

Whatever the reason, the viceroy's attack on the horrors of the city was frontal. He lighted the streets, four or five lamps to the block so that on dark nights the straight rows of lights elicited the admiration of even European visitors. He revitalized the system of night watchmen, increased the night patrols until they went on without ceasing, ferreted out and punished criminal hangers-on, and drove others into honest work. Adulteries, frays, and drunken brawls came quickly to a halt. Sanitary carts came every night between dawn and 8:30 to haul off the excrement and garbage (*inmundicia*) and on certain days of the week the cleaning of the streets and plazas went forward until not a particle of trash could be seen on them. Revilla Gigedo summarily ordered the obstructing carriages and their clumps of draft animals from the patio of the palace. In the plaza, in place of dirty fountains to dip from, he installed spouts with stopcocks within easy reach and completely renovated the atrium of the cathedral, ruined by abuse from people coming in from the square.

Some of this work went beyond mere surface cleaning and undertook to correct conditions decades in the making. Bands of men tore up the black, encrusted lead water pipes, laid terra-cotta pipes in their stead, and firmly repaved the streets over them; they also built sidewalks and covered the drains. His first step in cleaning up the city was the publication of a ban, brief, broad in scope, and reinforced by stinging penalties.[4] In a city of, say, 150,000, resting on the bed of an ancient lake, cupped in by mountains, sanitation problems were rendered formidable both by the nature of man and by the nature of the terrain. Following the practice of old Spain, the engineers had graded the streets to the center to carry off the water in single streams. These, however, were often clogged with mud and trash and led into drainage ditches that, because they were all but level, in turn did not have the force to wash away the obstructions that accumulated between the biennial cleanings. Even if they did, there was no place for this polluted drainage to go—no proper sewer (*recipiente*).

With no way to get the excrement and urine from the houses except by throwing it into the streets—a system more and more favored—Revilla Gigedo ordered the filth carried off in one type of cart and the garbage in another. Those carrying the former appeared an hour before sunup and remained out until 8:30 a.m.[5] People who could not meet the early carts with their inmundicia might go out with it between nine and eleven at night. That no one might plead ignorance, the carts carried a bell. Anyone who elected to remain in a warm bed and then, having leisurely arisen and stretched, to empty his chamber pots into the street faced this schedule of penalties: twelve reales for the first offense, double for the second, and triple for the third (articles 1 and 2).[6] To make the order perfectly clear, Revilla Gigedo stipulated that the owners of establishments and not the city were responsible for disposing of manure from the stables, of building scraps, and of refuse from tanneries and slaughterhouses for swine. That he warned these owners, however, not to throw the waste into the street reflects what was to be expected. Disposing of rubbish from construction and repair of public buildings and works was a duty of the lieutenant corregidor (article 3).

Throwing "the least thing into the streets" and shaking and beating sleeping mats, rugs, or other household effects fell under the same penalties. So did those who cleaned carriages and operators of tippling houses, pastry cooks, bottlers, or any other person who scoured his utensils in the streets or washed his clothes in the canals. Neither teamsters, farriers, shoemakers, nor anybody else might work in the streets. And fruit and food dealers might not operate outside assigned places. Shearing mules and horses and leaving horseless carriages in the open street would result in the same fine (article 4). The sanitary cartmen had only the responsibility of disposing of dead animals killed by the night watchmen. The owners of all others had to dispose of them at the assigned place within twelve hours on pain of a ten-peso fine for leaving them in the streets (article 5).

Not even churches and convents escaped the obligation of cleaning and sprinkling in front of their premises by six or seven in the morning. If they failed to do so or did not pile their garbage neatly for the cartmen, the penalty was a twelve-peso fine for the first offense, double for the second, and triple for the third, assessed against the owner and not the domestic. Those who could not pay money paid with three days' solitary confinement for the first offense, six for the second, and six for the third along with twenty-five lashes, administered in two turns within the jail (article 6).

The "most indecent abuse of both sexes," as Revilla Gigedo put it, was in "dirtying the streets and plazas," to him the most revolting aspect of the sanitary decline if not collapse in Mexico City. The patrols and other officers had orders to arrest all males committing "this abominable excess" and put their arms and legs forthwith in the stocks set up for this purpose at the doors of jails and police stations. A first offender got twenty-four hours, a second offender forty-eight, and for a third offense the prisoner got the same forty-eight hours but with his head in the stock this time. For this same offense the police carried a white woman to the "court jail" and an Indian woman to the ordinary public jail, suffering three days' confinement for the first offense, three days for the second, and three days for the third plus twenty-five lashes in two turns within the jail. Owners of pulque shops, "where this excess was most frequently committed," were made responsible for cleaning up the area within fifty yards of their establishment on pain of a six-peso fine for the first offense, twelve for the second, and eighteen pesos for the third. What the hygienic conditions were in the schools is implied in the requirement that the masters have toilets there and not allow the children to go out to dirty the streets. Moreover, this was "an essential part of training in good manners." Loss of license was the price schoolmasters and mistresses would pay for disregarding this regulation (articles 8 and 9). Besides all this, all houses on the streets had to have privies within three months, and all masters of building projects, as the first step, had to build a latrine on pain of paying for it themselves (articles 12 and 13).

The preoccupation with loose dogs so evident in this half-century came to the surface again in Revilla Gigedo's order that mastiffs of the largest kind, bulldogs or the large wolflike dogs used in bull fighting (*alanos*), and ferocious dogs of any kind not be allowed to run loose in the city or its environs without a secure leash. In case of violation, the police were to seize the dog, sell it, and apply the proceeds to the police-men's fund. In any case, the police would kill all dogs loose after curfew "as having no owner to look after them" (article 10). In all matters covered in this edict, the enforcement was rigorous and grounds of ap-peal narrow.

The dourest creole member of the protomedicato and the most re-cent arrival from Spain all agreed upon the benefits wrought by Revilla Gigedo's efforts. When they could catch their breath, they said that this insufferable squalor had caused not only disease but epidemics.[7] Dr. Gar-cía Jove, president of the protomedicato, informed the viceroy that the reports received from hospitals and from the parish churches revealed a sharp decrease in illnesses and deaths. Vicente Cervantes, who heard of the degeneration in sanitation and police before he came out from Spain to head the Royal Botanical Garden in 1788, remarked the same de-crease. As no one quite fully appreciated, Revilla Gigedo had done what Spanish administrators could never bring themselves to do; he had levied taxes on tender spots: first upon the Indians' pulque, the traditional way to turn, and second upon the owners of houses, the forbidden way to turn.

So completely dedicated did Revilla Gigedo appear that Mexicans turned upon him with a rare and pathetic affection. "Never," said the physician Matías Antonio Flórez, "can Mexico and its inhabitants pay the homage due his government." "So long as there is tongue to praise him and the sensibility to bless him," exclaimed Vicente Cervantes, Mexico could never forget his "geniality, his benevolence, his disinter-estedness, his uprightness, and all the rest of his eminent qualities."

But the stolid mass is hard to change. In less than a year into the government of the next viceroy, the Marquis of Branciforte, and at the very time that the protomédicos were praising Revilla Gigedo for his cleanup of the city, Pedro de Basave, the secretary of the viceroy who received these plaudits, wrote bitterly to the rector of the University of Mexico that, with animal-like abandon, the people were so befouling the city, especially at night, that to approach the university through the streets and plazas was a nauseating, suffocating experience.[8] Basave, who was bound to know that his master Revilla Gigedo detested the incumbent viceroy, might be accused of charging him with neglect were it not that Branciforte himself, on the occasion of renewing the new sanitation contract six months earlier, had repeated Revilla Gigedo's decrees on street cleaning and the removal of filth and garbage and even modified the 1790 regulations. With the design of keeping the cart drivers from skipping their rounds, he simply had the carts numbered so that the people and authorities could fix the blame and report any fault.[9] Reprinting old measures, however, did not necessarily revitalize the cleanup of a city with such extraordinary problems as Mexico City had.

When other conditions were just right, the sluggish drainage of Mexico City could all but suffocate the population and nearly did so fourteen years later. During the late night of March 23 and the early morning of March 24, 1810, a bare half-year before the uprising under Hidalgo, a great stench swelled up over Mexico City that left both the town council and the viceroy in a state of alarm. As the man surest of his authority, the viceroy responded by appointing Oidor Guillermo Aguirre as commissioner to investigate the cause of the horrible odor, urging him, "without loss of time," to set up a commission composed of physicians and engineers (*maestros mayores*).[10] So quickly did Aguirre move that the very next day, in his own house, he assembled a commission composed of the first protomédico, Dr. and Master José García Jove, Dr. Luis Montaña, Dr. Mariano Asnares, Antonio de Velásques, master of architecture, and Ignacio Castera, master builder of Mexico City. Their purpose was to suggest measures to avoid the "doleful consequences to the inhabitants of this immense city" of such miasmas as they had just experienced.

In a case such as this, where the whole sanitary situation of the Valley of Mexico might figure in any conclusion, the commission could only make distinctions and eliminate possible causes—most of them logical enough. The cleaning of the sewage canals, which somebody had evidently suggested as the cause of the all-pervasive fetor, could not be the cause as no such bad odor had ever before followed this routine procedure. The commission therefore fixed the blame on the polluted lakes, advised against draining them, and recommended planting trees to purify the atmosphere—a method surely not likely to afford immediate relief. In addition, the commissioners advised a special type of cart for hauling off all the garbage and "filthiness." To make sure that the conduit to Lake Tezcoco was not stopped up, they crowned their advice by reverting to the steps taken by the second Count of Revilla Gigedo, even though the archbishop viceroy had already posted notices reinstituting those measures. The viceroy now designated Master Builder Ignacio Castera and Dr. Luis Montaña to make a personal inspection. In the expansive way characteristic of him when dealing with a prime political question, Dr. Montaña summed up the inspection in thirty-four points. As a physician, he noticed many dead fish—which added their own effective element to the general fetor—and informed the viceroy that families gaining a living from fishing should be obliged to give up this occupation. As a medical man, he also noticed that there were fevers in the villages near the lake affected by the odor, but he did not profess to understand their nature. Dr. Montaña's engineering companion made some technical corrections in the report, urged redirection of the aqueducts bringing fresh water into Mexico City, and recommended the completion of a drainage project, which had been started in 1786 but left in abeyance because of the lack of funds. The last cry that went up concerning the problem was from a frustrated accountant, who said that only the Superior Government could provide the monies needed to finish the work, and in 1810 monies were scarce.

In Lima, another of the cities of colonial Hispanic America praised for its cleanliness by Salvador de Madariaga, sanitary conditions were no better than in Mexico City. In the administration of Viceroy Francisco Gil de Taboada (1790–96), which overlapped those of Revilla Gigedo and Branciforte in Mexico, Lima suffered from the same sanitary neglect. In 1796, the year that the Mexican physicians were so strongly testifying about the miserable sanitation, Hipólito Unánue, in ghostwriting the report of the outgoing viceroy, noted the foul air resulting from the filthiness of the streets in Lima. There, however, poor drainage in a lake bed was not to blame; the streets were well planned and the streams brought plenty of water with adequate fall, although drainage pipes and canals were no cleaner than in Mexico. What was lacking, said Unánue, was proper sanitary practice and policies. Viceroy José Fernando Abascal, who arbitrarily made Unánue chief protomédico in 1807, immediately took Unánue's advice by creating a sanitary commission (*junta de policía*). Among other things the commission aimed to get rid of was rubbish and fetid stagnant water that forced the people of Lima to breathe a noxious air charged with microbes, which Unánue believed caused continuous epidemics. Compared to the thirty-six sanitary carts authorized by Revilla Gigedo in Mexico City nearly two decades earlier, Lima had only six carts pulled by plodding oxen, although there was some increase in these after Abascal became viceroy. That Unánue was close to Abascal helped improve conditions somewhat, but sanitation remained a problem in Lima as well as in Mexico until independence came—and after.

Governmental Promotion of New Cures and Remedies

Improvement in sanitation was primarily the responsibility of viceroys and local administrative officials, who had both the money and the authority to make needed improvements, at least at times. The protomedicato was normally on the fringes of such efforts as advisers. For other public health matters, however, the protomédicos had more to say. One of these was control over dissemination of new medical knowledge, which, if allowed to go unchecked and uncensored, may have had disastrous results for the population. First by invitation and then by custom, the protomedicato came to censor any general work on medicine, and with a hypercritical eye to scrutinize any that proposed a drastic departure from orthodox practice, especially one proposing a new, radical treatment for an ancient scourge. Most new remedies were scarcely more than mere fancies, but they often appeared in print without having run any critical gauntlet whatsoever. In the age when the Enlightenment made useful knowledge the mark of progress, a paternalistic but progressive government such as that in Spain naturally put the power of authority behind the circulation of significant medical discoveries. Jealousy of the printed word, however, did not extend to the infinity of untried and exotic remedies that were now touted in magazines, essays, and special correspondence.

The chaos that resulted in the handling of new medical claims was owing in part to the fact that the protomedicato, though the official censor of medical works, often found itself working in a consultative capacity. Just as the government found the problem of smallpox, especially after the discovery of vaccine, entirely too big to dodge by leaving it to the protomedicato, so too it assumed control over the circulation of the authentic, newly discovered remedies for tropical afflictions. Thus some medical pamphlets and broadsides came to the public from the protomedicato, some came from the bishop, and still others from governors and viceroys. The one thing all these sponsors had in common was a desire—hard enough in those days when unction and pomp too often went side by side with learning—to put medical instructions in terms so simple that anyone who could read or get someone to read to him could make use of them.

Children were the great sufferers from such ignorance. They were peculiarly liable to neonatal tetanus, died with pathetic regularity from digestive disorders, and every few years offered themselves up as another non-immune generation to the ravages of epidemic diseases. Both creole and peninsular Spaniards had a great tenderness for their children and stood in constant dread of fatalities, especially when a long time had elapsed since a major epidemic. Eighteenth- and early nineteenth-century documents on social questions thus often touched on the care of infants. Doctors, who put great stress on good and plentiful food in the cure of the sick, knew that intestinal upsets somehow had something to do with feeding. Spanish medical literature is thus liberally punctuated with tracts and broadsides dealing with the care of infants. These concluded, naturally, that not nursing one's own infants was a special evil. Since the chances of infection in breast feeding were slighter, their argument seemed amply borne out.[11]

In the West Indies one of these diseases—one that sometimes seemed to afflict infants alone—was neonatal tetanus, called the "seven days' sickness." The Spaniards thought of this disease as "a kind of epilepsy" that struck the newborn so invariably within seven days that any child reaching the eighth day was safe. Rarely did an infant once attacked escape, and those who did, superstition had it, invariably died, either at the age of seven or at twenty-one, when the disease recurred. Climatic and sanitary factors in Cuba were such that serious commentators regarded the "seven days' disease" as one of the principal causes of the depopulation of that island. Cutting the umbilical cord with dirty knives and scissors probably was responsible for this awesome affliction.

Yet, even in those days when the pathogenic bacillus was not dreamed of, some astute person noticed that immediately after the umbilical cord was cut when the midwife anointed the navel with balsam of copaiba (*aceite de palo* or *aceite de canimar*) "as is sold in those dominions for half a real," the disease did not attack the child. In fact, there was not a single case of neonatal tetanus among infants so treated— a discovery worth bringing to the attention of the king himself! The government then printed a placard describing this simple and marvelously efficacious prophylactic, dispatched it to American officials for publication, and asked them to report on the results "if the specific were adopted."[12] This discovery made such a profound impression that within a decade it became common knowledge among those professing medicine throughout the Spanish empire. In fact, José Manuel Valdés, working under the direction of Dr. Hipólito Unánue in Lima, published a bachelor's thesis in 1807 that definitively introduced this amazing preventive to South American medical literature.[13]

In Mexico the protomedicato played its typical part. There in 1797, a year of much trial in the public health of Mexico, Viceroy Branciforte received a royal order calling attention to this preventive for tetanus. Although in New Spain innumerable children continued to die every year from a "species of convulsions" coming just one week after birth, he learned that not one death had occurred in Cuba among infants after the application of balsam of copaiba when the umbilical cord was cut. Practitioners in Mexico told the viceroy informally that the "seven days' disease" was not so common in Mexico, but Branciforte nevertheless passed the royal order over to the protomedicato in Mexico City, asking the doctors on that tribunal to set out "what they liked in the cases, manner, and quantity of the dose" to be used. The protomédicos, to their credit, rendered a thoughtful report after they analyzed the balsam, strongly endorsing the "specific." Then they even went on to say, and with more reason than usual, that it could be used in other cases such as wounds "to prevent corruption" and facilitate healing. Thereupon Branciforte published a ban throughout the kingdom and enjoined the protomedicato to make every effort to see to it that midwives and surgeons attending at childbirth should use this discovery in place of the "tallow, ash, salt, grease, or other useless or dangerous ingredients" then customary.[14] Though they prevented the disease, these men did not understand invisible bacteria any more than they grasped the idea of the insect vector of disease.

In another sphere no scientific explorer ever came out of the American tropics without a greater fear of small insects than of big animals. Mosquitoes were of two types—those that attacked by day and those that came on by night. Yet if we are to heed explorers like Im Thurn and Theodore Roosevelt, an ordinary attack of the black pium flies was worse than the best assault the mosquito could mount. To the Spanish colonial, though, these afflictions seemed a mere part of life ordered for them in the beginning. It was not so with the chigger fleas (*niguas*) who could leave a man with something more than a rash. These strange creatures burrowed under the nails, generally the toenails, or simply penetrated the skin, and deposited eggs that, when they hatched into larvae, became very dangerous. Even today the most careful person cannot be sure that, at the end of the day, he has properly searched himself for punctures. Neither can he be sure, once the sac has developed to the size of a pea, that he can pierce it with a needle and lift it out before it ruptures and causes infection and, for the unlucky ones, gangrene. Since this diabolical little insect lives in the ground, a person carelessly lying down in an infested place may run the risk of losing his life. Poor people and barefooted workers in the colonial epoch—and now—therefore suffered most. But a discovery made in Cuba brought the possibility of relief to them and increased the productivity of the island. A priest reported that if each nigua perforation were simply covered with olive oil, the sac would not develop. As simple in conception as putting nail polish over an ordinary chigger bite, this olive oil sealed off and smothered the eggs, a matter quite important enough for an official royal circular on November 20, 1786.[15]

In the case of epidemic diseases such as measles that never yielded to spectacular preventives as did neonatal tetanus and smallpox, the authorities in some American capitals could count on their local gazettes to carry warnings and instructions. Also, in places where there were no news magazines, some simple outline of a regimen for treatment was indicated whenever epidemics began to rage. This occurred in Puebla during an outbreak of measles in 1784. The initial steps were marked by prayer, religious processions, and petitions to various saints, followed by steps a bit more earthly. Physicians and surgeons of the town came together to make recommendations and issue instructions on how to deal with the epidemic. Finding the air contaminated, they called upon the people and local officials to throw all garbage out of the city, to keep the streets clean, to burn aromatic wood nightly, and to sprinkle everything with sulfur water. Doctors would be available at various parts of the city to give advice and, if needed, to dispense medicines to the poor free of charge.[16]

In times of extreme crisis it was the viceroy who usually acted first, not the protomedicato, although sometimes his first step was to consult the tribunal. In such cases he might instruct the protomédicos to draw up medical rules for circulation during an epidemic, rules so simple that everyone could understand them and the people could treat their own sick.[17] Smallpox, in particular, when it reached the proportions of a viceregal disaster, or when vaccine for its prevention was discovered, enjoyed all possible publicity. One has only to look back on the minute instructions provided for performing cesarean operations to determine that both the viceroy and the protomedicato were active in promoting new cures or new practices.

Control of Private Medical Publicity

Either a great menace or a fortunate discovery was necessary to bring the government into medical publicity, but private individuals voluntarily engaged in it all the time. At its worst, this activity amounted to passing superstitious lore from person to person. Very little better, though, was the unregulated boosting of an unapproved drug of a "secret, mysterious" specific with the aim of establishing a monopoly and making quick money. These phases of medical discussion produced an anarchy that was agitated by the nervous expectancy of the Enlightenment—a kind of optimistic hopefulness for more discoveries like smallpox vaccine and electricity. The point had not yet been reached when these discoveries were expected primarily from chemistry, but from nature—the nature that could produce the remedy if it could produce the sickness.

The magazines that appeared in the second half of the eighteenth century, with emphasis upon the useful knowledge characterizing the Enlightenment, often carried specifics and concoctions of such extraordinary promise that they passed to the most distant points in the empire. Described first in its native country in 1769, the pepper tree of Peru got a handsome promotion in New Spain eighteen years later. The husks of the leaves relieved the "cold humors" and swelling of legs and muscles; the twigs served to clean the teeth; the resin mixed in milk worked to destroy "clouds and cataracts of the eyes" and clean ulcers; and "the vinous liquor of its fruit" relieved kidney trouble. Immediately after partaking of this vinous liquor, a youth of "sixteen to eighteen" got relief from a persistent diarrhea while a woman immediately recovered from hysteria. The perfecter of all these remedies—leaf, twig, resin, and "vinous liquor"—must have been the owner of a grove of pepper trees, and an economist besides. All these claims and much more, said the *Gazette,* proved that the virtues attributed to this tree by the Peruvian natives were not illusory.[18]

Though it had authority to pass upon the purity of a drug already in the pharmacopoeia, the protomedicato apparently did not regularly certify new drugs. In consequence, many items, especially semi-medical ones such as teeth cleaners, made their own way through the incipient advertising of the eighteenth century. Upon occasion, though, energetic druggists advertised these, indicating they had been approved by the protomedicato.[19] One issue of the *Gazeta de México* played up a "True water for whitening and strengthening the teeth" that not only would leave them in their "natural state" but also would cure scurvy.[20] Two numbers later, however, the periodical reported candidly that the *"licor"* was nothing more than sulfuric acid diluted with water. It might, the slightly repentant editor reflected, clean the teeth, but it would also dissolve them "in short order."[21] Mark Twain's "Duke," traveling companion of Huckleberry Finn, never hawked a concoction better calculated to take the enamel off with the tartar.[22]

This increasing volume of irresponsible advertising had already attracted the hostile attention of the royal protomedicato. In February 1787 the *Gazeta de México*[23] carried an advertisement from Francisco Xavier Angulo offering two "liquors": one "to clean, preserve, and protect" the teeth and another to stop toothache, or, as Angulo put it, the "ache of molars and teeth."[24] As this was the first of a series to appear that year, the protomedicato, outraged that the advertisement of a new drug had appeared without its authorization and always fearful of the monopoly of a vital drug, met to launch an investigation and forbid any sale unless the drug met its standards. The first step was to determine the ingredients of the concoction offered. Under oath, the apothecary Angulo had a persuasive argument for the need of a dentrifice. In a printed broadside he had insisted that the reason for such early loss of the teeth by the majority of people was "the total neglect" of "such a necessary and precious adornment of nature. . . ." Thus, he offered a preparation (*opiata*) that would preserve the gums, hold the teeth firmly in their sockets, and keep them all healthy.

The reaction of the protomedicato was quick. Meeting the very next day, it decided to require Angulo to disclose the ingredients, exhibit his product, and present a printed statement setting forth his method. When put under oath, Angulo, eager not to offend the tribunal but equally eager to preserve his secret, gave the vague answer that the licor was made from *guaiacum* and brandy and the "opiate" of mollusks and gums with lemon syrup, honey of roses, and some drops of the essence of clove. When pressed for particulars on the mollusks and gums, he replied that the gums were myrrh and dragon's blood, the mollusks were pumice-stone, coral, "and such," all in a printed statement.[25] Satisfied about the ingredients, the protomédicos then had to determine the price. They accordingly asked the opinion of two respectable druggists, and though their opinions ranged from one-half to four or five pesos for two ounces of this new concoction, they ruled that the proper price for the "opiate" should be four reales and the licor one peso.[26] There was never any doubt that the price of drugs had to be fixed.

This problem of "secret remedies" for all kinds of illnesses did not end with the Angulo case. In fact, for a long time before and often after the decision of the protomedicato in 1787, gazettes went on advertising remedies with no indication whatsoever that they had passed the scrutiny of the protomedicato as required. Sorely troubled with the epidemic that raged in his time, Viceroy Branciforte was the man to make short shrift of this irresponsible practice. In 1797 he summarily ordered the editor of the *Gazeta de México* to announce no new drug unless the promoter first presented the endorsement of the protomedicato.[27]

There was apparently no basis for the censorship of advertising of medicine except the general authority that Spanish law gave to the protomédicos over spices, aromatic drugs, and medicines introduced into trade. Hence, there was bound to be some smarting under this uncertainty of jurisdiction. At the end of the eighteenth century, with the protomedicato seemingly firmly in charge of censoring new drug advertisements, a challenge arose over where the protomedicato got this power. In 1800 the viceroy required the protomedicato either to substantiate its claim or give up its censorship powers.[28] Seven years later Viceroy Iturrigaray went so far as to exempt the editors of both the *Gazeta* and the *Diario* in Mexico from the obligation of notifying the protomedicato before publishing an advertisement for a new drug.[29] Although this seemed like a real setback to the powers of the protomedicato, the pages of the *Gazeta* and *Diario* did not explode with a mass of outrageous claims for new cures by greedy promoters, at least no more outrageous than some that had met the approval of the protomedicato.

Finding new cures for persistent diseases and making them known was sometimes a private enterprise initially but later found endorsement from the protomedicato. Though a disease often considered to have afflicted seamen only, scurvy provoked many advertisements for "antiscorbutic" concoctions.[30] When in 1770 the ship *Oriflame* was lost just short of Callao, Dr. Vicente Lardizábal, a physician of San Sebastián, set to work to find a medicine to cure this seamen's sickness. What he came up with was a "cooked salad" of "seaweed or sargasso." To his work on this subject he gave the striking name of seaman's salad (*ensalada de los navigantes*).

Dr. Lardizábal had an aggressive and ingratiating background. His customs were "moral and Christian" and, despite a slight deafness, at thirty-six the Caracas Company of Guipúzcoa engaged him as its inspector of surgeons and drugs at San Sebastián and physician attending seamen arriving ill from overseas. For this honorific post he had ample preparation in medicine and botany, having received the doctor's degree in France. His first publication had reflected his preoccupation with scurvy,[31] and in the year before the loss of the *Oriflame* he had published a work for the direction and instruction of ships' surgeons.[32]

His seamen's salad was an idea so sweeping that if it had been realized, he would have changed the course of eighteenth-century history. No wonder that Juan Bautista de Gorzueta and Vicente Rodríguez de Rivas, directors of the Guipúzcoa Company, besought the Minister of the Indies, Julián de Arriaga, to take Dr. Lardizábal's work under his protection and see to it that, upon examination by the protomedicato, the king issue a royal order to open up the way for the greater prestige and usefulness of this discovery.

The protomedicato had plenty to say.[33] It remarked that Lardizábal had reasoned thus: seaweed is aperitive, has "absorbent virtues," and as many remedies for scurvy are aperitive and absorbent, seaweed was likewise curative. But since the "medical forest" contained many aperitive and absorbent plants that were antiscorbutic and others that were not aperitive and absorbent that were remedies, the logic was fallacious. Hence, the author should make the necessary experiments and if his conjecture was sound, not only would the protomedicato give him a license to publish but also, in all likelihood, the king would decorate him for a find so long concealed and so anxiously sought. Moreover, in the mood of newly converted laymen, the directors of the Caracas Company undertook to quiet the sarcastic misgivings of the protomedicato.[34] They thought it impossible for anyone to doubt "the simplicity and solid erudition" with which Lardizábal satisfied all "doubts and perplexities."

Inevitably, especially in the hands of nonscientists of those days when science still hovered between logic-chopping and experimentation, seaweed was not limited to scurvy but would cure other ills "such as constipation of the bowels, stubborn obstructions, nephritic symptoms, hypochondria, and whatever calls for diuretic and absorbent remedies." For support, Lardizábal fell back upon the experience of Cristóbal de Acosta whose *Book of Plants and Vegetables,* though published 193 years before, had endorsed seaweed as a preventive of scurvy. That book, Lardizábal contended, had been neglected, something that often happened as in the long neglect of Jacob's ladder as a remedy for epilepsy. He concluded, however, that new experiments such as those asked for by the tribunal would not take place because scurvy was infrequent where he was, and the experiments would require much of the surgeons' time aboard ships in voyages to America and Asia. Lardizábal then had the directors of the Caracas Company ask Arriaga to return his manuscript. That minister had it put in an envelope with no answer except that he wished to avoid being bothered further with such "useless projects."[35]

The right of the royal protomedicato to examine and approve or disapprove the publication of medical books did not extend to the issuance of patents. In fact, overtures for the exclusive use of any element of nature or any invention went directly to the viceroy, whether it pertained to something as surprising as a proposal to develop a flying craft[36] or another to develop an air-conditioning unit. In 1791 William White sent a paper to the *Mercurio peruano* of Lima dealing with such a machine. If not an air-conditioning device, this machine at least supplied "constant, fresh and regulated air" in the most trying climates. The Englishman stressed its usefulness in such crowded and confined quarters as ships, hospitals, prisons, and mines. The editor of the *Mercurio,* though, foresaw more domestic uses. He published the communication with the hope that the device—at ten to twenty guineas—might relieve the "slight ventilation" in Peruvian houses "in summer." In Lima, where the French advice to stop the burial of the dead in the walls and floors of churches had had no success, he advocated an air machine in every church to expel "the cadaverous and pestilential effluvia" that would eventually rid the country of the "Tertial Plague." Any man who has seen the monstrous contrivances sticking from the windows of modern buildings will appreciate White's prescience in recommending his invention as "an adornment."[37]

Of a more purely medical nature in Mexico, however, was an application that went to Viceroy Félix María Calleja (1813–16) early in 1816. José Miguel Muñoz, "honorary first assistant" of the surgical corps, and much affected by the wounded seen in five years of bloody civil war, wanted the exclusive ten-year privilege of manufacturing and selling an artificial leg that had all the movements as well as all the uses of the natural limb. To succeed, Muñoz had first to establish himself as a well-deserving figure in surgical circles and, then, to show that he had a useful and original invention. His claim upon favorable attention he based upon a six-year record (1804–10) of administering smallpox vaccinations and upon having perfected and presented to the Royal College of Surgery a surgical chair for use in cataract operations that combined "the comfort of the patient with that of the operator" and made a quick operation possible. With this chair he had performed operations upon eight poor persons who had completely recovered their sight. For this, as became a man seeking viceregal favors, he made no charge at all. And, now, he was about to manufacture an artificial leg of his own invention so good that it could be "used up to the point of dancing." No nuisance of a crutch was necessary, and, under a fine silk stocking, one could not tell the artificial leg from the original flesh. He hoped that the "enormous labor" that had gone into its perfection could be seen in the case of Prudencia Gutiérrez, "who is now enjoying one in this capital." The privilege of exclusive manufacture would make it possible for the poor, such as his majesty's soldiers, to profit from the creation.

The viceroy turned to Fiscal Ambrosio Sagarzurieta, pointing out that Muñoz's bent was in the direction of "useful inventions" such as the surgical chair he had perfected. An especially competent and perceptive man, Sagarzurieta observed that it only remained to prove that the invention functioned as Muñoz claimed and that it was Muñoz's work and not copied from one in use in Europe. For satisfaction on these two points, the viceroy should appoint two surgeons of his own choice to conduct an examination. He concluded by suggesting that Muñoz state what he would charge the "truly poor" and asking him to supply a sketch and to break down the costs to the public. Those appointed to make the investigation, Drs. Rafael Sagaz and Antonio Ceres,[38] concluded that the leg, after the most careful examination, showed the greatest mechanical ingenuity and in every respect justified the claims of the applicant. Its strong points, as they saw it, were that "it looked exactly like the natural leg," permitted wearing of a shoe, allowed "flection to the point of kneeling," perfectly maintained the balance of the body, and obviated the use of a crutch. Even looked upon as a simple imitation, the metal leg was more durable and economical than wooden ones of Europe publicized in Mexico. While the latter secured movement at the "expense of the stump," that of Muñoz, with the mechanism confined to the heel only, avoided interrupting movement and prevented the bad effects produced by pressure on the stump, which was left completely free! The "impulse to movement" the inventor secured by a "circular insertion" three fingers from the stump. In other artificial legs the pressure upon the stump prevented perspiration, which, in turn, led to inflammation that forced the user to put the limb aside for days at a time, whereas in that of Muñoz the heat given off by the stump was dissipated through small perforations along the entire length of the leg. The consultants concluded that, though they could not be absolutely sure that Muñoz was not guided by some model, they did think that only two European models had "been known on this continent up to now" and that use had exposed the defects of these. A strong argument for Muñoz was that the creators of other artificial legs were content to hide their secret discoveries, use them as monopolies, and prevent the public from profiting from them.

With his sketch and item-by-item explanation, Muñoz sent in an appeal for a patent, but he was careful to point out that the sketch was made from a leg created for a specific person and for that reason showed only the lower part of the leg. It should not be inferred, therefore, that the leg could not be used for persons with amputation at other places. By same mechanism that produced the movement in the ankle, that of the knee could also be produced, leaving the hip, knee, and foot free for movement. As for the price, Muñoz could not give a round figure. The materials for a leg that included the ankle alone cost twenty pesos and if the knee was included, forty-six pesos, though he asked to be allowed to graduate his price upward if the cost of materials should rise. Disclaiming greed or ostentation and protesting his love of humanity, he promised to sacrifice nothing in making artificial legs for soldiers. To reinforce the idea that he was a benefactor, Muñoz emphasized the cataract operations he had performed among the poor with such "happy results, and at no inconsiderable expense." In view of the favorable opinion of the two surgeons, Fiscal Ambrosio Sagarzurieta advised the viceroy to give Muñoz his patent,[39] provided that the king approve and that no extensions beyond the original term be granted.[40] The general assessor concurred, pointing out that if Muñoz's invention was not absolutely original he had, at least, brought the leg to its greatest degree of perfection.[41] Viceroy Calleja not only granted the ten-year patent but also ordered the concession "published in the papers of this capital."[42] In this whole business the surgeons, whose status had been much improved by the Royal College of Surgery and by the important role of the surgeon in the war going on, supplied the advice that in earlier times the royal protomedicato, speaking for both medicine and surgery, would have supplied.

Control of Epidemic Disease: Paying the Costs

When an epidemic reached the state of a catastrophe, it was no more under control of the doctors than a disastrously defeated army in full flight was under the control of its general. There was, however, an unwritten law plainly stated by the Spanish protomedicato in 1785 that one of the "most sacred institutes" of that tribunal was to watch over whatever disturbed the public health, to see to cure of diseases, and by coming to understand their causes, to prevent their perpetuation.[43] Yet this ideal, rarely expressed by a working protomédico, could hardly be expected to survive in America if it could not in Spain. After all, the members of the protomedicato were practicing physicians without public funds at their disposal and without authority to take official action in an epidemic. Also since this was the moment when their private practice was most needed and their income at its peak, they had no disposition to take charge of combating the epidemic, even if it were a good work that could be listed in their dossier of "merits and service." Besides, only the viceregal government had the means to deal with such disasters as epidemics.

Put a finger down upon the record of any epidemic from the seventeenth century to the cry of independence and the story is the same: the lack of adequate financing to prevent or stop them. Inevitably the responsibility for combating the spread of an epidemic fell to the viceroy or governor, not the medical authorities, and often they used measures that did not demand funds. In 1764 the governor of Cumaná heard that an epidemic in Caracas had wrought "unutterable calamities" for the lack of anybody to care for the multitude of sick people. To prevent the spread of the disease to Cumaná, Governor José de Diguja closed the ports and cut off all communication with the "infested province." When this failed to curb the epidemic, Diguja had to spend money: he set up a hospital to isolate those infected and prevent or slow down the spread of the disease. His measures were so effective that by the end of January 1765 the hospital had released eight hundred patients who were completely well and could return to the city to take care of others. Of the 8,396 who had contracted the disease, 2,005 died. To protect the Indian towns, he set watches on the mountain roads leading to them and allowed passage only to those driving their herds. All corregidores got strict orders that these advance guards allow no outsiders into these native villages and no Indians out.

In the small, infested native towns conditions were always bad. In these places people abandoned their houses, often leaving those suffering from the disease to die. Though there were few Spaniards in these towns, these people evidently threw themselves "with inexpressible charity" into the care of the sick. At the beginning of the epidemic in eastern Venezuela, the Bishop of Puerto Rico came to Barcelona on the coast west of Cumaná to take steps for the pastoral care of the patients, allotting them clerics and religious who had smallpox "to administer the holy Sacraments" and work night and day in the hospital and private houses helping the most needy, even attending to the burial of those who died. In all this the governor had no means beyond the alms collected, some offerings from patients, and two hundred pesos from the city properties (*propios*). Instead of drawing upon the royal exchequer—always the last resort—the governor reserved these funds against the further outbreak of the disease in the Indian towns. Despite the narrowness of the means, the crown contented itself with approving what had been done—without a word to improve financing for either this or the next epidemic.[44]

When the smallpox epidemic suffered in Mexico City in 1779 spread into the Indian parishes of the viceroyalty, the viceregal treasury made no provision whatsoever to relieve them. When the curate of the partido of San Jerónimo de Amanalco made a strong representation to the viceroy about the condition of these parishes, the viceroy instructed the Indian hospital to provide the "medicine and other help necessary" for that district. Casting about for the money to provide the needed medicines, the assessor of the Indian Court (*Juzgado de Indios*) suggested that for San Jerónimo de Amanalco and other needy districts funds be taken from funds that were provided for legal representatives for the Indians (*medio real de indios*). The crown rejected the plan, however, and insisted that the problem be met with the half-real levied on the Indians for support of their Indian hospitals (*medio real del hospital*).[45] About the only relief the natives could hope for was relief from tribute payments, but this usually came after the epidemic had made its crushing sweep through their communities.

Because the objectives of public welfare were left to charity under the Spanish system, meeting a crisis that required charity was always behindhand. Thus, instead of providing government funds in New Spain to combat the smallpox epidemic of 1797 in its early stages, Viceroy Branciforte did the only thing that he could do without risking the king's wrath; he joined other individuals and corporations in making personal contributions after the spread of the disease had terrorized at least some of the authorities and "powerful" inhabitants into a mood of generosity. In a society where honors and preferment raised a man so high, he had to respond with a generosity equal at least to his high preferment in order not to suffer a disgraceful deflation of his prestige. Viceroy Branciforte accordingly donated 4,000 pesos, but Archbishop Alonso Núñez de Haro y Peralta, who headed the committee improvised to deal with the menace to the city, personally gave 12,000 pesos. The ecclesiastical chapter, merchant guild, and mining guild, in turn, responded with 12,000 pesos each. Despite its near constant state of ferment, the cabildo of Mexico City provided 6,000 pesos.[46] One private individual, Francisco de Zúñiga, matched these figures with a donation of 12,000 pesos. The smallest sum accepted from these "powerful subjects" was ten pesos. Also, Branciforte elicited funds from the 181 charitable societies in the eight wards of Mexico City. In all, of the 127,897 pesos collected to deal with the epidemic, the societies provided 52,653 pesos and the corporations and individuals 75,244 pesos.[47] A broadside, printed at the instigation of the viceroy, thanked all those contributing to the relief of the afflicted.[48]

Public Measures to Deal with Smallpox: Isolation and Inoculation

Though the epidemic of 1797 was not as severe as that of 1779, liberal financing was far more essential because Mexicans were trying to curb the epidemic by means of inoculation. In England inoculation had begun in the first quarter of the eighteenth century when Lady Mary Wortley Montagu brought the practice to London from Turkey. Practitioners in the English colonies had used it occasionally during the first half of the eighteenth century, but it was not until the second half that this preventive measure enjoyed sporadic trial in such widely separated places in the Spanish empire as Chile, Guatemala, and Mexico. In Chile during the bitter decimations of the epidemics of 1765 and 1774, Dr. Fray Pedro Manuel de Chaparro, in bitter competition with Dr. Antonio Ríos for the post of protomédico, undertook to inoculate at his own risk. Although the earlier epidemic of 1765 carried off one-third of the Chileans contracting smallpox, in 1774 none of the five hundred people inoculated died. That Chaparro was still inoculating during the epidemics of 1785 and 1789 indicates that his work had been successful, and incidentally, that he preceded those who brought the blessings of this technique to New Spain.[49] In Guatemala José Felipe de Flores, the professor of prima of medicine, had campaigned for inoculation in 1780, and before leaving for Spain in 1796 he was able to boast that of 14,000 persons inoculated in Guatemala, only forty-six had incurred smallpox and died.[50] In Mexico the epidemic of 1797 forced the authorities to endorse inoculation that they had not adopted in the epidemic of 1779 when the terrible fears of the population about the dangers of the new practice, the contentiousness of the doctors, and the quibbling of the protomedicato all worked to stop the widespread use of the vaccine in New Spain.[51] In 1784 the backwardness of Mexico in accepting the new measure was readily apparent when the first volume of the *Gazeta de México* carried an item drawing upon French sources that recommended wearing a shirt dipped in sulfur solution as protection against typhus, smallpox, and measles.[52]

Still, despite the resistance in Mexico to inoculation, there was in the Spanish and Spanish colonial mentality a penchant for accepting inoculation. In the first place there was a confidence in the possibility of the discovery of a remedy, particularly a botanical remedy, for the most devastating disease that kept the minds of the people open to such an extraordinary thing as vaccination. To be sure, most of the "discoveries" brought forward, such as Dr. José de Flores's use of newts to cure cancer or another physician's insistence that the begonia was good for syphilis and scrofula, were silently passed over and left behind. So if the most renowned physicians were caught up in this almost otherworldly hope, acceptance and a willingness to try a new remedy could be expected from the ordinary man.

Even so, it required the cruel stimulus of an epidemic to advance the cause of inoculation, not because of scientific opposition to the principle, but because of a certain fear of the common people that in some parts of the world makes them elude vaccination even today. At the time of the smallpox epidemic of 1779, for example, the city of Mexico published a notice of the opening of a Hospital of Inoculation (*Hospital de Inoculación*) in the Convent of San Hipólito, where the attending surgeon would be a man "practiced and expert in the matter," but at that juncture the public had not been prepared, and there was virtually no response. Other efforts went toward helping people with no access to doctors to care for themselves. In Mexico City the viceroy sponsored an eight-page pamphlet written by Dr. José Ignacio Bartolache on how to recognize and treat smallpox,[53] and the cabildo paid the expenses of publication.

Other large cities of the viceroyalty, such as Puebla, could not expect the same prompt aid from the viceroy and did not even have a formal protomedicato to offer official medical advice. When, therefore, an epidemic really "ravaged" the city, the natural response often came from the bishop, who next to the viceroy himself commanded both the organization and the means to take effective countersteps. During the smallpox epidemic of 1779 Bishop López Gonzalo of Puebla decided to publish a set of instructions for those not prepared to treat this disease.[54] This pamphlet set out the various stages in the development of smallpox in such everyday and graphic language that any person who could read would be able to follow instructions and descriptions, running through the "invasion," the "eruption," "suppuration," and "desiccation." The language was plain enough to enable any nurse to recognize eruptions of "good" (benign) and "bad quality" (malign) eruptions, those showing the eruptions connected at the base and those fatal ones vulgarly called "flat-bottomed boats [*chatas*]," because they did not rise at the center.

Between the smallpox epidemics of 1779 and 1797 in New Spain, Spanish authorities began looking for some means of countering smallpox that aimed at its very extinction. For such a noble purpose they brought together pamphlets, booklets, and broadsides in French, German, and English that put them in an excellent position to recommend measures enjoying the most general approval. In contrast to the French, who were slow and indifferent to inoculation and finally suspended it, the Spaniards showed the same hopefulness and some of the alacrity that marked their quick use of vaccination. Francisco Gil, surgeon of the Royal Monastery of San Lorenzo and member of the Royal Medical Academy of Madrid, prepared the 172-page work[55] that the Minister of the Indies, José de Gálvez, and his associates hoped would point the way to the eventual extinction of this periodic scourge. Gálvez accordingly saw to the publication of this treatise and fired off copies to the Indies, among them a large number to the viceroy of New Spain.[56] By calling upon parish priests and doctors, and anybody else suitable for the purpose, he hoped to persuade the people of America of the great value and negligible risk in the method. Since Gil based his primary proposal—the pest house, the "house in the fields"—upon a vigorous measure enforced in Louisiana by the Conde de Gálvez, the nephew of José de Gálvez, Gil's system was thus a combination of isolation and inoculation. Quarantine alone had been a failure, even when a military cordon was thrown up to break off all intercourse with an infected region. The Indian population was bunched together in villages—highly useful for the purposes of conversion and work, but not suitable for the prevention of the spread of smallpox. Disease could run through a whole village, sometimes leaving it totally bereft of human beings. Because the Indians constituted the work force in New Spain, a severe epidemic among them could paralyze the country, whereas in the English colonies the deadly pest that "cleared the

those suffering from this disease. Provided with daily reports on the increase of the epidemic, the tribunal passed the information on to the viceroy with its advice upon the proper countermeasures—measures that in its judgment stayed the march of this fearful disease.[60]

The isolation method prescribed by Francisco Gil continued to hold sway. In his response to the outbreak of smallpox in the orphanage of Mexico City in the fall of 1790, Viceroy Revilla Gigedo ordered that the method set out in the *Disertación físico-médica . . .* be followed. The corregidor accordingly ordered that all those coming down with the disease be taken to the Hospital de San Antonio,[61] but the measures suggested by the protomedicato and instituted by Viceroy Branciforte in February 1797[62] developed some refinements.[63] They forbade ordinary communication with the "house of isolation" and even required the "fumigation" of letters emanating from there. Of the thirteen points developed in this order, however, the eighth calling for inoculation was the crucial one.

The smallpox epidemic of 1797 brought out still another set of instructions for inoculating against and curing smallpox. The viceroy's imprimatur reveals that this publication was a combination of practices suggested in a report of the protomedicato in Mexico and of information on a successful method laid down by Dr. José Celestino Mutis in New Granada, all severely edited for the purposes of simplicity and clarity. Sometimes the recommendations, as in the emphasis upon keeping the air fresh and the diet bland at critical points, have a curiously modern ring. Lamenting the disposition to multiply remedies and to favor the most severe in proportion to the mortality produced by the disease, they supported the course of assisting nature in the cure of smallpox by inoculation.[64] The actual inoculation would take place between the first and second fingers, where with a lancet or needle the operator would prick the skin, just short of drawing blood—or at least "no more than a drop or two"—and then open a pustule and transfer the pus to the pricked place. Despite the need to immunize the total population, those inoculated had to be carefully chosen. Female children in their menstrual periods, or approaching it, would not be inoculated.

As smallpox in Mexico City reached epidemic proportions in the fall of 1797,[65] the rich and the powerful in the city and neighborhoods began to organize informal groups to combat the disease and to contribute special funds for medicines, inoculations, and doctors. To make the most of these and coordinate their efforts, Viceroy Branciforte appointed a Chief Council of Charity (Junta Principal de Caridad) on October 26, composed of the highest figures in the audiencia, city, and chief corporations to serve under him in combating the crisis.[66] At the head of this junta of distinguished officials, he placed Archbishop Alonso Núñez de Haro y Peralta, a man who had been interim viceroy in 1787 and whose zeal for the well-being of the people had long before fixed their trust in him.[67] He had already justified this confidence by setting up the Hospital de San Andrés to care for those suffering from smallpox and allotting monies for the care of the indigent sick outside the hospital. As head of the junta he put pressure on doctors reluctant to serve those ill with smallpox, collected additional funds to deal with the epidemic, organized the work of those doctors willing to render help, promoted inoculation, and in every way attempted to deal with the epidemic as effectively as possible.[68]

This Junta Principal in no way superseded the royal protomedicato for the very good reason that the protomedicato had never had the authority required to deal with such a crisis. Its members did take a number of responsibilities, however. One of these was the assignment of doctors to care for those who came down with the disease.[69] Members of the protomedicato also met with members of the Junta Principal to make reports on the progress of the epidemic. Charged with making weekly statistical reports, the president of the protomedicato, García Jove, submitted figures not only on deaths from smallpox but also his opinions on whether the disease was increasing or waning and whether or not countermeasures were effective. Although not all his district reporters were faithful in providing their weekly figures, García Jove's weekly summary of November 12, 1797, reported 9,621 cases of smallpox.[70] A week later these had dropped to 6,320 cases. Not a man to show jubilation, García Jove commented that the epidemic had begun to subside.[71] That by December 4 there were only 2,896 ill with smallpox gave him the chance to observe that the capital, in the main, "is free of the whip of the epidemic."[72] A week later the figure had decreased dramatically by over half to only 1,242 cases.[73]

As if uniquely aware of the lessons that systematic compilation of statistics had taught them, the district or ward societies and the Junta Principal de Caridad had the satisfaction of seeing in February 1798 a published summary of their work.[74] They had expended 128,897 pesos. Of this sum, 22,643 pesos went to pay "doctors and barbers," while expenditures for medicines came to 23,553, and food to 45,834. They had assisted 44,516 patients, of whom 4,451 had died.[75] A general statistical table showed only 5,951 deaths among the 56,169 who had contracted the disease.[76]

In 1798 Mexicans thought that the measures for dealing with smallpox suggested in part by the protomedicato and instituted by the

Junta Principal and viceroy, and the more general acceptance of these measures by the public, explained why nearly twice as many of those contracting smallpox died in the 1779 epidemic as in that of 1797. For one thing the public showed a more general acceptance of the epidemiological advances recommended.[77] Acceptance of paramedical help was certainly one of these steps forward. The ward charitable societies, the Junta Principal, even the protomedicato accepted the use of barbers to assist during the epidemic with barbers in all eight districts of the city being paid for their services alongside the physicians.[78] What the viceroyalty needed, evidently, was not a few more physicians who could recite the prognostics of Hippocrates, but a greater number of men trained in the rudiments of medicine such as the admission of the barbers to practice, now shown to be possible. Moreover, though it still sanctioned such nonsense as bonfires, sprinkling vinegar, and fumigating with sulfur, the protomedicato did hit increasingly upon sound advice. The clamor to avoid the resale of the contaminated clothes of smallpox victims enjoyed not only the endorsement of the protomedicato but also the Junta Principal and the viceroy himself.

Support of inoculation by the royal protomedicato, the Junta Principal, and the viceroy also played some role.[79] The Junta Principal de Caridad had not only approved inoculation but also set up places in each of the eight wards for the performance of this operation, although the viceroy made it plain from the beginning that this practice should be voluntary.[80] Schoolmasters and parents could not be forced to present their wards or children for inoculation.[81] Inoculation undoubtedly cut down on the mortality figures, but it is difficult to determine how much. Of those inoculated in Valladolid in Michoacán, only 2.5 percent died, while 15 percent of those getting natural smallpox died.[82] For Mexico City a general table submitted by Superintendent Cosme de Mier showed that between September 10 and October 21, 1797, there were 1,908 cases of natural smallpox and ninety-eight deaths; of the 728 inoculated, only five died. Since inoculation was voluntary, there was a great variation from ward to ward in Mexico City. In Ward One there were 186 inoculations in the house where the prestigious Dr. Luis José Montaña practiced on the street called Puente de Santo Domingo, and 253 in the ward itself for a total of 439. Ward Two had five inoculations during the same period; Ward Three, 75; Four, 134; Five, only three; Six, 53; Seven, ten; and Eight, nine. During the last week of this report, October 14–21, there were only forty-three inoculations listed. Surely, then, an average of a bit over six inoculations a day as the epidemic rose to its height was hardly enough to impede the epidemic substantially.[83]

Vaccination and the Control of Smallpox

During the epidemic in Mexico City in 1797, authorities took a number of measures to control the spread of smallpox and to treat those afflicted, which helped to reduce fatalities and to lift public awareness of ways to treat the dread disease. Inoculation was one of these, and after it was first tried in 1779 had come into more general use, even for the indigent. But inoculation was dangerous and not generally accepted except by the most advanced medical practitioners. Unknown to these enlightened doctors in Mexico City and elsewhere, however, a revolutionary new discovery for controlling smallpox was in the offing. Virtually at the same time the epidemic was raging in Mexico, Edward Jenner was developing his new method of artificial implantation of the living virus of cowpox in order to immunize a person against smallpox.[84] This use of Jennerian vaccination began in earnest in England in the first decade of the nineteenth century and quickly spread to other parts of Europe and America.

In Spanish America adaptation of new techniques, new ideas, and new learning from Europe often took a generation or two to take hold. In the case of Jenner's revolutionary new discovery, however, there was no lag. Throughout the Spanish Indies the enthusiasm for immunization immediately manifested itself, and in Spain authorities without hesitation organized an expedition to bring the vaccine to the entire Hispanic world. Headed by Francisco Xavier de Balmis, this expedition carrying vaccine to America between 1803 and 1807 held out promise of lasting, undiluted glory for its director. Having served as an army doctor in New Spain some two decades before, Balmis envisioned himself as the first to bring the ineffable boon of the vaccine to America. He would impress his old colleagues and neighbors and put proud viceregal governments at his beck and call. And the expedition did immortalize him. "Nothing like it," says one observer, "had ever been attempted by any government, any country, or any man."[85]

The story of the Balmis Expedition has been well told elsewhere,[86] but less well known are the massive public efforts he stimulated to immunize the populace against smallpox. In Mexico these had been started—much to Balmis's surprise and disappointment—even before his arrival with the vaccine in 1804. A year earlier Viceroy José de Iturrigaray, most likely eager to impress his new constituency, had brought the vaccine in his baggage, and upon his arrival in Mexico City had his personal physician, Alejandro Arboleya, perform a vaccination in the presence of the members of the royal protomedicato and Dr. Antonio Serrano, director of the Royal School of Surgery. But sadly, the long voyage had robbed the fluid of its virtue. Later, however, Florencio Pérez

Comoto, the subdelegate of the Mexican protomedicato resident in Vera-cruz, notified Iturrigaray by courier that the vaccine had arrived on the frigates *Anfitrite* and *O,* and the viceroy responded with a summary order to send the fluid on to the capital immediately. It arrived at nine o'clock on April 25, 1804. So precipitately did Iturrigaray now proceed that Dr. Arboleya took as a witness the first physician he could find—Licentiate Joseph María Navarro—and vaccinated five orphans without waiting to locate either the protomédicos or Dr. Serrano. When it was certain that the vaccine had taken, Iturrigaray had his twenty-one-month-old son, Vicente, accompanied by the principal personages of his household, brought in a carriage to the orphanage, where Dr. Arboleya vaccinated him also.[87] By attending the poor orphans first, the viceroy gained credit for charity and humanity, and by bringing his son next, he did much to dispel horror of the new vaccine among the populace.[88]

When Balmis arrived in Mexico—after getting over his shock that the vaccine was already there—he immediately took steps to insure the preservation of the vaccine and stabilization of its production that he believed was the most critical measure needed at that moment. For this purpose he wrote the viceroy, proposing a new Junta Central of sixteen members under the protection of the Superior Government and the archbishop.[89] Eight of these sixteen were to come from honored and distinguished secular or lay persons who had shown the greatest zeal for the public welfare, electing one as president. They would be joined by six distinguished doctors and the senior regidor of the town council and city attorney serving ex officio. Although all would serve without salaries, Balmis provided that the personnel in the junta be changed annually to distribute the sacrifice of time equitably. He proposed that for Mexico City two doctors be named to vaccinate, arranging their schedules in such a way so that each doctor would have only three brief periods of duty each month. When smallpox broke out in a distant town, the Junta Central was to commission a qualified vaccinator to go there; his payment would come from the public funds of the town. The junta was also to see to it that each district had doctors on the lookout for cowpox. With a view to the vaccination of the whole population, the Junta Central required parish priests to cooperate in keeping records of those who were or needed to be vaccinated. He also recommended a "Public House of Vaccination," with a conspicuous sign bearing those words. Such a house, he said, should be clean, cheerful, and centrally located. So that the Junta Central not take total responsibility for vaccination in Mexico, he also believed central juntas should be formed in Puebla, Valladolid, Guadalajara, and Guanajuato. Interestingly, the Junta Central not the protomedicato was the principal promoter of vaccination in Mexico.

In Guatemala a similar junta was created. A royal order called upon the president of Guatemala, after the arrival of Balmis or a member of his expedition, to draw up and put in practice ordinances governing small-pox vaccination in the kingdom.[90] When Balmis himself sent a report to Guatemala from Mérida de Yucatán and Francisco Pastor actually brought the vaccine to Guatemala City, Dr. José Antonio Córdoba, the interim protomédico of Guatemala, drew up an elaborate plan for a Junta Central.[91] The goals of this Junta Central were propagation of the vaccine in the entire kingdom, keeping the vaccine alive with its virtue undiminished, and observation and recording all discoveries resulting from vaccination of possible benefit to the public.

The composition of this junta was a sensible combination of traditional political, ecclesiastical, and medical authorities. It consisted of six members and a secretary. Three of these—the archbishop, regent of the audiencia, and protomédico of the kingdom—were ex officio and perforce perpetual members. Three more members served two-year terms; these were to be elected one from the ecclesiastical chapter, one from the town council, and a third—not the protomédico—from among licensed physicians and surgeons. Elected by the Junta Central, the secretary served in perpetuity. No member might refuse to serve, and none might have salary or any other gratification; the honor was "equal to the importance of the work."

The organization and functioning of the junta reflect both the formality of the times and the seriousness of the vaccination process. The archbishop presided over sessions in his own palace, and when he could not be there, the regent of the audiencia took the gavel, or, in literal terms, the bell. At the outset, until the majority of the people in and around Guatemala City were vaccinated, regular meetings were weekly. Thereafter, they were held at least every fifteen days. Any problem, whether medical or economic, came under review of the junta: correspondence with the provincial juntas was read, commissions were issued, vaccinators named, and methods discussed to achieve "stability" of the vaccine.

The desire to keep abreast of the latest developments in vaccinating against smallpox was both intense and pathetic. The secretary not only had a blank book for the minutes, but he also kept two others—one in which he extracted all private books and papers appearing on the subject outside Guatemala and the other in which he recorded observations within the kingdom itself. Since the success of the vaccinating campaign depended upon keeping complete and accurate records, the secretary of the junta had the obligation of keeping a special book of the statistical tables turned in by each of the persons charged with vaccinating and of combining these for the use of the junta. Every six months the secretary of the junta informed the Superior Government of the number vaccinated and provided a statistical abstract and a summary of its minutes. These were then published in Guatemala City.

Although Dr. Córdoba, the protomédico, and his colleagues on the Junta Central might succeed in vaccinating enough people in and around Guatemala City to curb smallpox, there yet remained not only the other towns and villages in the kingdom but also the three episcopal cities of León in Nicaragua, Comayagua in Honduras, and Ciudad Real (now San Cristóbal de las Casas) in Chiapas. In each of these three the Guatemalan junta resolved to establish a Provincial Committee for Vaccine (*Junta Provincial de Vacuna*). The composition, as far as possible, would be in imitation of the Junta Central, composed of the bishop, the governor-intendant, a member of the ecclesiastical chapter, a member of the town council, and, "if there is one," a practitioner of medicine, and a secretary. Only the bishop and governor-intendant were ex officio and permanent. Since there was no town council in Comayagua to supply a member as in Guatemala City, the junta was expected to elect an honorable, respected, and propertied inhabitant or a secular priest not charged "with the cure of souls." Plainly recognizing the all but absolute lack of examined doctors in the kingdom outside Guatemala City, the Junta Central was called upon to name a specific vaccinator in each of these three places. As in nearly all colonial institutions, the secretary was the man who kept the juntas functioning. In the capital he conducted the correspondence with the provincial juntas, which kept the capital informed of every step to vaccinate the population and to keep the "fluid" alive. In all these matters the local juntas were subject to the orders of the central organization in Guatemala City.

When the vaccine reached Guatemala City, the royal protomedicato under the direction of Dr. Córdoba began weekly vaccinations to insure that somebody would be carrying the live virus at all times. The practice of weekly vaccinations was thus incorporated in the rules governing the Junta Central. In order to be thorough about this procedure, the rules of the Junta Central required the justice of the peace in each ward (*alcalde de barrio*) to form within two months a roll of the inhabitants, uniform in all the wards, listing clearly those in each house who had been vaccinated and those who had not. To avoid fraud and deception by a fearful population, a priest named by the archbishop would accompany the alcalde to inspire confidence, to instruct the people on the purpose of vaccination, and to disabuse them of the false ideas that always flew ahead of the vaccinator.

To carry out and conclude the actual vaccination, some extraordinary decisions were necessary. First, whereas the old-style inoculations had always been voluntary, compulsory vaccination of the entire population became so urgent it could not wait for the completion of the rolls being drawn up by the justices of the peace. It thus fell to the Junta Central to name a vaccinator and assistant commissioner for each ward to proceed from house to house vaccinating, keeping exact records of their progress, and making a follow-up visit to see how this work had turned out. All the vaccinators in the city were to be doctors or to have the approval of the protomedicato. Far from being persons just able to hand instruments to the operator, assistants were priests, aldermen, or well-to-do citizens. From these responsibilities the protomedicato might exempt no one, not even members of the junta—except, of course, the secretary. The name of any person refusing vaccination was turned over to the regent of the royal audiencia for prosecution. When the work in a ward was complete, the vaccinator submitted a report to the Junta Central showing not just those vaccinated, but those for whom vaccination was postponed and those in whom it did not take.

If it took Mexico until this century (1951) after some thirty years under a very public-health-minded government to eliminate smallpox,[92] the fight against the disease in Guatemala a century and a half earlier in 1805 faced the same problems. To "extinguish" smallpox, or even to aspire to do so, required that vaccination be carried out immediately and as systematically as possible in all towns. Once outside Guatemala City, assistance of churchmen became increasingly necessary. The archbishop thus ordered all curates, either themselves or through Indian chiefs or mestizo mayors, to draw up a list of those who were medically qualified for vaccination. These people then came to the capital for vaccination and returned immediately, accompanied by the alcalde, regidor, or some other person. Once back home in their native towns, the curate kept an eye upon those vaccinated, listing any upon whom the vaccination did not take, those that were false, or those having any special peculiarity. In case nothing untoward happened at the end of two weeks, these priests submitted their statistical reports to the commissioner appointed in the district. Such information went to the Junta Central just as it did in the capital.

Special commissioners undertook to vaccinate the people in the remoter provinces. Approved by the Superior Government, these men worked according to instructions supplied by the protomedicato. Their records went both to the protomedicato and to the provincial junta. The procedure in these places, insofar as possible, followed the routine in the capital, but the provincial juntas, once they were established, could decide what rules were not adaptable in their territories.

The aim of the Guatemalan authorities was to perpetuate the vaccine and keep it at a dependable level. Despite all the talk of vaccinating cows, sheep, and mules, arm-to-arm vaccinations at the proper intervals and on a competent number of people were the methods these people had to depend upon. The junta therefore had to begin with a list of those unvaccinated—those exempted in the first round and the priest's list of those still under five—in order to decide how many should be vaccinated in each district and at what intervals. This served two purposes: immunization of those vaccinated and the regular and dependable perpetuation of the vaccine. In consequence, vaccinating everybody at one time in a given place was forbidden.

The commissioner from the municipal council was responsible for maintaining the lists of those vaccinated in the campaign that followed the arrival of the Balmis vaccine. It was therefore necessary for private families, when they had a doctor in to vaccinate them, to keep the commissioner informed so that he could maintain the proper proportion of vaccinations. Any person who appeared voluntarily to be vaccinated was advanced in the line ahead of those there under compulsion. Outside Guatemala City, in particular, when a general vaccination took place, the priest was as conspicuous as the operator and the Indian musicians, who by special decree, played the same music that marked their other solemn ceremonies.

If, despite these precautions, the live vaccine was lost, the local junta appointed two persons to go to the closest place where the "fluid" was alive and to return, both vaccinated. The regulations required that in such cases a report be made promptly to the Junta Central in Guatemala City. In those hamlets, especially small or remote ones where the chances of keeping the vaccine going were slight, the Junta Central dispatched the vaccine arm-to-arm from the closest town. If it were lost in the capital, the junta brought it from the closest source. No village, no matter how small, might go more than five years without a general vaccination. Under such rules, if the juntas were alert and vigilant, it was logical to hope that the vaccine might be preserved indefinitely and smallpox stamped out.

No matter how great had been the horrors of epidemics, vaccination, one of the great miracles of medicine, could not stand alone; it required both propaganda and compulsion. These came first from the priest and then from Spanish judges. Copies of the *Reglamento* drawn up and printed in Guatemala and the treatise by Moreau de la Sarthe,[93] either a complete printing or a simplified extract of it, were placed in the hands of all Guatemalan curates and judges in order that they might "comply with religious scrupulosity to the charges which have been vested in them." Specifically, it was "the obligation of the curates to explain to their parishioners from the pulpit and even in chats "the marvelous efficacy of the vaccine fluid" to immunize "against pestilential smallpox." Thus, the blame for delay and obstruction fell heaviest upon the shoulders of the curates and judges. If they did not perform properly, the diocesan prelates and the Superior Government saw to it that they did. Nothing had more weight in the list of "merits and services" upon which promotion and honors depended than a good record in enforcing vaccination.

After the first round in this tremendous effort of 1805, vaccination in Guatemala City was confined to the hospital in a room set aside for this purpose. Only licensed practitioners had the authority to sanction vaccinations in private houses. Outside the capital the permanent organization being set up required that, before withdrawing, district commissioners should teach the techniques of vaccination in all main towns of the parish, preferring Spaniards of good reputation, education, and public spirit to do this. In exclusively Indian towns the vaccinator was required to teach his skill to the schoolmaster. The provincial junta would then issue a printed certificate of appointment to one or more vaccinators for the towns and no more than one for each Indian parish town. No one else might then vaccinate in his district without his consent. Since the medical profession had to be represented in the juntas, both provincial and local, the vaccinator took his post where there was no legal practitioner of medicine. In case there were two vaccinators and neither was a doctor, the junta selected one of the two to participate in discussions and vote in its sessions.

A similar Junta Central was established in Caracas to promote vaccination,[94] but in other areas of the Indies both governmental and private individuals were responsible for introducing the vaccine when it became available. In New Spain, for example, when the vaccine brought in by Balmis reached San Luis Potosí, the bearer found that six months before it had been put in use by Dr. Pedro de Puglia, a Swiss physician practicing there. In faraway Chile before the arrival of Balmis, the captain general commissioned Dr. José Antonio Ríos, the protomédico, and Dr. Pedro Manuel Chaparro to propagate the "fluid" and vaccinate the populace. With the assistance of the town council, they began vaccinating free of charge all those called in by means of public placards posted in Santiago announcing the service. In Chile, instead of transferring and keeping the vaccine alive in the arm of a vaccinated person, they claimed that by dissolving the scab in water, it lasted months without losing its virtue. Hence, the vaccine jumped from Santiago to the other important towns of Chile where salaried surgeons vaccinated gratis.[95] In 1805, the year before the South American branch of the Balmis expedition reached Lima, Dr. Pedro Belomo, chief surgeon of the naval base at Callao, with vaccine brought from Buenos Aires, succeeded in raising such an imposing and welcome pimple upon a Limeño boy that the event brought out the viceroy and the town council to give thanks to the Almighty.[96]

How much effect did these efforts have in foiling the deadly march of the next smallpox epidemic? Could the flurry of activity created by the coming of the Balmis expedition to Spanish America curb the dread disease? A summary of the innumerable documents on the expeditions made for the government at Cádiz show that as the branches of the expedition passed along, they had vaccinated 439,289 persons by the end of 1805.[97] But the number was far greater. For Mexico, where the expedition and the Junta Central had worked long and hard, only 12,744 were listed as being vaccinated in Puebla with no one else noted down in any other area of Mexico. For Peru, where Balmis was just getting started, only 22,000 were set down as having received the vaccine, and these only in some northern towns. Activity in such centers as Lima, Arequipa, and Cuzco was not listed. Also since the figure for Guatemala reached 200,000, the numbers vaccinated in Mexico and Peru surely should have been much higher. Even so, within a year and a half or two years (1803–5), more than 440,000 had been immunized. Under the tutelage of overseas experts with the latest scientific directives in their hands, the general populace had started with a flourish upon that long, long process of education that was not to be complete until the twentieth century. With the vaccine established, however, there was no reason beyond sloth and neglect why epidemics should not now be controlled if not prevented altogether.

As noted, the creation of a new and unprecedented movement to disseminate and preserve the vaccine in America was an exuberant response to the most extraordinary situation in the history of medicine in Spanish America. The pattern was dictated in great part by Balmis and his agents and by the enlightened figures in the juntas centrales and in political office who promoted vaccination throughout the Indies. As might be expected, however, when the sense of urgency faded away and the initial enthusiasm waned, vaccinating juntas, both provincial and local, died out. Sometimes the vaccine itself was lost. In fact, when Balmis returned to New Spain later in the decade, he attempted to insure the continuation of the vaccination process and methods to keep the vaccine alive, also for financing the operations, clear evidence that the initial fervor had died.[98] Still, by any standard, despite this loss of enthusiasm and the later neglect and failure to maintain the impetus Balmis had provided, the most massive public health effort ever launched in the Spanish Indies had turned out to be an unqualified success.

In all this what was the role of the protomedicato? Since the anti-smallpox movement had to be permanent, why did not the government in Spain entrust this effort to a medical organization that had been in existence for centuries in both Spain and the colonies? Why was it handed over to Balmis? For one thing, Balmis lived in an epoch in which the protomedicato in Spain was being periodically abolished and then restored. But even if the protomedicato had never come under this shadow, Balmis's personal ambition and quest for historical immortality was enough to make him the key figure. For another, to repeat once again, the protomedicato had no funds and no possibility of management of the vaccination process on the scale called for after Jenner's discovery. Even the viceregal government was not really adequate to this undertaking. Besides, the protomedicato seldom sought a role that it knew it could not properly play. In the end, it was the highest civil and ecclesiastical authorities who interrupted their own work to deal with public medical and sanitary questions for which they were fitted only because they had power and controlled money, good enough reasons for virtually any emergency. The protomedicato thus functioned not as officers with prime authority in medical matters and emergencies, but as mere consultants.

❧ *Glossary*

Abandono. Neglect.

Acenso. Promotion.

Acuerdo. Agreement, usually of a viceroy and the *audiencia* resulting in a vice-regal ban.

Alcalde de barrio. Ward leader or supervisor.

Alcalde de cuartel. Ward magistrate.

Alcalde mayor. Mayor of a town or city, also chief administrator of an *alcaldía mayor.*

Alcalde mayor examinador. Chief examiner.

Alcalde ordinario. Alderman of a city council.

Alférez real. Ensign, standard bearer, community official.

Alguacil. Constable or sheriff.

Alguacil mayor. Bailiff.

Ama. Nurse.

Ama de confianza. Nurse or confidant sworn to secrecy.

Amanuense. Scribe.

Aprobado. Passed, approved as in an examination.

Arbitrariedad. Arbitrary or illegal act.

Asesor letrado. Legal assistant.

Audiencia. High court of appeals, also an advisory council to viceroys and governors.

Auditor de guerra. Literally auditor of war, a high-placed royal or viceregal lawyer and adviser.

Auto de aprobación. Act of certification.

Auxiliatoria. Order of compliance.

Avería. Convoy tax on overseas trade.

Ayuntamiento. City council, city hall.

Barbero. Barber, bleeder.

Bachiller. Holder of a bachelor's degree.

Battalón fijo. Regular battalion garrison.

Boticario. Licensed pharmacist.

Boticario mayor. Chief pharmacist.

Bubas. Buboes.

Cabildo. City council or town council.

Cámara. Room, executive committee.

Casa de Contratación. House of Trade.

Casa de expósitos. Orphanage.

Cátedra. Proprietary chair at a university.

Catedrático. Holder of a proprietary chair at a university.

Cédula. Royal order-in-council.

Celosia. Latticework screen, a symbol used by phlebotomists for their shops.

Censo. Money deposited in trust paying a fixed annual interest, usually five percent.

Censuras. Censures, usually by the Inquisition.

Chino. Cross between an Indian and an Indian-Black mixed blood (*lobo*).

Chino moreno. Brownish *chino*.

Cirujano mayor. Chief surgeon.

Claustro. University cloister made up of university professors and holders of higher degrees in the university city.

Comadre. Midwife.

Composición. Obligatory monetary assessment placed on foreigners, free mulattoes and blacks, land sales, etc.

Compuesto. Legal recognition as a proper immigrant, usually acquired for a fee payment.

Concurso. Assemblage.

Conjuez. Associate judge.

Consulta. Written opinion of a full royal council such as the Council of the Indies, sent to the king to help resolve a problem at issue.

Consultor. Consultant.

Convictorio. Jesuit college.

Corregidor. Chief royal administrator in a province (*corregimiento*).

Corregimiento. A province governed by a *corregidor*.

Cortina. Curtain, screen.

Corto. Poor (in examinations).

Curandero. Literally curer, illegal practitioner of medicine, quack.

Decano. Dean, senior man.

Despacho auxiliatorio. Official approval by a royal council.

Diputado. Deputy, inspector.

Ducado. Ducat, usually valued at 375 *maravedís*.

Ensalmador. Enchanter.

Escribano. Notary public.

Escritura. Deed.

Escudo. A unit of currency of one *peso* of eight *reales* in Cuba.

Especiero. Dealer in drugs and aromatic spices.

Espurio. Bastard, child of an unknown father.

Estudio general. A university that offered degrees in the major faculties of theology, law, canon law, and medicine.

Expediente. File of papers on a specific subject.

Factor de las boticas. Drug buyer.

Facultativo. Faculty member.

Familiar. Lay member of the Inquisition.

Fiel executor. Inspector of weights and measures.

Fiscal. Crown attorney.

Fiscal de lo civil. Legal adviser of the civil *sala* of the *audiencia.*

Fuero. Special privilege.

Fuero militar. Special privilege accorded to a member of the military.

Gazeta. Gazette, newspaper.

Gracias al sacar. Royal certificate granting a privilege or exemption, usually obtained by payment of a fee.

Grado de indulto. University degree sold for a fee.

Guardafaroleros. Keepers of the streetlights.

Hernista. Surgeon specializing in hernias.

Hoja de archivo. Archival cover sheet.

Información de limpieza. Proof of blood purity.

Informe. Report.

Imundicia. Excrement and garbage.

Intruso. Literally intruder, quack.

Jubilación. Retirement.

Jubilado. Retired, superannuated.

Juez conservador. Legal judge of a hospital.

Juez de competencia. Arbiter in a conflict of jurisdiction.

Juez de residencia. Judge conducting a judicial review of an official's tenure in office.

Juez en torno. Literally judge taking a turn; in Mexico a judge of the royal *audiencia* appointed annually to sit with the royal *protomedicato* as legal representative.

Juez privativo. Judicial protector.

Junta. Temporary governing committee.

Junta de guerra. Council of war.

Junta de policía. Sanitary commission.

Justicia. Magistrate, justice.

Juzgado de Indios. Indian court.

Lagartijas. Newts.

Licenciado. Licentiate, holder of a master's degree.

Limpieza de sangre. Purity of blood.

Llagas. Generic term for sores of all sorts.

Lobo. Cross between an Indian and a Black.

Maestrescuela. Member of the cathedral chapter with royal and pontifical authority to confer higher degrees and to validate documents looking toward the incorporation of degrees in the university, chancellor.

Maestro mayor. Master builder.

Maravedí. A basic Spanish unit of money and account.

Matlazahuatl. Disease in Mexico with symptoms resembling those of typhus.

Matrona. Midwife.

Mayordomo. Superintendent, overseer.

Media anata. A tax of one half of the first year's salary levied on all Spanish officials.

Médico. Licensed doctor.

Médico primero. Chief doctor.

Medio real de indios. Half-*real* tax paid by Indian tributaries to support their legal protector.

Medio real de hospitales. Half-*real* tax paid by Indian tributaries to support hospitals for Indians.

Mestizo. Cross between white and Indian.

Ministro executor. Agent of the court, bailiff.

Montepío. Pension.

Montepío militar. Pension for a military person.

Naturas. Sores.

Niguas. Chigger fleas.

Noche fúnebre. Literally funeral night, the night of an examination for a licentiate.

Oficial mayor. Public official.

Oidor. Civil judge of a royal *audiencia*.

Oidor doctor. Doctor of laws sitting on the royal *audiencia* as a civil judge.

Opiata. Drug or herb preparation.

Oposición. Trial lecture and competition for a university chair.

Opositor. One who competes in an *oposición*.

Papel sellado. Stamped legal paper.

Pardo. Mulatto (in a military context).

Partera. Midwife.

Partido. District.

Pasante. University student filling a residence requirement.

Pasantía. Required student residence time at the university.

Pase. Written permit.

Peña de cámara. Court fine.

Périto. Expert.

Peso. Coin valued at eight *reales* or 272 *maravedís* in the Indies. (See also *peso fuerte.*)

Peso fuerte. A Spanish American coin of eight *reales* or 272 *maravedís*, as distinguished from a Spanish *peso de vellón* of fifteen or twenty *reales*.

Pobre de solemnidad. Destitute.

Plazas sencillas. Simples.

Practicante. Intern.

Prima de medicina. First chair of medicine in the university.

Procurador. Agent.

Procurador general. Chief city attorney.

Procurador mayor. Chief attorney.

Promotor fiscal. Prosecuting attorney.

Propinas. Gratuities, tips.

Propio. City property, tax on city property.

Protobarbero. Expert examiner in phlebotomy.

Protoboticario. Expert examiner in pharmacy.

Protocirujano. Expert examiner in surgery.

Protofarmacéutico. Expert examiner in pharmacy.

Protoflebotomiano. Expert examiner in phlebotomy.

Protomedicato. A board usually composed of three doctors to examine and license physicians, surgeons, and other practitioners and to perform other administrative, judicial, and scientific duties related to medical practice.

Protomédico. Medical examiner, member of the board of medical examiners.

Protomédico general. Official appointed to oversee medical research and medical examinations in the Spanish Indies prior to 1646 when the *protomedicato* was established.

Provisor. Ecclesiastical judge to whom a bishop delegated legal authority.

Purga. Purge.

Puro adulterino. Total bastard.

Rapista. Unlicensed practitioners of medicine.

Real. Royal; also one-eighth of a peso valued at 34 *maravedís*.

Realtor. Clerk of court, reporter.

Recipiente. Sewer.

Recopilación. Compilation or compendium, usually of laws.

Regente. Regent, high official of the royal *audiencia* whose function was to expedite the work of the *audiencia*.

Regidor. Town councilman, alderman.

Relación de méritos. Vitae.

Reprobado. Failed, as in an examination.

Romancistas. Licensed surgeons taking their training by apprenticeship rather than at the university, contrasted with Latin surgeons who were university trained and knew Latin.

Rúbrica. Sign or initials, official signature.

Ruego y encargo. Writ of mandamus.

Sala. Room or section as in the criminal and civil sections of the royal *audiencia*.

Señoría. Lordship.

Síndico procurador. Official chosen or elected by a group or village to look after its interests.

Sin réplica. Without reply, usually ordered by the king to insure prompt enforcement of royal law.

Situado. Military subsidy.

Sobresaliente. Outstanding, as in an examination.

Solar. House lot.

Solimán. Corrosive sublimate, mercuric chloride.

Sub-delegación. Subcommission.

Sub-delegado. Subdelegate, subcommissioner.

Sumaria. Deposition in the preparatory process of a legal case.

Supernumerario. Extra official appointed to fill a future opening in a post, usually granted for a fee.

Suplente. Substitute.

Tabardillo. Typhoid.

Terna. List of three submitted for nomination to a civil or clerical office.

Tierras, solares, e caballerías. Real property.

Título de grado. Diploma.

Tostón. One-half peso.

Tratamiento. Treatment, mode of address.

Tribunal de Cuentas. Tribunal of Accounts, auditing bureau.

Tribunal facultativo. Faculty tribunal.

Vecino. Citizen, freeman, legal white resident.

Vellón. Spanish currency, usually copper or some alloy, not of pure gold or silver as the coins minted in the Indies.

Visita. Inspection.

Visita de sanidad. Ship inspection by a licensed doctor.

Visitador. Inspector.

Visitador médico. Medical inspector.

Vísperas. Literally vespers, second chair of medicine in a university.

Zambo. Afro-Indian mixed blood.

ACB.	Archivo Colonial, Bogotá, Colombia.
AEAM.	Archivo del Ex-Ayuntamiento de México, Mexico City, Mexico.
AGG.	Archivo General de Gobierno, Guatemala City, Guatemala.
AGI.	Archivo General de Indias, Sevilla, Spain.
AGNC.	Archivo General de la Nación, Caracas, Venezuela.
AGNM.	Archivo General de la Nación Mexicana, Mexico City, Mexico.
AHFM.	Archivo Histórico de la Facultad de Medicina de la Universidad de México, Mexico City, Mexico.
AHIAH.	Archivo Histórico del Instituto Nacional de Antropología e Historia, Mexico City, Mexico.
AHNB.	Archivo Histórico Nacional, Bogotá, Colombia.
AHNM.	Archivo Histórico Nacional, Madrid, Spain.
ARAQ.	Archivo de la Real Audiencia de Quito, Quito, Ecuador.
BNB.	Biblioteca Nacional, Bogotá, Colombia.
BNP.	Biblioteca Nacional, Lima, Peru.
s.f.	*sin fecha* (no date listed).
s.l.	*sin lugar* (no place listed).
S.M.	*Su Majestad* (Your Majesty).
s.p.	*sin pagina* (no page number).

❧ Notes

Editor's Preface and Acknowledgments

1. *The Diplomatic History of Georgia: A Study of the Epoch of Jenkins' Ear* (Chapel Hill, 1936); *The Spanish Missions of Georgia* (Chapel Hill, 1935).
2. *Dr. Narciso Esparragosa y Gallardo: Varón ilustre de Venezuela* (Caracas, 1953).
3. The protomedicato was a board, usually composed of three *protomédicos* or licensed medical examiners, appointed by the king to examine and license physicians, surgeons, phlebotomists, etc., and to perform other administrative, judicial, and scientific duties. In the Indies the protomedicato was first established in 1646 in Lima and Mexico City.
4. "The Illicit Practice of Medicine in the Spanish Empire in America," in George P. Hammond and Ernest J. Burrus, eds., *Homenaje a José María de la Peña y Cámara* (Madrid, 1969): 141–79; and "Legitimacy and *Limpieza de Sangre* in the Practice of Medicine in the Spanish Empire," *Jahrbuch für Geschichte von Staat, Wirtschaft und Gesellschaft Lateinamerikas* 4 (1967): 37–60.

Author's Preface

1. *Anuario de Estudios Americanos*, III (1946): 1040–46. (Hereinafter Schäfer, "Los Protomedicatos en Indias.")
2. Archivo General de Indias, Sevilla (hereinafter AGI), Buenos Aires, 335.
3. *Historia de la medicina peruana*, 3 vols. (Lima, 1951); *La medicina en el virreinato*, II, 60. (Hereinafter Lastres, *La medicina en el virreinato*.)
4. AGI, México, 2260. D. Silvestre Collar a D. Antonio Porcel, Madrid, 13 de abril de 1803.
5. Ibid., 2260. D. Antonio Porcel a D. Silvestre Collar, Madrid, 24 de mayo de 1803.
6. In minor and local crises, and sometimes in major and general ones, the town council was among the first to feel concern and act upon it.
7. Donald B. Cooper, *Epidemic Disease in Mexico City, 1761–1813: An Administrative, Social and Medical Study* (Austin, 1965). (Hereinafter Cooper, *Epidemic Disease*.)

1. *The King's Physicians Follow Columbus*

1. Aníbal Ruiz Moreno, *La medicina en la legislación medioeval española* (Buenos Aires, 1946), p. 188ff, 197–202. (Hereinafter Ruiz Moreno, *La medicina.*)

2. In Spanish terms, the archiater was the "Physician of the King's Bedchamber," and when he assumed municipal duties, he was more like the protomédico in Spanish and American towns before the creation of the tribunal of the protomedicato.

3. Miguel Eugenio Muñoz, ed., *Recopilación de las leyes, pragmáticas, reales decretos, y acuerdos del Real Proto-Medicato* (Valencia, 1751), Cap. II, Art. 1, pp. 32–33. (Hereinafter Muñoz, *Recopilación.*)

4. Ibid., Cap. II, Art. I, p. 34, gives examples of.the emperor's deference to the rulings of the archiaters.

5. Ibid., Cap. II, Art. I, pp. 32–36.

6. For the various Spanish codes of this epoch, see Ruiz Moreno, *La medicina,* pp. 21–29.

7. Schäfer, "Los Protomedicatos en Indias," p. 1040.

8. Ibid.; see also Lastres, *La medicina en el virreinato,* II:56.

9. Ricardo Benavente Garcés, *El protomedicato en Chile* (Santiago de Chile, 1928), p. 15. (Hereinafter Benavente Garcés, *El protomedicato en Chile.*)

10. Ruiz Moreno, *La medicina,* pp. 24–25.

11. Muñoz, *Recopilación,* pp. 37–38.

12. Ruiz Moreno, *La medicina,* pp. 24–29, offers convincing citations.

13. *Fuero juzgo,* Libro XI, Ley VI (antigua), cited in Ruiz Moreno, *La medicina,* p. 30. This principle was also incorporated in the *Siete partidas,* Partida 7, Tít. 15, Ley 9, and included in Muñoz, *Recopilación,* Cap. XIII, Art. VIII, p. 165.

14. *Las siete partidas del sabio rey, Don Alfonso el IX* . . . , 4 vols. (Barcelona, 1843–44). (Hereinafter *Siete partidas.*) Partida 2, Tít. 9, Ley 10. This famous code, drawn up as a model, was not put into force until 1348.

15. Ibid., Partida 7, Tít. 8, Ley 6; Muñoz, *Recopilación,* Cap. XIII, Art. VIII, p. 164.

16. Antonio Hernández Morejón, *Historia bibliográfica de la medicina española,* 7 vols. (Madrid, 1842–52), VI:346–47. (Hereinafter Hernández Morejón, *Historia bibliográfica.*)

17. The medical legislation of this reign, notably the ordinances of 1477, 1491, and 1498, came into the permanent Spanish code. *Nueva recopilación (Recopilación de las leyes destos reynos* . . .), 3 vols. (Madrid, 1640), Lib. III, Tít. VI, Ley 1. (Hereinafter *Nueva recopilación); Muñoz, Recopilación,* Cap. II, Arts. III, IV, pp. 39–50.

18. *Nueva recopilación,* Lib. III, Tít. XVI, Ley 1, Art. 3; Muñoz, *Recopilación,* Cap. XVII, Art. I, p. 317.

19. "hacer justicia en sus personas, y bienes por los tales crimenes, y delitos. . . ." Muñoz, *Recopilación,* Cap. XVII, Art. II, p. 318.

20. Ibid., Cap. XVII, Art. III, pp. 319–20.
21. Hernández Morejón complains that Miguel Eugenio Muñoz did not give the names of the members of this board, which, after *"esquisitas diligencias,"* he himself did supply (*Historia bibliográfica,* I:256). Of course, Muñoz, working in the middle of the eighteenth century, much of the time no doubt in Valencia, would have had to resort to the same "exquisite" and painstaking search that Hernández Morejón was so proud of.
22. *Nueva recopilación,* Lib. I, Tít. VII, Ley 14; Muñoz, *Recopilación,* Cap. IX, Art. II, III, pp. 120–21.
23. Muñoz, *Recopilación,* Cap. IX, Art. IV, pp. 121–22.
24. Thomas W. Palmer, Jr., *Guide to the Law and Legal Literature of Spain* (Washington, D.C., 1913), p. 35. For an example of the perplexity this situation might cause in the colonies as late as the eighteenth century, see John Tate Lanning, *The Eighteenth-Century Enlightenment in the University of San Carlos de Guatemala* (Ithaca, N.Y., 1956), p. 107. (Hereinafter Lanning, *The Eighteenth-Century Enlightenment.*)
25. Sebastián del Castillo, in his "Aprobación," put the case, no doubt, as he had heard it from his friend Muñoz: "Mas como las Pragmáticas, Decretos, y Leyes pertenecientes a este importante primario objeto de la salud pública, ley entre todas la suprema, que divulgadas en diversos tiempos, se hallavan confussamente comprehendidas entre los difusos cuerpos de nuestro patrio derecho, eran muchas, sobre muy antiguas; y no era menos, ni en el número, ni en el aprecio las posteriores Reales providencias, que sin colación fixa andavan separadas, y dispersas, por averlas hecho assí precisas la mutación de los tiempos." Muñoz, *Recopilación,* Aprobación, s.p.
26. Ibid., Advertensias, s.p. The Cuaderno of the Mesta was the legal guide to regulations of the sheep-raisers' guild.
27. Ibid., Cap. XIII, Arts. I–IX, pp. 158–69.
28. Ibid., Cap. XXII, Arts. I–III, pp. 368–74.
29. "Este médico sevillano [Dr. Chanca] fué el primero que echo una mirada de observación sobre la naturaleza, producciones y costumbres de aquel país. . . ." Hernández Morejón, *Historia bibliográfica,* II:198.
30. For the entire text of this letter, see Martín Fernández de Navarrete, *Colección de los viages y descubrimientos que hicieron por mar los españoles desde fines del siglo XV . . . ,* 5 vols. (Madrid, 1825–37), I:347–72.
31. AGI, Indiferente General, 418. Real cédula al Almirante D. Cristóbal Colón y a D. Juan de Fonseca, obispo de Badajoz, Medina del Campo. s.l., s.f., 1497.
32. Ibid., 418. Real cédula para que el Bachiller Gonzalo Velloso sea cirujano en la Española y la señalen de repartimiento 100 indios, Sevilla, 6 de junio de 1511.
33. Ibid., 419. Real cédula al licenciado Figueroa en favor del Bachiller Velosa, Zaragoza, 29 de octubre de 1519. The internal evidence strongly indicates that Velloso and Velosa were the same individual. In the text of this document Velloso is dubbed "licentiate," but the title of the cédula refers to him as "Bachiller Velosa." Even so, extracurricular promotion from degree to degree was natural and even common in the early settlements.

34. Fray Luis de Figueroa, Fray Alonso de Santo Domingo, and Fray Bartolomé de Manzanedo.

35. Ibid., 419. Real cédula para que el licenciado Barreda, médico, tenga 50,000 maravedís de salario por médico de la isla Española, Madrid, 22 de julio de 1517. Schäfer says that Barreda "or Barrena" remained on the island where he died just before 1540. Schäfer, "Los Protomedicatos en Indias," p. 1042.

36. Benavente Garcés, El protomedicato en Chile, p. 37.

37. Schäfer, "Los Protomedicatos en Indias," p. 1041. Schäfer names "Dr. Torbissimis" as the other protomédico.

38. For the respect accorded the ensalmador in the sixteenth century, see John Tate Lanning, Pedro de la Torre: Doctor to Conquerors (Baton Rouge, La., 1974), pp. 49, 50, 96–97. (Hereinafter Lanning, Pedro de la Torre.)

39. AGI, Indiferente General, 420. Real cédula al licenciado Rodrigo Figueroa para que los protomédicos y boticarios no usen de sus oficios, Barcelona, 26 de julio de 1519.

40. Schäfer, "Los Protomedicatos en Indias," p. 1042.

41. Actas de cabildo del ayuntamiento de México, 54 vols. (México, 1889–1916), I, 115. Cabildo de 11 de enero de 1527. (Hereinafter Actas de cabildo de México.)

42. It was not this Pero López but another Pedro López who, at a much later date, founded the famous Hospital de los Desamparados in Mexico City.

43. Lastres, La medicina en el virreinato, II:57–58.

2. The Municipal Protomedicato

1. J. García Icazbalceta, Obras de D. J. García Icazbalceta, 10 vols. (México, 1896–99), I:86, citing Bernal Díaz del Castillo, Historia verdadera de la conquista de la Nueva España, caps. 174, 183. (Hereinafter García Icazbalceta, Obras.)

2. Ibid., I:86–87.

3. The phrase was "syn amor ni desamor."

4. Actas de cabildo de México, I:115. Cabildo de 11 de enero de 1527. His appearance before the council on January 8, as some historians have it, would have made this action on January 11 unnecessary, and as there was no meeting on January 8, a feat distinctly magical.

5. See chap. 1, pp. 21–22.

6. On August 8, 1533, the cabildo appointed "Licentiates Barreda and Alcázar" to examine the apothecary Alonso Núñez, "there being no protomédicos to examine him." Actas de cabildo de México, III:49.

7. Schäfer, "Los Protomedicatos en Indias," p. 1042, says that Barreda died in Española just before 1540. This position, however, does not mean absolutely that Barreda did not accompany López to Mexico, where nearly everybody with ambition and prospects was going, and return to the island to die. As Schäfer attributed the founding of the Hospital de Desemparados in Mexico City to this Pero López—an event that took place at least thirty-two years after

his death—there is no reason to assume that, moving with such a broad sweep as he did move, he was not also wrong about Barreda. Francisco A. Flores, *Historia de la medicina en México desde la época de los indios hasta la presente,* 3 vols. (México, 1868–88), II:168, suggests from a dubious source that Barreda appeared at the cabildo of January 8, 1527, to be sworn in as the first protomédico in Mexico, but does not explain the difficulty that no meeting was held on that day. The phrase "in substitution for Licenciate Barreda," which would suggest Barreda's physical presence and priority as protomédico, can be explained by López's use of papers issued to him and Barreda by the Spanish protomédicos some eight years before. Besides all this, most experienced paleographers cannot be sure that what is in the record as Barreda was not Barrera or Herrera. (Hereinafter Flores, *La historia de medicina en México.*)

8. See n. 1, p. 4, *Actas de cabildo de México,* III:49. Cabildo de 8 de agosto de 1533.

9. Ibid., IV:31. Cabildo de 4 de agosto de 1536. As set out in 1563, the duties of these protomédicos—"like those in Spain"—were "to inspect apothecary shops and medicines, examine persons who wish to qualify as physicians, surgeons, barbers, apothecaries, midwives [*comadres, parteras*], and dealers in spices and aromatic drugs." Ibid., VII:103. Cabildo de 29 de enero de 1563.

10. García Icazbalceta, *Obras,* I:87, n.1.

11. *Actas de cabildo de México,* I:115, 158; II:21, 30; III:49, 61; IV:31, 154; V:191; VI:58, 285; VII:103, 413, 468.

12. Ibid., IX:85. Cabildo de 9 de diciembre de 1585.

13. "Since the land was won. . . ." See ibid., VII:103. Cabildo de 29 de enero de 1563.

14. See, for example, ibid., VI:285; VIII:327. On one of those days when they "conversed" about the damages that flowed from practicing without a license, the aldermen of Mexico City agreed that the remedy was to appoint a protomédico. Why, after making ten separate appointments for this purpose, they should have spoken of "the need of a protomédico" they did not say. Perhaps they merely had a temporary vacancy. The man they appointed, however, was Dr. Juan de Alcázar, ibid., VI:285. Cabildo de 14 y 17 de mayo de 1557. The paleographers of the printed edition of the *Actas* entered this name as "Dr. Alcaraz," but there was no such doctor revolving in Mexican medical circles at the time, and besides, the original manuscript says "Dr. Alcázar," a man well known in the history of the University of Mexico.

15. Ibid., VII:103; VIII:327. Cabildos de 29 de enero de 1563 y 3 de marzo de 1578.

16. The second by this name.

17. Ibid., VIII:374–75. Cabildo de 9 de enero de 1579.

18. Ibid., XI:17. Cabildo de 25 de julio de 1592.

19. Ibid., XIV:68. Cabildo de 21 febrero de 1600.

20. See ibid., VIII:20. Cabildo de 28 de febrero de 1572.

21. Ibid., VIII:282. Cabildos de 15 y 19 de abril de 1577.

22. Alvaro Manrique de Zúñiga, Marquis of Villamanrique.

23. AGI, México, 1091. Real cédula al Dr. Luis de Porras, Barcelona, 2 de junio de 1585.

24. Título de Luis de Porras para protomédico, 3 de diciembre de 1585. *Actas de cabildo de México,* IX:86.

25. Ibid., IX:84–86. Cabildo de 9 de diciembre de 1585.

26. This angry assertion was not in strict conformity with the law, for a pragmatic of Philip II (1563) required even royally appointed protomédicos to present their titles to the cabildos for confirmation.

27. The city itself had followed this custom.

28. According to his commission, the new medical officer would name a druggist to assist him when he inspected drugstores and a *"protobárbero"* to assist him when he examined a phlebotomist.

29. AGI, México, 1091. Real cédula al virrey de la Nueva España, San Lorenzo, 4 de junio de 1586.

30. It named Dr. Pedro López and Dr. de la Fuente. *Actas de cabildo de México,* IX:242. Cabildo de 4 de enero de 1588.

31. Ibid., XV:106. Cabildo de 11 de noviembre de 1602.

32. Ibid., XV:165–66. Cabildo de 26 de mayo de 1603.

33. Two years after claiming his post Sepúlveda asked the city to give him a license to return to Santo Domingo for his wife and, while he was gone, to maintain his status as a *vecino* and keep his real property intact (*tierras e solar e cavallerías*), Libros de cabildos de Lima, 20 vols. (Lima, 1935–62), I:359. Cabildo de 26 de julio de 1539. (Hereinafter *Libros de cabildos de Lima.*)

34. Ibid., I:141. Cabildo de 20 de abril de 1537.

35. See chapter 3, p. 60.

36. Ibid., IX:452. Cabildo de 10 de noviembre de 1581.

37. Ibid., IX:452. Cabildo de 17 de noviembre de 1581.

38. Ibid., IX:562. Cabildo de 17 de agosto de 1582.

39. See chapter 3, p. 60.

40. The commission, dated 31 de diciembre de 1588, is published in ibid., XI:290–91.

41. This act of formal obedience took place on January 11, 1590. Ibid., XI:292.

42. Ibid., XI:293–95. For a summary of the 1568 instructions, see chapter 3, p. 60.

43. Ibid., XVI:401. Cabildo de 2 de mayo de 1620.

44. See Lanning, *Pedro de la Torre,* pp. 18–19.

45. Francis Borgia Steck, ed. and trans., *Motolinía's History of the Indians of New Spain* (Washington, D.C., 1951), p. 149.

46. For use of this term, see R. C. Padden, *The Hummingbird and the Hawk* (Columbus, O., 1967), p. 250.

47. In colonial days llagas was a generic term and included *"llaga corrosiva, virulenta, sordida, fistulosa, cavernosa, etc." Diccionario de la lengua castellana, compuesto por la Real Academia Española* (Madrid, 1783), p. 601.

48. *Actas de cabildo de México,* I:154–55. Cabildo de 23 de diciembre de 1527.

49. Ibid., II:30–31. Cabildo de 24 de enero de 1530.

50. Ibid., II:145–46. Cabildo de 17 de noviembre de 1531.
51. F. Fernández del Castillo, *La Facultad de Medicina según el Archivo de la Real y Pontificia Universidad de México* (México, 1953), pp. 79–80. (Hereinafter Fernández del Castillo, *La Facultad de Medicina.*)
52. *Actas de cabildo de México,* VI:116–17. Cabildo de 10 de noviembre de 1553.
53. Bartolomé Rivera (1607), Alonso García (1608, 1609, 1610, 1612, 1615, 1617, 1618, 1619), Francisco Urieta (1621, 1622, 1623), Mateo Hinojosa (1624), Francisco Ordóñez (1625, 1626, 1629), Gerónimo Ortiz (1636, 1637, 1638, 1639, 1640, 1641, 1642). Ibid., XVI:436; XVII:151, 296, 453; XVIII:242; XX:78, 251; XXI:150; XXII:8, 215; XXIV:118, 364; XXV:86, 220; XXVI:84; XXVII:36; XXX:107; XXXI:8, 171, 311; XXXII–XXXIII:6, 163, 274, 426.
54. Ibid., XVI:436; XVII:296; XX:78, 251; XXI:150; XXI:215; XXIV:225; XXV:86.
55. Ibid., XVII:453; XVIII:37; XXI:436; XXII:215; XXIV:42, 225, 364; XXV:200; XXVI:84; XXX:107. In addition, it entered into a contract with San Juan de Dios for surgical care between 1626 and 1636.
56. Ibid., XXIV:118. Cabildo de 30 de julio de 1621.
57. Ibid., IX:345; XII:111; XVIII:359–61. Cabildos de 11 de septiembre de 1589, 10 de enero de 1595, y 18 de junio de 1612.
58. Ibid., XII:241. Cabildo de 2 de enero de 1596.
59. Real cédula al virrey de Nueva España, El Pardo, 24 de noviembre de 1607. Ibid., XVIII:360.
60. Ibid., XVIII:361. Cabildo de 8 de junio de 1612.
61. Ibid., XX:98, 107. Cabildos de 30 de enero y 5 de marzo de 1615.
62. Herrera in fact got his appointment from the city on January 11, 1589. Ibid., IX:316.
63. Ibid., XXIII:198. Cabildo de 17 de agosto de 1620. The name of Marcos Falcón appears in the acts of the Mexican cabildo until 1626 and, then, in 1629, the name Martín Sánchez Falcón reappears, either because a kinsman took his place, or because the clerk reverted to the old habit of referring to the father, Martín Sánchez Falcón.
64. See chapter 6, pp. 153–57.
65. Ibid., XXI:99. Cabildo de 4 de noviembre de 1616.
66. *Batir cataratas. . . .*
67. *Actas de cabildo de México,* XXI:103. Cabildo de 11 de noviembre de 1616.
68. Ibid., XXIV:42. Cabildo de 4 de marzo de 1621.
69. Ibid., XXIV:381. Cabildo de 17 de febrero de 1622. See also, XXIV:356, 381; XXV:30, 93, 119, 208, 242.
70. *Libros de cabildos de Lima,* IV:452, 516. Cabildos de 28 de septiembre de 1551 y 1 de febrero de 1552.
71. Ibid., V:195, 196, 197, 239, 245, 320. Cabildos de 17 y 20 de agosto de 1554, 4 y 14 de enero, y 26 de agosto de 1555.
72. This election, in 1572, was in violation of the Spanish custom barring physi-

cians from being rectors of universities. See John Tate Lanning, *Academic Culture in the Spanish Colonies* (New York, 1940), p. 20. (Hereinafter, Lanning, *Academic Culture.*)

73. *Libros de cabildos de Lima,* V:464. Cabildo de 8 de junio de 1556.

74. Ibid., V:520. Cabildo de 4 de septiembre de 1556.

75. Ibid., VI, Part I:223. Cabildo de 20 de octubre de 1559.

76. Ibid., VI, Part I:431. Cabildo de 31 [*sic*] de junio de 1561.

77. Ibid., VI, Part II:433; VII:166. Cabildos de 1 de julio de 1566 y 22 de octubre de 1571.

78. In those early years, especially when there was disagreement in the cabildo, the royal audiencia reviewed and approved outlays such as this one.

79. Ibid., VII:360, 384. Cabildos de 6 y 17 de octubre de 1572.

80. Ibid., VII:542; VIII:685; IX:267. Cabildos de 15 de diciembre de 1573, 28 de noviembre de 1578, y 1 de julio de 1580.

81. Ibid., IX:573; X:81. Cabildos de 14 de septiembre de 1582 y 22 de mayo de 1584.

82. Ibid., XIV:127; XIX:651. Cabildos de 5 de julio de 1602 y 11 de agosto de 1623.

83. Ibid., XX:234, 309. Cabildos de 9 de diciembre de 1625 y 16 de marzo de 1626.

84. *Libros de cabildos de la ciudad de Quito,* 26 vols. (Quito, 1934–60), VI:284–85. Cabildo de 10 de diciembre de 1574. (Hereinafter *Libros de cabildos de Quito.*)

85. Ibid., XVII:74–75. Cabildo de 8 de noviembre de 1593.

86. Ibid., XIII:33–34. Cabildo de 12 de septiembre de 1597.

87. Ibid., XIV:157–59. Cabildo de 30 de abril de 1601.

88. If he had had any academic degrees, these would have been mentioned before his character and reputation.

89. Ibid., XX:443–44. Cabildo de 5 de diciembre de 1608.

90. Three hundred *patacones* of 8 reales each.

91. Ibid., XX:487. Cabildo de 27 de julio de 1609.

92. Ibid., XXVI:11. Cabildo de 2 de agosto de 1610.

93. Ibid., XXVI:81–82. Cabildo de 13 de junio de 1611.

94. Ibid., XXVI:84–88. Cabildo de 30 de junio de 1611.

95. "porque libremente puedan venir los médicos famosos a curar a ellas, por saber que ninguno esta asalariado por la ciudad que les haya de preferir de más de que esta tan pobre que cuando se va a hacer alguna relación a la real audiencia, toman el libro en prendas no tener con que pagarla. . . ." Ibid., XXVI:288. Cabildo de 12 de julio de 1613.

96. Ibid., XXVI:500. Cabildo de 29 de octubre de 1615.

97. Ibid., XXX:10–12. Cabildo de 5 de noviembre de 1638.

98. *Libros de cabildos de Lima,* IV:511. Cabildo de 18 de agosto de 1556.

99. Ibid.

100. Ibid., V:678; VI:72. Cabildos de 22 de octubre de 1557 y 3 de junio de 1558.

101. Ibid., VII:160; IX:266–67. Cabildos de 5 de octubre de 1571 y 28 de abril de 1580.
102. *Actas del cabildo de Caracas,* 1 vols. (Caracas, 1943–69), VII:85–86. Cabildo de 12 de febrero de 1651. (Hereinafter *Actas del cabildo de Caracas.*)
103. *Libros de cabildos de Lima,* I:191. Cabildo de 16 de marzo de 1538.
104. Ibid., II. Cabildo de 4 de abril de 1539.
105. Ibid., V:339, 341; VI:287, 531. Cabildos de 1 y 3 de enero de 1561, 1 de enero de 1565 y 1 de enero de 1568.
106. Ibid., VI:20–21. Real orden, Lima, 8 de febrero de 1562.
107. Ibid., VI:382. Cabildo de 7 de enero de 1566.
108. Ibid., VII:238. Cabildo de 28 de febrero de 1572.
109. Ibid., XIII:117. Cabildos de 8 de junio y 3 de julio de 1598 y 5 de abril de 1599. By a "straw" or "cane" of water the Peruvians mean as much water as, flowing continuously, could come in through a straw or a cane. In other places, Guatemala, for instance, such terms as "half a *real*" or a *"real"* were used.
110. Ibid., VI:481; VIII:201. Cabildos de 20 de febrero de 1567 y 24 de febrero de 1576.
111. Ibid., I:310. Cabildo de 10 de marzo de 1539.
112. *Actas de cabildo de Caracas,* V:158. Cabildo de 25 de enero de 1623.
113. Ibid., V:227. Cabildo de 12 de septiembre de 1627.
114. Ibid., IX:196; X:33, 56–57. Cabildos de 13 de enero de 1657, 28 de enero y 2 de mayo de 1658.
115. *Libros de cabildos de Lima,* VII:236. Cabildo de 22 de febrero de 1572.
116. Ibid., VII:583; VIII:33, 149, 336. Cabildos de 1 de marzo de 1574, 3 de diciembre de 1574, 23 de diciembre de 1575, y 23 de noviembre de 1576.
117. *Esclavo cuadrillero.*
118. *Libros de cabildos de Lima,* VIII:245. Cabildo de 14 de mayo de 1576.
119. *Actas de cabildo de México,* XVI:436 (1607); XVII:151 (1608); XVII:453 (1610); XVIII:242 (1612); XX:78 (1615); XXI:150 (1617); XXII:8 (1618).
120. See, for example, the *Actas de cabildo de Caracas,* VIII:18. Cabildo de 24 de enero de 1650.
121. Pascual Iborra, "Memoria sobre la institución del Real Protomedicato," *Anales de la Real Academia de Medicina,* VI (Madrid, 1885):190.
122. *Actas de cabildo de México,* III:61. Cabildo de 7 de noviembre de 1533.
123. *Libros de cabildos de Lima,* I:161. Cabildo de 30 de agosto de 1537.
124. Ibid., I:181–82. Cabildo de 25 de enero de 1538. The Lima council on the eighteenth of the same month had licensed Juan López on the condition that, in cases of importance "mucha que tome acompañado que sea persona de esperiencia. . . ."
125. Ibid., IV:305. Cabildo de 1 de diciembre de 1550.
126. Ibid., IV:616. Cabildo de 11 de noviembre de 1552.
127. Ibid., IV:624. Cabildo de 27 de noviembre de 1552.
128. Ibid., VI:423. Cabildo de 7 de junio de 1566.

129. Ibid., XIII:185. Cabildo de 6 de noviembre de 1598.

130. *Actas de cabildo de México,* XX:223. Cabildo de 13 de noviembre de 1615.

131. *Libros de cabildos de Quito,* II:40–41. Cabildo de 20 de abril de 1548.

132. Ibid., XIV:44–45. Cabildo de 6 de marzo de 1600.

133. *Actas de cabildo de Caracas,* V:83. Cabildo de 28 de agosto de 1621.

134. *Actas de cabildo de México,* I:158. Cabildo de 22 de enero de 1528.

135. Ibid., II:87. Cabildo de 3 de febrero de 1531.

136. *Libros de cabildos de Lima,* I:256. Cabildo de 5 de diciembre de 1538.

137. Ibid., XVIII:157–58. Cabildo de 31 de octubre de 1617.

138. Guillermo S. Fernández de Recas, *Medicina: Nómina de bachilleres, licenciados y doctores, 1607–1780 y guía de méritos y servicios, 1763–1828* (México, 1960), p. 63. (Hereinafter Fernández de Recas, *Medicina.*)

139. *Actas de cabildo de México,* XXIV:73. Cabildo de 21 de mayo de 1621.

140. Ibid., IV:154. Cabildo de 3 de diciembre de 1538.

141. Ibid., IV:214. Cabildo de 5 de octubre de 1540.

142. Ibid., II:21, 30. Cabildos de 12 de noviembre de 1529 y 24 de enero de 1530.

143. Ibid., IV:154. Cabildo de 3 de diciembre de 1538.

144. Ibid., VI:58. Cabildo de 4 de julio de 1552.

145. Lanning, *Pedro de la Torre,* pp. 86–87, nn. 95 and 96.

146. *Libros de cabildos de Lima,* I:387. Cabildo de 16 de octubre de 1539.

147. Ibid., III:416. Cabildo de 24 de julio de 1551.

148. Ibid., VII:268, 270. Cabildos de 28 de abril y 1 de mayo de 1572.

149. Ibid., VIII:226. Cabildo de 9 de abril de 1576.

150. July 7, 1959. Luis Antonio Eguiguren, ed., *Diccionario histórico cronológico de la Real y Pontificia Universidad de San Marcos y sus colegios,* 3 vols. (Lima, 1940–51), II:459. (Hereinafter Eguiguren, *Diccionario histórico.*)

151. *Libros de cabildos de Lima,* IX:73–74. Cabildo de 3 de agosto de 1579.

152. Ibid., IX:408. Cabildo de 14 de julio de 1581.

153. Ibid., XIII:84–85. Cabildo de 6 de noviembre de 1598.

154. Ibid., XIII:204. Cabildo de 15 de enero de 1599.

155. Ibid., XIV:561. Cabildo de 10 de noviembre de 1603.

156. *Actas de cabildo de Caracas,* V:42. Cabildo de 10 de enero de 1621.

157. *Actas de cabildo de México,* IV:214. Cabildo de 5 de octubre de 1540.

158. Ibid., IV:153. Cabildo de 19 de noviembre de 1538.

159. Ibid., VI:127. Cabildo de 26 de enero de 1554.

160. Ibid., VI:274. Cabildo de 15 de febrero de 1557.

161. The protomédicos were Dr. Jerónimo de Herrera and Dr. Bravo and the surgeon to serve with them was Dr. Contreras. Ibid., XI:58. Cabildo de 4 de enero de 1593.

162. Ibid., XI:59. Cabildo de 8 de enero de 1593.

163. Ibid., XI:60. Cabildo de 12 de enero de 1593.

164. Ibid., IV:95. Cabildo de 14 de septiembre de 1537.

165. Ibid., IV:202. Cabildo de 18 de junio de 1540.

166. Ibid., IV:221. Cabildo de 17 de diciembre de 1547.

167. Probably the dread *matlazahuatl,* a disease with symptoms remarkably like those of typhus.

168. Ibid., V:191. Cabildo de 10 de octubre de 1547. Licentiate Pero López, Dr. Juan Alcázar, and Licentiate Juan Aguilera composed the commission.
169. *Libros de cabildos de Lima,* I:181. Cabildo de 18 de enero de 1538.
170. Ibid., I:254. Cabildo de 6 de diciembre de 1538.
171. Ibid., I:256. Cabildo de 6 de diciembre de 1538.
172. Ibid., IV:109. Cabildo de 17 de noviembre de 1553.
173. *Actas de cabildo de Caracas,* VI. Cabildo de 4 de septiembre de 1649.
174. *Actas de cabildo de México,* IV:43. Cabildo de 13 de octubre de 1536.
175. *Libros de cabildos de Lima,* XV:279. Cabildo de 4 de diciembre de 1606.
176. Ibid., XX:272. Cabildo de 23 de enero de 1620.
177. *Actas de cabildo de Caracas,* VII:99. Cabildo de 11 de noviembre de 1651.
178. *Libros de cabildos de Lima,* XV:905. Cabildo de 16 de octubre de 1609.
179. Luis A. Eguiguren, *Catálogo histórico del claustro de la Universidad de San Marcos, 1576–1800* (Lima, 1912), p. 53. (Hereinafter Eguiguren, *Catálogo histórico.*)

3. *Organization and Practice*

1. For the confusion resulting from a misunderstanding of the office of the protomédico general, see chapter 2, pp. 25–26.
2. Archivo Histórico Nacional, Madrid (hereinafter AHNM), Cedulario Indico, tomo 33, f. 342, No. 277; Archivo General de la Nación, México (hereinafter AGNM), Reales cédulas (Dup.), 47:262, fs. 157v–158r. Instrucción al Doctor Francisco Hernández, Madrid, 11 de enero de 1570.
3. AGNM, Reales cédulas (Dup.), 47:262, Arts. 1–6.
4. Ibid., 47:262, fs. 157v–158r, Arts. 6–12.
5. The term was *audiencia y chancillería.*
6. Ibid., 47:262, Arts. 7–8.
7. Ibid., 47:262, fs. 157v–158v.
8. Ibid., 47:262, f. 156–156v. Título del Protomédico General, de todas las Indias, Islas e tierra firme del Mar Océano, al Doctor Francisco Hernández, médico de su Magestad, Madrid, 11 de enero de 1570.
9. Since the law *Nueva recopilación,* Lib. III, Tít. XVI, Ley 4, states that the protomédicos might not send commissaries beyond the five-league limit round the city, the inference is that subordinates did actually operate.
10. Muñoz, *Recopilación,* Cap. IV, Art. I, pp. 53–55.
11. Pragmática de Felipe II, San Lorenzo, 2 de agosto de 1593.
12. Muñoz, *Recopilación,* Cap. IV, Art. II, p. 58.
13. *Nueva recopilación,* Lib. III, Tít. XVI, Ley 9, Arts. 1 y 2. In America the audiencia took the place of the council and made this determination.
14. Ibid., Lib. III, Tít. XVI, Ley 9, Art. 3.
15. One key each in the hands of the senior protomédico, the secretary, and one of the examiners. The examiners were paid per diem.
16. Muñoz, *Recopilación,* Cap. IV, Art. IV, pp. 59–60.
17. Ibid., Cap. IV, Art. V, p. 61.

18. Those beyond the number allowed by law and, presumably, by custom were called supernumeraries (*supernumerarios*).

19. His main condition was that the appointments made in Mexico be sent to him for confirmation.

20. AGI, México, 780. Copia de un capítulo de la respuesta de las cartas del Sr. Juan de Palafox, siendo obispo de Puebla, y visitador de la Nueva España, [Madrid], de 18 de febrero de 1646, sobre los protomédicos de la Ciudad de México.

21. AGI, Indiferente General, 551. Real cédula al Conde de Salvatierra, virrey de la Nueva España, Madrid, 18 de febrero de 1646. This cédula can also be found in AGI, México, Legajos 36, 389, and 7890; AGI, Buenos Aires, 20, and in AGNM, Protomedicato, 1:1. John Tate Lanning, ed., *Reales cédulas de la Real y Pontificia Universidad de México de 1551 a 1816* (México, 1946), No. 174 bis, pp. 241–42. (Hereinafter Lanning, *Reales cédulas*.)

22. AGI, México, 36. Informe del Dr. D. Juan de Molina, residente en esta Corte . . . s.f., s.l. Thus when the explosive cédula of 1646 dropped into their midst, the protomédicos were Dr. Pedro de los Arcos Monroy, Dr. Francisco de Toro Morejón, and Dr. Juan de Melgarejo.

23. AGNM, Reales cédulas (Dup.), 24:37, f. 49–49v. Real orden, México, 24 de marzo de 1665.

24. Dr. Alonso Fernández Osorio, who held the first chair, became first proto-médico and president, while the senior doctor (*decano*) of the faculty of medicine, Dr. Rodrigo Muñoz de la Zorca, became second protomédico. However, Salvatierra took Dr. de Toro with him to Peru—a very slight reduction in the number of protomédicos. As a royal order of 1665 mentions Dr. de Toro as a member of the tribunal when Salvatierra transferred to Lima in 1648, the conclusion is inevitable that his master had salvaged the third post for him.

25. Doctors of law sitting as judges (*oidores*) of the royal audiencia.

26. AGI, México, 36. El Virrey Salvatierra a S.M., México, 18 de mayo de 1647.

27. Ibid., 36. El Consejo de 10 de octubre de 1647.

28. Dr. de los Arcos Monroy on October 23, 1635, and Dr. de Melgarejo on August 14, 1643.

29. Ibid., 36. Los doctores Pedro de los Arcos Monroy y Juan de Melgarejo piden confirmación de sus títulos . . . s.f., s.l.

30. Zaragoza, 9 de junio de 1646. The law based upon these two cédulas is *Recopilación de leyes de los reynos de las Indias. . . .* 3 vols. (Madrid, 1681), Libro V, Título VI, Ley 3. (Hereinafter *Recopilación de Indias*.) AGI, México, 1771. Informe de la Contaduría General, Madrid, 10 de febrero de 1783. See AGI, Lima, 543, *Constituciones de la Universidad de San Marcos de Lima* (Lima, 1735), Tít. VI, Const. 86, fs. 35v–36. (Hereinafter *Constituciones*.)

31. AGI, México, 36. Juan Bautista Sáenz a D. Juan de Solórzano, Madrid, 17 de noviembre de 1645.

32. Archivo Nacional del Perú, Lima (hereinafter ANP), Protomedicato, Legajo Unico, passim.

33. AGNM, Reales cédulas (Dup.), 14:695, f. 425–425v. Real orden a la Universidad de México, México, 12 de junio de 1647.
34. AGI, México, 36. Informe del Sr. D. Juan de Solórzano, s.f., s.l.
35. AGNM, Reales cédulas (Dup.), 24:37, f. 49–49v. Real orden para que se publique y cumpla la cédula de su Magestad, en razón de que se consuman las plazas de los Protomédicos como fueren vacando hasta que queden tres, México, 24 de marzo de 1665.
36. After 1676 the law *Recopilación de Indias,* Lib. I, Tít. XXII, Ley 4, merely by endorsing the statutes of the University of Mexico, provided that the archbishop, the senior oidor of the royal audiencia, the inquisitor, the rector, the maestrescuela, dean of the cathedral, the professor of prima, and the senior doctor should vote.
37. AGI, México, 397. Real cédula a la Universidad de México, Madrid, 8 de agosto de 1699. For a printed version, see Lanning, *Reales cédulas*, No. 83, pp. 112–13.
38. AGI, México, 776. El arzobispo de México a S.M., México, 4 de agosto de 1722 (2 fols., 6 folios anéxos); el rector de la Universidad a S.M., México, 5 de agosto de 1722 (5 folios); el Virrey de México, el Marqués de Valero a S.M., México, 6 de agosto de 1722 (6 folios, 38 folios anéxos).
39. The statutes did not, as the viceroy claimed, make any such provision.
40. AGI, México, 776. Memorial del Dr. D. Marcos Salgado, protomédico, a S.M., s.f., s.l.
41. Ibid., 776. Informe del Señor fiscal, Madrid, 22 de enero de 1723.
42. Ibid., 776. Acuerdo del Consejo, Madrid, 25 de enero de 1723. Ibid., 416. Real cédula al Arzobispo de México, Buen Retiro, 20 de marzo de 1723.
43. In 1754 one of the opositores for the post of substitute for the chair of prima of medicine challenged the vote of the professor, the father-in-law of an opponent. The board would not allow the professor of vísperas to take his place. As this question had arisen in 1746, the king threw out the election and ruled that in such cases the senior professor in the faculty or, in want of him, the senior graduate should vote in place of the retired professor of prima. Lanning, *Reales cédulas,* No. 136, pp. 182–83. Real cédula a la Universidad de México, Aranjuez, 11 de mayo de 1754. See also AGI, México, 446 and 776. Real cédula al arzobispo de México, Aranjuez, 11 de mayo de 1754. Also AGI, México, 446. Certificaciones de la acordada por el Consejo sobre la votación de la Cátedra de prima de medicina, Madrid, 22 de febrero y 30 de junio de 1754.
44. The Council of the Indies immediately put the reform of 1646 into practice. The appointment of Dr. Alonso Fernández Osorio in 1647 as "perpetual protomédico" and president of the tribunal got royal confirmation within three months—prompt dispatch of business in that day. AGI, México, 1097. Real cédula de confirmación de título de primer protomédico de la Nueva España al Dr. Fernández Osorio, Madrid, 22 de febrero de 1648.
45. AGNM, Reales cédulas (Dup.), 173:252, f. 346–346v. Títulos de presidente del protomedicato, Madrid, 11 de agosto de 1799.
46. AGI, México, 1079. Real cédula al Fiscal de lo civil de la Audiencia de

México, Madrid, 15 de noviembre de 1709. AGI, Indiferente General, 1551 contains the confirmation of the letter of the following protomédicos in Lima: Dr. Franciso Bermejo (Madrid, 3 de octubre de 1694), Dr. Joseph de Avendaño (Madrid, 23 de diciembre de 1714), Dr. Francisco de Vargas y Machuca (San Lorenzo, 17 de agosto de 1720), Dr. Bernabé Ortiz de Landaeta, Dr. Isidro Joseph de Ortega y Pimentel (San Ildefonso, 31 de julio de 1766). The same legajo contains seven confirmations of protomédicos of New Spain between 1759 and 1799.

47. Ibid., 36. Acuerdo del Consejo de Indias, Madrid, 29 de junio de 1647.

48. See, for example, AGNM, Reales cédulas (Dup.), 40:41, fs. 37–38. Título de protomédico primero de la Nueva España, al doctor Francisco Antonio Jiménez, catedrático de prima de medicina, México, 28 de mayo de 1693. AGI, México, 403. Confirmación del título de Protomédico primero de la Nueva España, que el Virrey de ella dió a Dr. Juan Brizuela, Madrid, 31 de diciembre de 1709 (minuta). AGI, México, 419. Confirmación del título de primero Protomédico de la N.E. que el Virrey de ella dió a J. Marcos José Salgado, El Pardo, 2 de marzo de 1726.

49. AGI, Indiferente General, 1551. Títulos de los empleados del Tribunal del Protomedicato de la Nueva España, desde 1759 hasta 1799. Doctors Juan Gregorio de Campos (1759), José Tomás García del Valle (segundo protomédico 1769), Ignacio de Segura (tercero, 1773), Juan de la Peña Brizuela (segundo, 1778), José Ignacio García Jove (1781), Joaquín Pío Antonio de Eguía (1797), José Ignacio García Jove (protomédico pérpetuo, 1799).

50. Some of those who took this post were Dr. Rodrigo Muñoz de la Zorca. AGI, México, 1097. Real cédula de confirmación del título de segundo protomédico de la Nueva España al Dr. Rodrigo Muñoz, Madrid, 18 de enero de 1648; Dr. Jerónimo Ortiz, AGNM, Reales cédulas (Dup.), 24:62, fs. 87–87v. Nombramiento de segundo protomédico de la Nueva España al decano de la facultad de medicina, Dr. Jerónimo Ortiz, México, 8 de octubre de 1665; Dr. José Díaz Brizuela, AGI, México, 389. R. C. concediendo título de protomédico segundo de la N.E. a Dr. José Díaz Brizuela, Madrid, 20 de febrero de 1680; Real cédula concediendo confirmación de tercer protomédico de la N.E. al Dr. D. Pedro de Soto de Acuña, Madrid, 20 de febrero de 1680, AGI, México, 393; AGNM, Reales cédulas (Dup.), 33:348, fs. 381–82. Real cédula concediendo confirmación del título de Segundo Protomédico de la N.E. que el virrey de ella dió en virtud de cédula real al Dr. D. Félix Vela del Castillo, Madrid, 15 de marzo de 1690; Dr. Ignacio de la Vega, AGI, México, 399. Confirmación del título de Protomédico segundo en propiedad de la Nueva España, que el virrey de ella dió, en virtud de R. C. al Dr. Ignacio de la Vega Salazar, Madrid, 19 de noviembre de 1703; Dr. Joseph Valentín del Guijo, AGI, México, 432. By the death of Dr. Ildefonso de Rotas. Real cédula concediendo confirmación del título de Protomédico segundo en propiedad del Tribunal de Protomedicato de la N.E. que el virrey de ella dió al Dr. D. Joseph Valentín del Guijo, Buen Retiro, 15 de julio de 1740.

51. For the formula in appointment and confirmation in this seat, see AGI, México, 391. Real cédula por la que se concede confirmación del título de

tercer protomédico de la N.E. que el Virrey de ella dió en virtud de R.C. al Dr. D. Diego Osorio y Peralta, Buen Retiro, 15 de noviembre de 1685; AGI, México, Legajo 394. R.C. concediendo título de tercer Protomédico de la N.E. para el Dr. D. Francisco Antonio Ximénez, Madrid, 30 de diciembre de 1692; AGNM, Reales cédulas (Dup.), 40:29, fs. 24v–25v. Nombramiento al doctor José Montaño como tercer protomédico de la Nueva España, México, 1 de enero de 1693; AGI, México, 401. Confirmación del título de Protomédico tercero de la N.E. que el Virrey de ella dió al Dr. Juan José de Brizuela, Madrid, 26 de marzo de 1705; AGI, México, 407. Confirmación del título de protomédico tercero de la N.E. que el Virrey de minuta ella dió al Dr. D. Marcos Salgado, Madrid, 26 de agosto 1715; AGI, México, 419. Confirmación del título de protomédico tercero de la N.E. que el Virrey de ella dió al Dr. D. Cristóbal de la Vega, El Pardo, 2 de marzo de 1726; AGI, México, 429. R. C. concediendo confirmación del título de protomédico tercero de la N.E. que el Virrey de ella dió al Dr. D. Juan Manuel de Báeza, San Lorenzo, 2 de diciembre de 1737. These documents often mention the predecessor and, for that reason, would be useful in establishing a complete list of the holders of each of the three seats.

52. For example, Dr. Diego Osorio y Peralta was appointed in 1681, AGNM, Real cédulas (Dup.), 33:36 y 173, fs. 26v–27, 162v–63; he was not confirmed until 1685—about a month short of four years.

53. For the specific struggle of the spokesmen of surgery and botany to be represented on the protomedicato, see pp. 275–79.

54. *Constituciones de la Real y Pontificia Universidad de México* (México, 1775), Tít. XI, Const. 133; Tít. XX, Const. 325. (Hereinafter *Constituciones de la Universidad de México.*)

55. AGI, México, 325. Real cédula a la Real Universidad de México, Madrid, 8 de agosto de 1799.

56. Instead of second and third protomédicos as in Mexico, in Lima the chief protomédico served with permanent examiners (*alcaldes examinadores*), to 1821.

57. Ibid., 36. Informe del Sr. Juan de Solórzano, s.f., s.l. Since Solórzano gave up his post as oidor in Lima in 1627 and returned to Spain to occupy first the post of fiscal of the Consejo de Hacienda and then that of the Indies, and since this question came after 1646, this document must date from the middle decade of the seventeenth century.

58. Thus, the viceroy had appointed José Sequiera and Hipólito Bueno de la Rosa, who were not professors of prima, as protomédicos generales.

59. AGI, Lima, 914, Expediente 68. Protomédico y Cátedra de Medicina, Aguirre, Iturrizarra y los Catedráticos, s.f. I am indebted to Dr. Richard Konetzke for my knowledge of the existence of this *expediente.*

60. Ibid., 914, Exp. 68. El virrey del Perú a D. José de Gálvez, Lima, 16 de noviembre de 1783.

61. Ibid., 914, Exp. 68. Los doctores y catedráticos de la Real Universidad de San Marcos al rey, Lima, 1 de diciembre de 1783. For the law referred to, see *Recopilación de Indias,* Lib. V, Tít. VI, Ley 3. The royal cédula of February

18, 1646, "annexing" the chair of prima to the presidency of the protomedicato was addressed to New Spain only, but the laws of the Indies extended the principle to Lima. The clerk of the protomedicato in Lima, for example, reported in 1758 that the professor of prima of medicine always held the post of protomédico general. Archivo Colonial, Bogotá (hereinafter ACB), Médicos y Abogados, 5, fs. 262v–63f.

62. AGI, Lima, 914, Exp. 68. Dictamen del fiscal, Madrid, 12 de agosto de 1784. Sala segunda.

63. Ibid., 914, Exp. 68. Juan José de Aguirre a S.M., Lima, 6 de septiembre de 1784.

64. Ibid., 914, Exp. 68. Dictamen del Consejo, Madrid, 23 de septiembre de 1784.

65. John Tate Lanning, *The University in the Kingdom of Guatemala* (Ithaca, N.Y., 1955), pp. 194–96. (Hereinafter Lanning, *The University in the Kingdom of Guatemala.*)

66. AGI, Lima, 914, Exp. 68. Petición de D. Juan Joseph de Iturrizara, Lima, 13 de marzo de 1786.

67. Eguiguren, *Catálogo histórico,* p. 54.

68. Two opinions of the Council of the Indies fiscal succinctly summarizing this controversy (Madrid, May 28, 1786, and August 9, 1786) appear in Richard Konetzke, ed., *Colección de documentos para la historia de la formación social de Hispanoamérica, 1493–1810,* 3 vols. (Madrid, 1953–62), II, no. 292: 597–601. (Hereinafter Konetzke, *Colección.*)

69. In 1789 the tribunal had a legal assistant (*asesor letrado*), fiscal, clerk, and porter, who generally also served as bailiff in judicial matters and inspections. AGI, Lima, 686; AGI, Buenos Aires, 20. Viceroy Teodoro de Croix a don Antonio Porlier, Lima, 30 de marzo de 1789, No. 80.

70. In that year the organization of the protomedicato in Lima was as follows: Protomédico general: Dr. Juan José de Aguirre; Alcaldes examinadores médicos: Dr. Miguel Tafur, Dr. José Vergara, and Dr. José Pezet, supernumerary; Examinador de cirujía: Dr. Pedro Belomo; Asesor: D. Gaspar Antonio Aguirre; Escribano: D. Jerónimo de Villafuerte; Alguacil mayor: D. Manuel Echevarría; Alguacil interino: D. José García del Real; Portero: Pablo Tello. H. Valdizán, *La facultad de medicina de Lima, 1811–1911* (Lima, s.f.), p. 75. (Hereinafter Valdizán, *La facultad de medicina de Lima.*) This list does not include any lieutenant protomédicos in the principal cities nor any protoboticarios, examiners in pharmacy, who varied from inspection to inspection.

71. The protomedicato of Lima came to have subdelegates in Trujillo, Huamanga, Tarma, Ica, and Arequipa. See John E. Woodham, "Hipólito Unánue and the Enlightenment in Peru" (Ph.D. dissertation, Duke University, 1964), p. 197. (Hereinafter Woodham, "Hipólito Unánue.")

72. The terms of an appointment might expressly exclude some of these functions.

73. ACB, Médicos y Abogados, 5, fs. 261v–62v. Informe de Luis Agustín Gon-

zález, escribano del Tribunal del Real Protomedicato, Lima, 18 de diciembre de 1758.

74. The most critical year was 1528. The official transfer of Castilian medical law to America took place in 1535.

75. The doctor of medicine did not submit to examination by the protomedicato to practice medicine; he had already as a rule secured a license upon the expiration of his two years' apprenticeship following his bachelor's degree.

76. The candidate might not use any of the time while studying arts to get ahead by taking a course in medicine.

77. Muñoz, *Recopilación,* Cap. X, Art. II, p. 139.

78. Ibid., Cap. X, Art. VII, p. 146, n. 7.

79. *Institutiones medicae.* . . . (Madrid, 1594) and *Institutiones chirurgicae jussi regio factae.* . . . (Madrid, 1594). Mercado also published *Instituciones que Su Magistad mandó hazer al doctor Mercado* . . . (Madrid, 1599).

80. Where the class lasted for one hour, the professor read for only forty-five minutes.

81. *Nueva recopilación,* Lib. III, Tít. XVI, Cap. II, Ley 11; Muñoz, *Recopilación,* Cap. X, Art. V, pp. 142–43.

82. See Muñoz, *Recopilación,* Cap. X, Art. IX, p. 147.

83. The *Recopilaciones de buen uso* included "all the remedies used by the faculty of medicine" and established by the protomedicato.

84. *Nueva recopilación,* Lib. III, Tít. XVI, Leyes 6 y 9; Muñoz, *Recopilación,* Cap. X, Art. X, p. 148.

85. Muñoz, *Recopilación,* Cap. X, Arts. III y IV, pp. 140–42; *Nueva recopilación,* Lib. III, Tít. XVI, Leyes 6, 7, y 9.

86. Presumably, the "rest" of the total fee of seventy-five pesos "deposited" for the examination, amounting to thirty-four pesos.

87. ACB, Médicos y Abogados, 5, fs. 259v–61f, 263v. Informe de Luis Agustín González, escribano de su majestad y del Tribunal del Real Protomedicato, Lima, 18 de diciembre de 1758.

88. Ordenanzas de 1588, Cap. 26. Muñoz, *Recopilación,* Cap. VII, Art. III, parra. 5, pp. 94–95. For the fees allowed in examinations conducted in Spain see *Nueva recopilación,* Lib. III, Tít. XVI, Ley 7.

89. AGI, Santo Domingo, 889. Real cédula al Protomedicato de la Habana, El Pardo, 18 de enero de 1766.

90. Muñoz, *Recopilación,* Cap. VII, Arts. I, II, pp. 91–92.

91. Ibid., Cap. VII, Art. III, p. 95.

92. For the protomédico, 100,000 maravedís, for the examiners 60,000, and for the assessor, 20,000.

93. Ibid., Cap. VII, Art. VII, pp. 96–99. Real cédula, San Lorenzo, 11 de septiembre de 1740. This cédula set the first protomédico's salary at 2,000 pesos provinciales, that of the second and third at 1,000 ducados vellón—figures that will give an idea of what the Spanish government thought a good salary for the most prominent physicians in the kingdom should be.

94. AGNM, Reales cédulas (Dup.), 47:262, Art. 10, fs. 157v–58.

95. ANP, Protomedicato, Legajo Unico, Cuaderno 19, fs. 1v–2. Constancia de pago que hiciera Fray Felipe del Carmen, procurador del Matriz Betelemitas . . . Año de 1806.

96. See, for example, AGNM, Reales cédulas (Dup.), 36:358, f. 295. Real decreto, 7 de junio de 1698.

97. Ibid., 18:436, f. 240.

98. Ibid., 88:98, f. 180–80v. Real orden al virrey de la Nueva España, Aranjuez, 30 de mayo de 1766.

99. AGNM, Protomedicato, 1:1. Francisco Xavier de Gamboa, México, 18 de julio de 1789 y Francisco Baso de Ibáñez al virrey, México, 29 de julio de 1789.

100. Fernando Dávila et al., *Aranzeles de los tribunales, juzgados, y oficinas de justicia, gobierno, y real hacienda, que comprehende la Ciudad de México, Capital de Nueva España* . . . (México, 1759).

101. *Aranzel de el Protomedicato* (México, 1759), p. 4.

102. In 1789 there was a professor of prima of medicine, 500 pesos; of vísperas, 235 pesos; of surgery, 100 pesos; of "method," 100 pesos; of mathematics, 100 pesos. AGNM, Protomedicato, 1:1. Ramón Gutiérrez del Mazo al virrey, México, 17 de julio de 1789.

103. In 1687 the viceroy, the Duque de la Palata, fixed this salary at 781 pesos and 2 reales. Eguiguren, *Catálogo histórico,* p. 53.

104. In 1758, the clerk of the tribunal del protomedicato of Lima, in an informe sent to Bogotá, gave fees at slight variance with those given by Viceroy de Croix in 1789. The deposit for examinations was 75 pesos, 4 reales for physicians and Latin surgeons; all others examined deposited 57 pesos, 4 reales, except Indians, who deposited only 47 pesos, 4 reales. ACB, Médicos y Abogados, 5, fs. 260v–61v. Informe de Luis Agustín González, escribano del Tribunal del Protomedicato, Lima, 18 de diciembre de 1758.

105. AGI, Lima, 686. Virrey Teodoro de Croix a D. Antonio Porlier, Lima, 30 de marzo de 1789.

106. King John II at the Cortes of Burgos (1429), Petitions 23 and 24, and the Cortes of Zamora (1432), Petitions 31 and 32. *Nueva recopilación,* Lib. VI, Tít. IV, Ley 7; Muñoz, *Recopilación,* Cap. XXII, Art. I, p. 368. (The dates of these cortes are so garbled in both these compilations as to place them in the time of Charles V.) The title of the law lists druggists as among those exempted, but in the text no mention of druggists appears.

107. Bobadilla, cited in Muñoz, *Recopilación,* Cap. XXII, Art. II, p. 369.

108. The *Constituciones imperiales* admitted these rights as common law so long as there was "no municipal law to the contrary." Muñoz, *Recopilación,* Cap. XXII, Art. II, pp. 370–72.

109. AGNM, Reales cédulas (Dup.), 170:189, f. 243. Real orden al virrey de Nueva España, Madrid, 26 de julio de 1798.

110. Ibid., 209:84, fs. 112–13. Real orden al virrey de Nueva España, Cádiz, 12 de agosto de 1813.

111. ANP, Protomedicato, Legajo Unico, Cuaderno 6, Año de 1818. Luis Ratera Mtro Flebotómico sobre que se le excepción del alistamiento.

112. As the American tribunals of the protomedicato did not have their own separate "constitutions," Dr. Pezet must have been referring to the compilation of Miguel Eugenio Muñoz published in Spain sixty-seven years before. (Dr. Pezet's ruling is dated August 3, 1818.)

113. What the military authorities did, however, is not clear. The cover sheet, prepared by the Peruvian archivist (*hoja de archivo*), says that the petitioners were exempted.

114. Lanning, *Reales cédulas,* No. 50, pp. 63–64. Real cédula al virrey de la Nueva España, Cuenca, 12 de junio de 1642. The cédula was incorporated in the university statutes and was still in force in 1775. *Constituciones de la Universidad de México,* Tít. XIX, Const. 276.

115. AGNM, Reales cédulas (Dup.), 40:28, f. 24. Parecer del Dr. don Juan de Escalante y Mendoza, México, 18 de octubre de 1692.

116. Bernardo Balbuena, *Grandeza mexicana,* in S. de Madariaga, *The Rise of the Spanish American Empire* (New York, 1947), p. 178. (Hereinafter Madariaga, *The Rise of the Spanish American Empire.*)

117. *Constituciones de la Universidad de México,* Tít. XVII, Const. 242; AGNM, Reales cédulas (Dup.), 33:237, f. 232. Real orden del Conde de Monclova, México, 21 de febrero de 1688; 40:31, fs. 26v–27.

118. A dignitary of the cathedral church with royal and pontifical authority to oversee and confer higher degrees.

119. Most applications for exemptions from passing the required time at the university came in the faculty of canon law, followed in order by law, theology, medicine, and arts.

120. AGNM, Reales cédulas (Dup.), 30:681, f. 248–48v. Real orden, México, 4 de agosto de 1677.

121. Ibid., 28:668, fs. 500v–501. Real orden del Marqués de la Laguna, México, 7 de agosto de 1686.

122. Though the 1775 *Constituciones de la Universidad de México,* Tít. XVII, Const. 54, require four years for the bachelor's in medicine, the internal evidence is that only three years were actually required in 1691.

123. AGNM, Reales cédulas (Dup.), 40:1, fs. 1–2.

124. Since the university had no grading system and the secretary did not keep the records of courses being taken, it was necessary for the student at the end of each course or year, to get a certificate from the professor that he had taken the course successfully and present this to the secretary of the university for the permanent record. At the same time, supported by two witnesses, he personally swore that he had had the course in question.

125. Ibid., 33:276, fs. 280v–81v. Real orden del Conde de Monclova, México, 19 de octubre de 1688.

126. Ibid., 17:230, fs. 243–44. El virrey dispensa al Bachiller Joseph de Armendáriz el tiempo que le falta de la pasante en la facultad de canones, México, 25 de agosto de 1657.

127. Ibid., 29:145, f. 282. Real orden del Virrey Mancera, México, 22 de junio de 1667.

128. Ibid., 29:30, f. 36. Real orden del Marqués de Mancera, México, 29 de junio de 1667. See also the case of Bachelor Juan Pacero, 33:228, f. 234. Real orden del Conde de Monclova, México, 2 de diciembre de 1687.

129. Ibid., 33:395, f. 450. Real orden, México, 17 de octubre de 1691.

130. Ibid., 24:68, f. 100. Real orden, México, 24 de octubre de 1665.

131. Ibid., 40:23, f. 21; 40:28, f. 24. Reales ordenes del Conde de Galve, México, 22 de octubre de 1692 y 1 de diciembre de 1692.

132. Ibid., 29:30, f. 36. Real orden del Marqués de Mancera, México, 22 de junio de 1667.

133. Ibid., 17:23, fs. 343–44. Real orden del Duque de Albuquerque, México, 25 de agosto de 1657.

134. Ibid., 33:235, f. 231. Real orden del Conde de Monclova, México, 13 de febrero de 1688.

135. Ibid., 44:517, fs. 430v–31. Real orden del Virrey Sarmiento de Valladares, México, 10 de marzo de 1700.

136. Ibid., 44:519, fs. 431v–32. El virrey dispensa de pompa y paseos en la recepción del grado de doctor en medicina del licenciado Nicolás Altamirano, México, 10 de marzo de 1700.

137. Ibid., 44:517, fs. 430v–31. Real orden del Virrey Sarmiento de Valladares, Conde de Montezuma, México, 17 de junio de 1702.

138. Ibid., 29:30, f. 36. Real orden del Marqués de Mancera, México, 22 de junio de 1667.

139. For example, the Duke of Albuquerque, granted such relief to Joseph de Armendáris, Bernardo de Aguilera, and Juan Yañez de Avila in 1657 and 1658. Ibid., 17:243, f. 361; 246, fs. 362v–63; 273, fs. 404–4v.

140. Ibid., 24:202, f. 135. Real orden del Marqués de Mancera, México, 14 de abril de 1667.

141. A course meant an entire year's study in a given faculty.

142. Constituciones de la Universidad de México, Const. 243, pp. 129–30.

143. AGNM, Universidad, 22. Libro de claustros, desde 1734–50, fols. 127–30; Alberto María Carreño, Efemérides de la Real y Pontificia Universidad de México, 2 vols. (México, 1963), II:513. (Hereinafter Carreño, Efeméridas.)

144. AGI, México, 1115. Real cédula para que la Universidad de México cumpla y observa lo prevenido en la constitución que se cita . . . , Villaviciosa, 22 de noviembre de 1758. This cédula appears in Lanning, Reales cédulas, No. 143, pp. 194–95.

145. He cited not only the cédula of June 12, 1642, but the Constituciones de la Universidad de México, Tít. XIX, Const. 276, and the Recopilación de Indias, Lib. I, Tít. XXII, Ley 30, explicitly forbade the viceroy to exempt students from requirements for degrees.

146. AGI, México, 395 y 1102. Real cédula al virrey de la Nueva España, Madrid, 1 de junio de 1695. These cédulas also appear in Lanning, Reales cédulas, Nos. 69 and 75, pp. 91–92, 102–3.

147. *Constituciones de la Universidad de México,* Tít. XIII, Const. 160. Three days for temporal chairs and thirty for proprietary ones.

148. AGI, México, 1102. Real cédula a la audiencia de México, 1 de junio de 1695. This document is printed in Lanning, *Reales cédulas,* No. 70, pp. 92–93.

149. In 1722, the situation had again so deteriorated that, at the behest of the University of Mexico, the king ordered express observance of the cédula of June 1, 1695, and of the *Recopilación de Indias,* Lib. I, Tít. XXII, Ley 3. Lanning, *Reales cédulas,* No. 111, pp. 146–47. Real cédula al virrey de la Nueva España, Balsain, 17 de julio de 1722.

150. Lanning, *Reales cédulas,* No. 125, pp. 162–66. Real cédula a la audiencia de México, El Pardo, 16 de febrero de 1739.

151. *Constituciones de la Universidad de México,* Tít. XVII, Const. 245, pp. 130–32.

152. AGNM, Protomedicato, 3:12. Dn. José Fulgencio de Araujo sobre dispensa para examinarse de médico. Año de 1799.

153. *Nueva recopilación,* Lib. III, Tít. XVI, Ley 8. This law, in force in Spain after 1579, was applicable in America, though it was not until 1695 that the king expressly extended Spanish law respecting examination and licensing, among other things, to New Spain. AGI, México, 1102. Nueva España, de partes, c. 42, fs. 428v–33v; AGNM, Reales cédulas (Dup.), 43:44, fs. 142–51v. Real cédula al virrey de la Nueva España, Aranjuez, 5 de mayo de 1695.

154. *Nueva recopilación,* Lib. III, Tít. XVI, Ley 7. This was an enactment of Philip II (1588).

155. AGNM, Reales cédulas (Dup.), 33:235, fs. 230v–31. Real orden, México, 4 de febrero de 1688.

156. Normally it fell vacant every four years.

157. Ibid., 18:146, fs. 130–36v. Real orden, México, 31 de mayo de 1651.

158. When the chair of prima of medicine was vacated by the death of the incumbent, Dr. Diego de Magaña, the viceroy, who had appointed Magaña, now named Dr. Jerónimo Ortiz also. Ibid., 17:248, f. 366. Real orden, del Conde de Alba de Aliste, México, 1 de enero de 1658.

159. See *Constituciones de la Universidad de México,* n. 22, p. 119. Because student voting made the candidates demagogic, the judges consisted of the archbishop, the senior oidor of the audiencia, the senior inquisitor, the rector of the university, the dean, the maestrescuela, the professor of the proprietary chair of prima in the faculty, and the senior professor in the faculty. After 1687, in case the senior inquisitor could not serve, the oidor immediately junior to the senior took his place. AGNM, Reales cédulas (Dup.), 34:144, fs. 381–82v. Real cédula al virrey de la Nueva España, Madrid, 12 de agosto de 1687.

160. AGNM, Reales cédulas (Dup.), 24:29, fs. 37–38v. Real orden del Marqués de Mancera, México, 25 de febrero de 1665.

161. Ibid., 24:36, f. 48v. Real orden del Marqués de Mancera, México, 23 de abril de 1665.

162. Ibid., 40:65, fs. 55–58v. Real orden del Conde de Galve, México, 10 de diciembre de 1695.
163. Real cédula al rector y claustro de la Universidad de México, Madrid, 9 de octubre de 1696. Lanning, *Reales cédulas,* no. 79, pp. 107–9.
164. AGI, Indiferente General, 668. Real despacho por el que se restablece el Tribunal del Protomedicato, Cádiz, 22 de julio de 1811.
165. Ibid., 668. Real despacho relativo a los profesores de que se ha de componer el Tribunal del Protomedicato mandado restablecer por decreto de S.M. de 22 de julio de 1811, Cádiz, 21 de septiembre de 1811.
166. AGNM, Reales cédulas (Dup.), 205:54, fs. 59–60. Real orden al virrey de la Nueva España, Cádiz, 26 de septiembre de 1811.
167. AGI, Indiferente General, 550, Expediente No. 3. Decreto de 11 de septiembre, 1814. *Gazeta* Núm. 138.
168. Archivo del Ex-Ayuntamiento de México, México (hereinafter AEAM), Médicos y Boticas, 1:10. Cabildo de 8 de agosto de 1814.
169. A thorough search of the files of royal orders and cédulas in the Archivo General de la Nación in Mexico does not turn up any such specific document. Neither did there appear any copy of the so-called "ley de tribunales," which was supposed to have ended the protomedicato in America.
170. AGI, Indiferente General, 673. Real despacho por el que restablece el Tribunal de Protomedicato, Madrid, 20 de mayo de 1820.
171. The twenty-five signatures included those of the celebrated physicians Hipólito Unánue, Miguel Tafur, Félix Devoti, and José Manuel Valdés. Juan B. Lastres, *Hipólito Unánue* (Lima, 1955), pp. 178–79. (Hereinafter Lastres, *Hipólito Unánue.*)
172. For an illustration of the confusion this process caused, even in the Council of the Indies, see AGI, Buenos Aires, 335. Dictamen del fiscal, Madrid, 29 de junio de 1804.

4. *Problems of Jurisdiction*

1. Muñoz, *Recopilación,* Cap. VI, Art. III, p. 87.
2. AGNM, Reales cédulas (Dup.), 40:2, fs. 2–4. Real orden del Virrey Conde de Galve, México, 24 de enero de 1692.
3. Archivo General de Gobierno, Guatemala City (hereinafter AGG), Al.4, 13779, 2004. Dictamen del Dr. Vicente Sorogastua y Carranza, Nueva Guatemala, 27 de junio de 1800.
4. ACB, Médicos y Abogados, 5, f.264. Dr. Juan José del Castillo, in a postscript to Luis Agustín González's description of the Lima protomedicato sent to Dr. Cancino in Bogotá, says he has heard a collection has come from Spain, setting out the "privileges, exemptions, and faculties" of the protomedicato edited by an oidor of Valencia. That he gives an inexact title is proof of his claim that he did not have it in hand.
5. Archivo Histórico de la Facultad de Medicina de la Universidad de México,

Mexico City (hereinafter AHFM), Protomedicato, 6:8, fs. 1–62. Manuel del Campo y Rivas al Real Protomedicato, 11 de agosto de 1815; Dr. Ignacio García Jove al juez en turno, 17 de agosto de 1815; Manuel del Campo y Rivas al Mro. y Dr. Ignacio García Jove, 21 de agosto de 1815.

6. *Nueva recopilación,* Lib. III, Tít. XVI, Ley 4.
7. Juan Ramón Beltrán, *Historia del Protomedicato de Buenos Aires* (Buenos Aires, 1937), p. 5. (Hereinafter Beltrán, *Protomedicato de Buenos Aires.*)
8. AGI, México, 1299, No. 122. Revilla Gigedo al rey, México, 26 de junio de 1791.
9. *Recopilación de Indias,* Lib. V, Tít. VI, Ley 1.
10. AGI, México, 1299. El Real Protomedicato al rey, México, 27 de junio de 1791.
11. *Recopilación de Indias,* Lib. V, Tít. VI, Ley 3.
12. AGI, Mexico, 1299. Certificación del escribano y receptor de la Real Audiencia, México, 30 de julio de 1791.
13. Ibid., 1299. Respuesta del Sr. Fiscal, Madrid, 9 de noviembre de 1791.
14. AGNM, Reales cédulas (Dup.), 151:145, fs. 65–68v. Real cédula al virrey de Nueva España, Aranjuez, 31 de enero de 1792. The viceroy gave the complementary orders on June 4, 1792.
15. Benavente Garcés, *El protomedicato en Chile,* pp. 73–75. See also *Recopilación de Indias,* Lib. V, Tít. VI, Leyes 5 y 6.
16. AHNM, Consejos, 51690. Real cédula a la audiencia de Chile, Madrid, 22 de diciembre de 1790.
17. AGI, Indiferente General, 1344. Consulta del Tribunal del Protomedicato de Madrid, 27 de julio de 1791. This consulta apparently had been brought on by the creation of a protomedicato in Buenos Aires.
18. Ibid., 1344. Consulta del Tribunal del Protomedicato de Madrid, 27 de julio de 1791. "A 17 de junio de 1798, S.M. no viene en ello."
19. Muñoz, *Recopilación,* Cap. VII, Art. X, pp. 102–5.
20. Ibid.
21. AGI, México, 1751. Real Protomedicato de Nueva España al rey, México, 30 de junio de 1792.
22. Ibid., 1751. Dictamen del fiscal, Madrid, 30 de noviembre de 1793; Auto decreto del Consejo de Indias, Madrid, 14 de enero de 1793.
23. AGI, Indiferente General, 1291. Minuta de consulta del Consejo de Indias, Madrid, 17 de noviembre de 1718.
24. ACB, Médicos y Abogados, 4, fs. 138–40. Pedimento de Manuel Maitin, Panamá, 21 de abril de 1760.
25. Ibid., 4, f. 140r–40v. Decreto del gobernador, Panamá, 22 de abril de 1760.
26. Ibid., 4, fs. 140v–45v. Informe del Dr. Francisco Ventivoglio de la Case, Panamá, 23 de abril de 1760.
27. *Recopilación de Indias,* Lib. V, Tít. VI, Ley 1.
28. ACB, Médicos y Abogados, 4, fs. 134v–35v. Título de protomédico para el Dr. Francisco Ventivoglio de la Case, Bogotá, 17 de diciembre de 1759.
29. *Nueva recopilación,* Lib. III, Tít. XVI, Ley 2.
30. *Recopilación de Indias,* Lib. V, Tít. VI, Ley 6.

31. ACB, Médicos y Abogados, 4, fs. 145v–46r. Pedimento del Dr. don Francisco Ventivoglio, Panamá, 12 de mayo de 1760.
32. Ibid., 4, fs. 146v–47r. Informe de Bartolomé Pinto de Rivera, Panamá, 13 de mayo de 1760.
33. Ibid., 4, f. 147r. Decreto del gobernador Guill, Panamá, 14 de mayo de 1760.
34. Ibid., 4, f. 147r–47v. Decreto del Gobernador Guill, Panamá, 28 de mayo de 1760.
35. Ibid., 4, f. 146v. Notificación, 2 de junio de 1760.
36. Ibid., 4, fs. 151An.–51Br., 151Cn.–51Cv., 151Er.–51Fv. Dr. Francisco Ventivoglio de la Case al virrey, Panamá, 20 de junio de 1760, 13 de noviembre de 1760, 13 de enero de 1761.
37. A certified copy of an entry in the Libro Capitular of the cabildo in Panama showed that the governors there had appointed protomédicos after the founding of the viceroyalty whenever there were vacancies. Ibid., 4, f. 150–50v.
38. *Recopilación de Indias,* Lib. V, Tít. VI, Ley 1.
39. AGI, Lima, 686. Virrey Teodoro de Croix a don Antonio de Porlier, Lima, 30 de marzo de 1789.
40. For a more detailed summary and review case, see AGI, México, 1139. El consejo de Indias pleno de dos salas a S.M., Madrid, 25 de junio de 1798, No. 12.
41. In Spain these were the only matters that could be appealed from the royal protomedicato.
42. Where there was no audiencia, the governor's assessor rendered the binding opinion.
43. This printed circular cédula (San Lorenzo, 27 de octubre de 1798) may be found in AGG, Al. 23, 10090, fs. 216–219; Al. 4, 13779, 2004; AHFM, Protomedicato VI, 8 and in John Tate Lanning, ed., *Reales cédulas de la Real y Pontificia Universidad de San Carlos de Guatemala* (Guatemala, 1954), pp. 247–57. (Hereinafter Lanning, *Reales cédulas de San Carlos.*)
44. Quoted at length in their exchange with the viceroy on their jurisdiction. AHFM, Protomedicato 6:8, fs. 1–5. Expediente sobre la jurisdicción y alcances de los Tribunales del Protomedicato (1805–15).
45. A "majestic and honorific" ornament made like the canopy of a bed and held out from the wall on a frame, with fringe hanging down from the front and sides and a curtain at the back separating it from the wall. Generally made of velvet or damask decorated with braid and sometimes bordered with gold or silver, it was exactly the same conception as the cover for a throne.
46. AHFM, Protomedicato 6:8. Virrey Iturrigaray a la real audiencia, México, 16 de septiembre de 1805; Decreto de la real audiencia, México, 17 de septiembre de 1805.
47. Ibid., 6:8, f. 8. Decreto y notificación, 1 de octubre de 1805.
48. Ibid., 6:8. Decreto de 11 de noviembre de 1805; notificación de 15 de noviembre de 1805.
49. Ibid., 6:8. Dictamen del fiscal, 24 de diciembre de 1805 y del asesor, 2 de enero de 1806.
50. Ibid., 6:8. Dictamen del fiscal, 10 de marzo de 1806.

51. Ibid., 6:8. Manuel de Campo y Rivas al virrey, s.f. (c. 1814–15).
52. Ibid., 6:8. Dr. y Mro. José Ignacio García Jove al Oidor Manuel del Campo y Rivas, México, 7 de agosto de 1815.
53. Ibid., 10:11. Expediente sobre la queja del doctor Manuel del Campo y Rivas, juez en turno, contra los miembros del Protomedicato, sobre su jurisdicción. Manuel del Campo al Dr. García y Jove, México, 11 de agosto de 1815.
54. The "Sor. Muñoz" referred to was Miguel Eugenio Muñoz. Ibid., 10:11. Dr. y Mro. José Ignacio García Jove a Manuel del Campo y Rivas, México, 17 de agosto de 1815.
55. Wherever there were audiencias, two oidores (accompanied by at least one alcalde del crimen, the crown attorney, the alcalde ordinario, alguacil, and jail clerk, and, if he so desired, the corregidor) visited and inspected jails every Saturday. At Christmas, in keeping with the tradition of humanity to prisoners at that season, the whole audiencia made a special inspection. Except in the case of men sentenced by the alcaldes del crimen and by the Tribunal of Accounts, those sentenced for cheating the crown in financial matters, and men arrested for deserting their wives, the oidores could legally release prisoners, especially those found jailed without sufficient cause. (*Recopilación de Indias,* Lib. VII, Tít. VII, Leyes 1–17.) Campo was legally correct in his position that those in jail on a writ of the protomedicato might be released by the visitation.
56. *Novísima recopilación de leyes de España,* 6 vols. (Madrid, 1805–7). Lib. VII, Tít. XI, Leyes 2, 3, 4, 5, 6, 8; Lib. VII, Tít. XII, Leyes 7, 12. (Hereinafter *Novísima recopilación.*)
57. *Recopilación de Indias,* Lib. V, Tít. VI, Ley 2.
58. Ibid., Lib. V, Tít. VI, Leyes 4 y 5.
59. AHFM, Protomedicato 6:8. Manuel del Campo y Rivas al Dr. y Mro. José Ignacio García Jove, México, 21 de agosto de 1815.
60. Ibid., 6:8. José Ignacio García Jove a Manuel del Campo y Rivas, México, 7 de septiembre de 1815.
61. Manuel del Campo had cited the *Recopilación de Indias,* Lib. V, Tít. VI, Ley 2, based upon a decree of Charles II, to show that the royal laws of Spain were applicable.
62. Ibid., Lib. II, Tít. I, Leyes 39 y 40. The law, based upon a cédula of Philip IV, Monzón, 8 de marzo de 1626, says that no "pragmatic" published in "these kingdoms" may go into force in America without a special cédula dispatched by the Council of the Indies.
63. AHFM, Protomedicato 6:8, fs. 32–56v. José Ignacio García Jove a Manuel del Campo y Rivas, México, 7 de septiembre de 1815.
64. Ibid., 6:8, fs. 57–58. Manuel del Campo y Rivas al Dr. y Mro. José Ignacio García Jove, México, 15 de septiembre de 1815.
65. Ibid. Decreto del Virrey Calleja, México, 27 de enero de 1816.
66. Ibid. José Ignacio García Jove al virrey, México, 17 de septiembre de 1815.
67. AGI, Indiferente General, 500. The law of October 9, 1812, applied to America by the decree of January 23, 1813.

68. *Siete partidas,* Partida 2, Tít. 31, Ley 7.

69. AGNM, Universidad, 52, fs. 139–40v. Published in Francisco Fernández del Castillo, *La facultad de medicina,* pp. 189–91. The record of this case is also carried in AGNM, Reales cédulas (Dup.), 33:174, fs. 278r–80. Real orden al Real Protomedicato, México, 19 de octubre de 1688.

70. AGNM, Reales cédulas (Dup.), 40:2.

71. *Recopilación de Indias,* Lib. V, Tít. VI, Ley 2.

72. AGI, México, 1754. Real cédula de [Aranjuez] 5 de mayo de 1695 para que en la ciudad de México, se guarde y cumpla el estilo y costumbre que se guarda en el Protomedicato de España, en los examenes de médicos, cirujanos, visitas de boticas y todo lo demás que le pertenece. This cédula also appears in AGNM, Reales cédulas (Dup.), 43: fs. 142–51v, and in J. M. Reyes, "Historia de la medicina. Estudios históricos sobre el ejercicio de la medicina," *Gazeta médica de México* I (1865):254–55.

73. AHNM, Consejos, 1018. "Consultas curiosas del Consejo," Tomo 3, N-V, Lib. 1018, Consulta no. 20. Consulta del Consejo a S.M., Madrid, 31 de julio de 1736.

74. AGI, Santo Domingo, 1607. Juan Manuel Cagigal a José de Gálvez, Habana, 28 de febrero de 1782, No. 186.

75. Ibid., 1458. Expediente tocante a la queja que José Rodríguez, cirujano de Cuba, da del Gobernador de aquella plaza. Año de 1766, Consejo, No. 23.

76. Ibid., 893. Real orden al Presidente de la Casa de Contratación, Madrid, 12 de abril de 1774.

77. Ibid., 874. Real cédula al Gobernador de Caracas D. Francisco Alberro, Aranjuez, 6 de abril de 1692.

78. He cited *Recopilación de Indias,* Lib. V, Tít. VI, Leyes 2, 3, 4, 5.

79. AGI, México, 1769. Dictamen del fiscal, Madrid, 21 de abril de 1779.

80. Ibid., 1767. Decreto de 22 de abril de 1779.

81. Ibid., 1776. D. Antonio Porlier al Gobernador del Consejo de Indias, Aranjuez, 15 de abril de 1790.

82. Ibid., 1776. Memorial de D. Mariano Aznares, Madrid, 30 de marzo de 1790.

83. Ibid., 1776. Dictamen del fiscal, Madrid, 17 de enero de 1791; Decreto del Consejo, 20 de enero de 1791.

84. AGI, Chile, 265. La real audiencia de Chile al rey, Santiago de Chile, 29 de abril de 1776.

85. Ibid., 265. Dictamen del fiscal, Madrid, 26 de febrero de 1777.

86. Ibid., 265. Expediente No. 35: Expediente respondido del Sr. Fiscal sobre la oposición hecha a la cátedra de Prima de Medicina de la Real Universidad de Santiago de Chile. It took 263 folios to record these trivial legal evasions.

87. AGNM, Universidad, 19, fs. 91–96v. Claustros de 13 y 30 de marzo de 1697. These incidents are summarized from this source by Carreño, *Efemérides,* I:370.

88. AGI, México, 398. Acuerdo del Consejo de 14 de mayo de 1700; Real cédula al rector de la Real Universidad de México, Madrid, 5 de julio de 1700; Real cédula a la audiencia de México, Madrid, 5 de julio de 1700. See also Lanning, *Reales cédulas,* No. 86:114–15.

89. Rómulo Velasco Ceballos, ed. *La cirugía mexicana en el siglo XVIII* (México,

1946), pp. 62–65. Bando del Virrey de Croix, México, 10 de abril de 1770. (Hereinafter Velasco Ceballos, *La cirugía.*)

90. Ibid., pp. 62–65.

91. Ibid., pp. 203–4. Informe del Real Protomedicato, México, 17 de diciembre de 1782.

92. Ibid., p. 206. Decreto del Virrey Mayorga, México, 31 de marzo de 1783.

93. Ibid., pp. 217–18. Manuel Antonio Moreno al Virrey Revilla Gigedo, México, 22 de enero de 1791.

94. Ibid., pp. 218–22. El Protomedicato (Dr. y Mro. José Giral; Dr. y Mro. José Francisco Posado) al Virrey Revilla Gigedo, México, 5 de abril de 1791.

95. Composed of the *regente* of the audiencia, an oidor, the civil fiscal, the senior regidor, the *síndico procurador,* and a member of the ecclesiastical cabildo.

96. AGI, Indiferente General, 2660. Real cédula circular, Aranjuez, 2 de marzo de 1804. AGNM, Reales cédulas (Dup.), 192:15; AGNM, Protomedicato 3:15 y 16.

97. Except, as in the case of surgeons, the media anata of 5 pesos, 2 reales, and 6 granos.

98. AGNM, Protomedicato 3:16. Informe del dn. Antonio Serrano al virrey, don José de Iturrigaray, México, 21 de septiembre de 1804.

99. Ibid. Antonio Serrano al Virrey José de Iturrigaray, México, 15 de diciembre de 1804.

100. AGNM, Reales cédulas (Dup.), 92:169, fs. 296–97. Real cédula al virrey de Nueva España, Aranjuez, 20 de mayo de 1768.

101. *Reales ordenanzas generales de los colegios y escuelas de cirugía* (México, 1799). (Hereinafter *Reales ordenanzas generales.*)

102. Ibid., Part. 5, Cap. 9, Art. 1, f. 240.

103. AGNM, Protomedicato 3:16. Antonio Serrano al Virrey Iturrigaray, México, 15 de diciembre de 1804.

104. The apprenticeship method, especially where the apothecary was more interested in free labor than in education, was not calculated to produce men who could vie with doctors and aristocrats in other professions.

105. The media anata of 5 pesos, 2 reales, and 6 granos.

106. This statement of the case for the reform of pharmacy is based upon ibid. Informe de Vicente Cervantes al Virrey José Iturrigaray, México, 21 de septiembre de 1804.

107. This, they said, was expressly against chapter 13 of the *Ordenanzas* of the protomédicos.

108. AGNM, Protomedicato 3:16. Informe del real protomedicato al Virrey José de Iturrigaray, México, 31 de diciembre de 1804. Velasco Ceballos, *La cirugía,* pp. 314–24.

109. AGNM, Protomedicato 3:16. México, 3 de febrero de 1805.

110. Ibid. Extracto del informe de José Ignacio García Jove y Luis Montaña al virrey, México, 12 de noviembre de 1814.

111. Ibid. Antonio Serrano al Virrey Félix María Calleja, México, 23 de febrero de 1815.

112. AGNM, Reales cédulas (Dup.), 171:184. Real cédula, San Lorenzo, 27 de

octubre 1798. Viceroy Azanza published this cédula by a bando, México, 21 de marzo de 1800. See AGNM, Bandos, 20, f. 186.

113. Lib. V, Tít. VI, Ley 1.

114. San Lorenzo, 10 de noviembre de 1797.

115. AGNM, Protomedicato 2:16. José Mesía al virrey, México, 11 de febrero de 1815.

116. AGI, Indiferente General, 640. Decreto de S. M. al Conde de Medellín, Madrid, 23 de enero de 1679; La Casa de la Contratación a S.M., Sevilla, 7 de febrero de 1679.

117. Ibid., 640. Acuerdo del Consejo, Madrid, 16 de febrero de 1679.

118. Earl J. Hamilton, "Wages and Subsistence of Spanish Treasure Ships, 1503–1660," *The Journal of Political Economy* 37 (August 1929):430–45.

119. AGNM, Reales cédulas (Dup.), 128: f. 60v–60r. Real orden, México, 10 de noviembre de 1771.

120. AGNM, Protomedicato 1:4. Sobre que los facultativos se rehusan a hacer los méritos a las embarcaciones. Años de 1808 a 1809.

121. Ibid., f. 4. Cabildo de 7 de febrero de 1806.

122. Ibid., fs. 4–5. Acuerdo del cabildo de Veracruz, 14 de febrero de 1806.

123. Ibid., fs. 5–7. Acuerdo del cabildo de Veracruz, 30 de diciembre de 1808.

124. One of them was from the "médico titular" of Veracruz and subdelegate of the protomedicato, José de Avila.

125. Ibid., fs. 9–10, 16–17.

126. Ibid., fs. 12–13.

127. Ibid., fs. 14–15. Miguel Sauch al gobernador intendente, Veracruz, 16 de enero de 1809.

128. Ibid., fs. 18–21. Francisco Hernández al gobernador intendente, Veracruz, 26 de enero de 1809.

129. Ibid., f. 23; 5, f. 29. The exemption took place, apparently, on January 31 as a result of Hernández's rebuttal.

130. AGNM, Protomedicato 1:5. Expediente promovido por el Dr. Florencio Pérez Comoto, en representación de otros facultativos, pidiendo no se exima de la visita de sanidad mal Dr. dn. Francisco Hernández. Año de 1809.

131. Ibid., fs. 25–28.

132. Of the doctors setting up in Veracruz as doctors, only "Bachelor Luna," Joaquín Alvanedo, and Juan Bautista Crivelli gave Pérez Comoto their power of attorney. As subdelegate of the royal protomedicato, Sauch could not join the others against Hernández, though he did not conceal his prejudice against his recalcitrant competitior. AGNM, Protomedicato 1:5. Miguel Sauch al cabildo de Veracruz, Veracruz, 3 de febrero de 1809.

133. Ibid., fs. 33–34v. Petición del Dr. Florencio Pérez y Comoto al virrey, s.l., s.f.

134. Ibid., f. 61r–61v. García Dávila al Virrey Pedro Garibay, Veracruz, 18 de febrero de 1809.

135. Ibid., fs. 47r–54r. Petición de dn. Ignacio de la Campa Coz, México, s.f.

136. Ibid. Dictamen del fiscal de lo civil, Ambrosio Zagarzurieta, México, 19 de junio de 1809; Decreto del virrey, México, 20 de junio de 1809.

137. Ibid. Dictamen del fiscal, México, 30 de junio de 1809.

138. Ibid. Decreto del virrey, México, 26 de julio de 1809.

139. Ibid. Dictamen del fiscal de lo civil, México, 31 de julio de 1809; Decreto del virrey, México, 27 de agosto de 1809.

140. Ibid. Informe del sub-delegado del protomedicato, Miguel Sauch, Veracruz, 5 de septiembre de 1809.

141. This doubling of the "faculties" was a violation of law and, in Veracruz at least, a violation of the royal dispatch of November 10, 1797.

142. This same dispatch required military chiefs to see to it that army surgeons not venture out of surgery and practice professions for which they did not have the proper qualification and license.

5. *The Illicit Practice of Medicine*

1. *Intrusos* (quacks). The *curandero,* though synonymous with *intruso,* especially in the cities and towns where there were Spaniards, became the pathetic and superstitious "curer" in the countryside and native villages.

2. AGI, México, 780. Real cédula al Virrey Conde de Alba de Liste, Buen Retiro, 6 de junio de 1652.

3. To piece together a decent income, however, even the most renowned physicians gladly accepted part-time appointment in the government-financed Indian hospital. There they went their well spaced rounds and then left their native patients, often in extremis, to their interns.

4. AGI, Indiferente General, 421. Real cédula que el Licenciado Barreda sea médico de la isla Española, Granada, 14 de septiembre de 1525.

5. Ibid., 421. Real cédula a la audiencia de Santo Domingo, Valladolid, 1 de junio de 1527.

6. AGI, Santo Domingo, 1123. Real cédula al gobernador de la isla de Cuba, Valladolid, 2 de abril de 1604.

7. Ibid., 889. Real cédula al gobernador de la Habana, Madrid, 11 de julio de 1765.

8. Ibid., 879. Real cédula a la ciudad de San Juan de Puerto Rico, Madrid, 4 de diciembre de 1709.

9. Ibid., 894. Real cédula al gobernador de Puerto Rico, San Ildefonso, 21 de agosto de 1777.

10. AGI, Indiferente General, 551. José de Limonta al Señor Capitán General de Puerto Rico, Cádiz, 4 de julio de 1813.

11. AGI, Santo Domingo, 893. Real cédula al gobernador de Caracas, El Pardo, 15 de marzo de 1776.

12. P. D. Rodríguez Rivero, *Historia médica de Venezuela hasta 1900* (Caracas, 1931), pp. 120–23.

13. He had laid claim to the degrees of licentiate and doctor of medicine from Padua, and, at least, presented a license with a doctor's name rubbed out and his own inserted—clumsily.

14. AGI, Justicia, 199. Autos fiscales con el Dr. Pedro de la Torre, médico, vecino

de México, sobre que no actue en su facultad por no tener el título corre-
spondiente. Sentencia dada y pronunciada, en la dicha ciudad de México en
28 de marzo de 1545.

15. Ibid., 199. Sentencia en grado de revista, México, 19 de mayo de 1545.

16. Ibid. Autos fiscales con el doctor Pedro de la Torre. . . .

17. As a man might begin the practice of medicine with the bachelor's degree, the
licentiate and doctorate (seven licentiates and 143 doctors between 1567 and
1820) were duplications except for a few overseas physicians whose degrees
were "incorporated." The number of degrees is based upon AGNM, Universidad, Grados de Bachilleres en Medicina, Tomos 279–83. See Fernández
de Recas, *Medicina,* pp. 273–79.

18. AGNM, Universidad, Libro de claustros, 1788–1801. Claustro pleno de 4 de
abril de 1791.

19. Archivo Histórico del Instituto de Antropología e Historia, México (hereinafter AHIAH), Protomedicato, T-4, 12. Legajo de expedientes relativos a
examenes en la facultad de medicina. Año de 1810.

20. AGG, Al. 3–12, 12766–861, 1912–38. See Lanning, *The University in the
Kingdom of Guatemala,* pp. 200–204, and John Tate Lanning, "Grados aca-
démicos en el Reino de Guatemala (ms., Duke University), pp. xiii–xxi, 100–
101, 123–24.

21. The proprietary professor had retired while continuing to draw three-fourths
of an inadequate salary—exactly the same as it was in 1820.

22. AGG, Al.4, 5824, 265. Plan que el Dr. Pedro de Molina formuló para
organizar el Real Colegio de Cirujía, Guatemala, 8 de abril de 1820.

23. Ninety years before, in 1660, the University of San Marcos was still without
the number of medical chairs that the Spanish law required for the accreditation of a degree in medicine. The faculty, in begging for a chair of medicine,
stressed the shortage of physicians. AGI, Lima, 337. El claustro de la Universidad de San Marcos al rey, Lima, s.f.

24. John Tate Lanning, "Legitimacy and *Limpieza de Sangre* in the Practice of
Medicine in the Spanish Empire," *Jahrbuch für Geschichte von Staat, Wirtschaft und Gesellschaft Lateinamerikas,* 4 (1967):46–52.

25. AGI, Caracas, 241. D. Lorenzo Campins a S.M., Caracas, 11 de julio de
1775. Primera representacion.

26. Ibid., 241. El rector y claustro de la Universidad de Caracas a S.M., Caracas,
21 de agosto de 1776.

27. Ibid., 241. El rector de la Universidad y Seminario de Caracas a S.M., Caracas,
24 de agosto de 1776.

28. ACB, Médicos y Abogados, 6, fs. 379–407. Autos de residencia sobre que se
haya protomédico en esta corte.

29. Ibid., 6, 407, bis.

30. Biblioteca Nacional, Bogotá (hereinafter BNB), Manuscritos, 169. Petición
de Sebastián José López Ruiz, Santa Fe, 27 de enero de 1779.

31. Ibid., 202. "Méthodo provisional e interino de los Estudios que han de observar los Colegios de Santa Fe por aora y hasta tanto, que se erige Universidad
pública, o su Magestad dispose otra cosa," fs. 17–18.

32. Ibid., 174.
33. ACB, Reales cédulas, 34, fs. 739–40f, 742–45. Real cédula a la Audiencia de Santa Fe, San Ildefonso, 2 de octubre de 1801; Real cédula al virrey de Santa Fe, San Ildefonso, 2 de octubre de 1801.
34. ACB, Médicos y Abogados, 4, fs. 653–56. Procurador General Juan Millán y Pinto al Señor Alcalde Ordinario Justicia Mayor, Guayaquil, 16 de julio de 1792.
35. AGI, Quito, 354. Don Francisco Calderón y Piedra a S.M., Quito, 18 de mayo de 1793.
36. Ibid., 354. Dictamen del fiscal, Madrid, 17 de enero de 1795.
37. ACB, Médicos y Abogados, 4, fs. 665–66. Gobernador José de Aguirre Irisarri al Virrey José de Espeleta, 6 de abril de 1795.
38. Archivo de la Real Audiencia de Quito, Quito (hereafter ARAQ), cuerpos docentes. Expediente relativo a la cátedra de medicina de la Universidad de San Fernando. Carondolet al rector de la Universidad de San Fernando, Quito, 13 de agosto de 1803; Fr. Felipe Carrasco al Presidente Carondolet, 26 de agosto de 1803.
39. AGNM, Protomedicato, 2:5, fs. 23–32. Respuesta y pedimento del procurador general, Querétaro, 31 de agosto de 1787.
40. Ibid., 2:5, fs. 26ff.
41. Ibid., 3:3. Quejas del Dr. don José Sánchez Camaño sobre los perjuicios que causan los curanderos que se consienten en el Valle de Santiago, intendencia de Santiago.
42. See, for example, ibid., 3:3. Juan Antonio Riano al virrey, Guanajuato, 23 de mayo de 1795.
43. Ibid., 3:3. Decreto del virrey, México, 3 de julio de 1795.
44. Ibid., 2:5–8.
45. Ibid., 3:6. El Real Protomedicato (Giral, Peña, García Jove) al virrey, México, 15 de marzo de 1788.
46. Ibid., 2:5, fs. 10–15. The commission is dated August 18, Viceroy Marqués de Croix's *pase,* September 17, and that of the cabildo of Querétaro, September 22, 1768.
47. Ibid., 2:5. Instructions dated August 19, 1768.
48. Returning to one of its original purposes, botanical research, the royal protomedicato instructed Díaz Chacón to look out for any "plant, fruit, flower, stone, soil, animal," or anything else whatsoever that might have medicinal properties, to classify the discovery as, for example, tree or herb, state the illness it was good for, and "describe the mode of application."
49. Ibid., 2:5. Representación del procurador de Querétaro, 6 de septiembre de 1787.
50. Ibid., 2:5. Informe del Tribunal del Protomedicato, México, 22 de octubre de 1787.
51. Ibid., 2:5. Tribunal del Protomedicato al Virrey Revilla Gigedo, México, 30 de abril de 1790.
52. Ibid., 2:10. El Bachiller don Miguel Chacón, sobre curanderos perjudiciales en Querétaro, 9 de octubre de 1790.

53. Ibid., 2:10. Informe del Real Protomedicato, México, 26 de marzo de 1791. Las abades de las Capuchinas al Superior Gobierno, Querétaro, 2 de julio de 1790.

54. Ibid., 2:10. José Félix Flores and José María de Estrada al virrey, s.f. Sent to the fiscal, May 19, 1791.

55. Ibid., 2:10. Decreto del Virrey Revilla Gigedo, México, 31 de mayo de 1791.

56. Ibid., 4:1. Declaración de los doctores D. Miguel Díaz Chacón y D. Ramón del Guante, Querétaro, 1 de febrero de 1794.

57. Ibid., 4:1. Real cédula de tolerancia y ámparo, San Lorenzo, 1 de diciembre de 1793.

58. Ibid., 4:1. Decreto del Virrey Revilla Gigedo, México, 9 de mayo de 1794.

59. *Recopilación de Indias,* Lib. V, Tít. VI, Ley 7.

60. AGNM, Protomedicato, 4:1. Don Pedro de Septién Montero y Austri al Virrey Revilla Gigedo, 3 de mayo de 1794.

61. Ibid., 4:1. Parecer del fiscal, México, 18 de septiembre de 1797; Decreto del virrey, 9 de octubre de 1797.

62. Ibid., 4:1. E.C.P. al Virrey Branciforte, México, 20 de diciembre de 1797.

63. Ibid., 4:1. Real Protomedicato al virrey, México, 5 de junio de 1798.

64. Ibid., 4:1. El virrey al Tribunal del Protomedicato, México, 11 de junio de 1798.

65. AHIAH, Protomedicato, T-4, 15, fs. 29–30v. Miguel Lemus y Tapia al Protomedicato, San Andrés, 19 de enero de 1723.

66. Ibid., T-4, 15, f. 59–59v.

67. AGI, México, 780. Dr. don Marcos José Salgado al rey, s.f.

68. Ibid., 416. Real cédula al virrey y audiencia de México, Madrid, 29 de mayo de 1723.

69. AHFM, Protomedicato, 4:17, fs. 1–2. Oficios de fray Antonio Nogueyra al Protomedicato, en los que informa sobre el traslado a México de lego Antonio Bera, conforme a los deseos del Tribunal. Año de 1795.

70. Ibid., 4:20, f. 1. El prior del convento del Carmen al Tribunal del Protomedicato, México, 8 de febrero de 1796.

71. Ibid., 3:12, fs. 1–17. Causa formada contra María Antonia López Rayón, por curandera. Año de 1791.

72. Ibid., 3:12, f. 1v. Deposición de José González y Mora, México, 10 de enero de 1791.

73. Ibid., 3:12, f. 1. The order is dated January 3, 1791.

74. Ibid., 3:12, fs. 1v–3. Deposición de Manuel José Bentemilla, México, 10 de enero de 1791.

75. Ibid., 3:12. fs. 3–4. Deposición de Juan María de Rivero, México, 14 de enero de 1791.

76. Ibid., 3:3, fs. 1–12. Causa formada de oficio del Real Tribunal del Protomedicato contra Dionisio Castellano por haber revelado una providencia secreta. Año de 1791.

77. Ibid., 3:12, fs. 8v–9v. Deposición de María Antonia López Rayón, México, 11 de febrero de 1791.

78. Ibid., 3:12, fs. 5v–6. Deposición de Joaquín Barrientos y Francisco Carabantes, México, 11 de febrero de 1791.
79. Ibid., 3:12, fs. 5v–6. Parecer del fiscal, México, 2 de marzo de 1791.
80. *Causa médico criminal* (Lima, 1764).

6. *Foreign Doctors in the Spanish Empire*

1. *Recopilación de Indias,* Lib. IX, Tít. XXVII, Ley 35.
2. Benito Gerónimo Feijóo y Montenegro, *Teatro crítico,* 2nd ed., 8 vols. (Madrid, 1773–81), I:110. (Hereinafter Feijóo, *Teatro crítico.*)
3. The following discussion is based on the *Recopilación de Indias,* Lib. V, Tít. VI, Leyes 2, 4, 5, 6; Lib. IX, Tít. XXVII, Leyes, 1, 6, 7, 9, 10, 21, 23, 25, 31, 32, 35, 36, 38; Lib. IX, Tít. XXXI, Ley 1.
4. "These kingdoms," in contrast to "those kingdoms" in the Indies, were Castile, León, Aragón, Valencia, Cataluña, Navarra, Mallorca, and Menorca.
5. *Nueva recopilación,* Lib. III, Tít. VII, Ley 13.
6. Muñoz, *Recopilación,* Cap. X, parra. xi, p. 149.
7. AGI, Santo Domingo, 874. Real cédula al gobernador de la Habana, Madrid, 24 de junio de 1682.
8. AGI, México, 780. Año de 1723. Sin lugar.
9. Ibid., 780. Parecer del fiscal, 8 de abril de 1723. Se vió en Consejo, 9 de abril, y se acordó: "Como lo dice el Sr. Fiscal."
10. AGNM, Reales cédulas (Dups.), 4:30, f. 29–29v; 4:38, f. 36–36v. Real cédula al presidente y oidores de la audiencia de México de la Nueva España, y arzobispo, Bentosilla, 17 de octubre de 1602.
11. *Recopilación de Indias,* Lib. V, Tít. VI, Ley 4.
12. AGI, México, 780. El Protomedicato de Nueva España a S.M., s.l, 1728; Resolución del Consejo de Indias, Madrid, 26 de abril de 1728.
13. Ibid., 780. D. José de Cárdenas, mayordomo del Hospital Real de Indios de México a S.M., s.l., 1741.
14. Ibid., 780. Acuerdo del Consejo de Indias, Madrid, 22 de enero de 1742.
15. D. Francisco Antonio Ledrán received authorization on February 8, 1715, and, when this was not executed, again on November 14, 1723.
16. Ibid., 381. S.M. al Consejo de Indias, Aranjuez, 21 de mayo de 1724.
17. *Nueva recopilación,* Lib. III, Tít. VII, Ley 11.
18. AGI, México, 381. Informe del fiscal, s.f. Se vió en el Consejo, Madrid, 9 de junio de 1724.
19. Ibid., 417. El Consejo de Indias a S.M., Madrid, 17 de julio de 1724.
20. Ibid., 1081. Real cédula al Virrey de la Nueva España, El Pardo, 2 de marzo de 1726. Also in AGNM, Reales cédulas (Dup.), 45:68, fs. 275–76.
21. AGI, Indiferente General, 36. Licencia a D. Santiago Estevanzos para que pueda volver a la N.E. y ejercer a aquel reino la facultad de medicina, Madrid, 19 de agosto de 1727.
22. Ibid., 7. Licencia para embarcarse D. Santiago Estevanzos, Madrid, 2 de septiembre de 1727.

23. *Recopilación de Indias,* Lib. V, Tít. VI, Ley 3.
24. AGI, Indiferente General, 7. El Consejo de Indias a D. Andrés de Elcorobarrutia, Madrid, 18 de septiembre de 1728. Resolución de S.M.: "Como parece." Publicose en 27 de octubre de 1728.
25. AGI, México, 16. Real cédula por que se concede al Dr. D. Juan de Ynglevi naturaleza en estos reinos y los de Indias, Aranjuez, 30 de mayo de 1739.
26. Ibid., 16. Real cédula concediendo licencia para embarcarse el Dr. D. Juan Ynglevi y pasar a la N.E. con un criado moreno, justificando haberlo traido de aquel reino, Alcalá, 19 de junio de 1739.
27. As stated in the *Recopilación de Indias,* Lib. IX, Tít. XXVII, Ley 31.
28. AGI, México, 1111. Real cédula concediendo licencia a D. Jorge Abercromby para que pueda residir en la Nueva España y ejercer su facultad de medicina, Aranjuez, 2 de junio de 1745. Real cédula concediendo licencia para que D. Jorge Abercromby se embarque con un criado y la ropa y libros de su uso, Buen Retiro, 28 de junio de 1745.
29. AGI, Indiferente General, 16. Real cédula por la que se concede a D. Jorge Abercromby naturaleza de los reinos de las Indias, San Lorenzo, 3 de noviembre de 1745. This document may also be found in AGI, México, 1111.
30. Ibid., 16. Real cédula por la que se concede a D. José Guillermo Bates naturaleza de los reinos de las Indias, Aranjuez, 22 de junio de 1785.
31. AGI, Ultramar, 733. Real cédula para que se publique el nuevo arancel con el aumento que se expresa de los servicios pecuniarios a las gracias llamadas al sacar, Madrid, 3 de agosto de 1801.
32. AGNM, Protomedicato, 2:9. Informe del Real Protomedicato, México, 13 de diciembre de 1790.
33. See chapter 5, pp. 145–48.
34. AGNM, Protomedicato, 2:9. El doctor Domingo Melica, solicita del Excmo. Sr. Virrey Conde de Revilla Gigedo, le conceda derecho de naturalización, México, s.f.
35. Ibid., 2:9. Dictamen del fiscal, México, 9 de mayo de 1790.
36. Ibid., 2:9. Informe del Real Protomedicato, México, 13 de diciembre de 1790.
37. See AHFM, Protomedicato, 4:3, f. 1. El Conde de Revilla Gigedo al Real Tribunal del Protomedicato, México, 1 de agosto de 1791.
38. Ibid., 4:3. Decreto del Real Protomedicato, México, 26 de octubre de 1791.
39. AGI, Indiferente General, 16. Informe del Consejo de Indias, Madrid, 2 de septiembre de 1793. Real cédula para que se concede a Dr. D. Domingo Melica pueda permanecer en su actual destino de médico en Querétaro, San Lorenzo, 1 de diciembre de 1793.
40. Ibid., 16. Real cédula por la que se concede a D. Juan Lucás Toniero, médico y cirujano, naturaleza en los reinos de las Indias, Aranjuez, 21 de mayo de 1739.
41. Ibid., 8. Real decreto de S.M., Aranjuez, 11 de junio de 1738. AGI, Indiferente General, 3. Real cédula para que D. Joseph Dumont, médico honorario de familia, pueda pasar al reino de N.E. y ejercer su facultad de medicina, San Ildefonso, 20 de agosto de 1738.

42. AGI, México, 571. D. Baltasar Rous, de nación francesa, cirujano en la Villa de Campeche, reino de N.E. a S.M., s.l., 1758.

43 Ibid., 571. Informe del Cabildo, Justicia y Regimiento de Mérida de Yucatán, 10 de noviembre de 1756; Informe del ayuntamiento de Campeche, 14 de julio de 1757.

44. *Recopilación de Indias,* Lib. IX, Tít. XXVII, Ley 10.

45. AGI, México, 571. Informe del fiscal, Madrid, 17 de julio de 1758.

46. Ibid., 571. Consejo de Indias, en Cámara, 19 de julio de 1758. Ibid., 1115. Real cédula para que D. Baltasar Rous ejerza libremente su facultad de cirujano, Villaviciosa, 16 de septiembre de 1758.

47. Ibid., 1115. Real cédula para que a D. Germán Ducruette no se le impida el mantenerse y ejercer su facultad de Cirugía, en el reino de N.E. sin embargo de lo mandado en la real cédula que se expresa, Buen Retiro, 12 de febrero de 1760.

48. AGI, Indiferente General, 1330. D. José Laporta al rey, Cádiz, 28 de diciembre de 1781.

49. Ibid., 1339. Expediente sobre D. Juan le Blond, médico recibido en los Protomedicatos de Santa Fe y Perú, solicita pasar al reino de N.E. Año de 1786.

50. The Council advised following, especially, *Recopilación de Indias,* Lib. V, Tít. VI, Leyes 4, 5, 6.

51. AGI, México, 1138. Consulta del Consejo de Indias en Sala Primera, México, 19 de abril de 1796.

52. AGI, Santo Domingo, 1122. Real cédula al gobernador de la isla de Cuba, Lisboa, 11 de junio de 1582.

53. Ibid., 889. El rey al Presidente de la Audiencia de la Contratación, Marqués del Real Tesoro, Madrid, 1 de julio de 1765, al gobernador de la Habana, 8 de julio de 1765.

54. Ibid., 890. Real cédula al presidente y oidores de la audiencia de Cádiz, Aranjuez, 17 de mayo de 1766; Real cédula al gobernador de la Habana, Aranjuez, 17 de mayo de 1766.

55. Ibid. Carta a la audiencia de Cádiz, Cádiz, 12 de diciembre de 1766.

56. Ibid., 898. Real cédula al gobernador de la Habana. Madrid, 10 de agosto de 1793.

57. Ibid., 885. Real cédula a la audiencia de Santo Domingo, Buen Retiro, 4 de mayo de 1749.

58. Ibid., 898. Real cédula al gobernador de Santo Domingo, Madrid, 3 de abril de 1789.

59. Ibid., 1123. Real cédula al gobernador de Puerto Rico, San Lorenzo, 19 de octubre de 1799.

7. *Legitimacy and Blood Purity*

1. *Siete partidas,* Partida 7, Tít. 6, Ley 1.

2. AGI, Lima, 308. Real cédula al arzobispo de Lima, Madrid, 21 de enero de

1594. Published in Konetzke, *Colección,* II, 1:14.

3. AGI, México, 776. Auto acordado del Consejo de Indias, Madrid, 30 de abril de 1728.

4. These papers, when they bear any dates at all, are dated between February and June 1741. AGI, Santo Domingo, 426.

5. *Constituciones de la Universidad de México,* prólogo, parras. 19 y 20.

6. Ibid., Const. 246.

7. AGI, México, 1769, Expediente No. 17. Año 1779.

8. Archivo Histórico Nacional, Bogotá (hereinafter AHNB), Cedulario de Ayala, 48, f. 171v. Real cédula al Consejo, San Ildefonso, 2 de septiembre de 1784, published in Konetzke, *Colección,* III, 2:539–40. A royal cédula of the same year, San Ildefonso, 27 de septiembre de 1795, enabled an *expósito* to be naturalized as white in order to take university degrees and practice medicine. He had been "well brought up in a private house"—the bastard of an "illustrious family." AHNB, Cedulario de Ayala, 85, f. 249v, published in Konetzke, *Colección,* III, 2:751–52.

9. AGI, Lima, 914. Dictamen del fiscal del Consejo de las Indias, Madrid, published in Konetzke, *Colección,* III, 2:597–601.

10. AGI, Buenos Aires, 273. Real cédula, Aranjuez, 19 de febrero de 1794; AHNB, Colegios, 1, published in the *Gazeta de México,* VI, (No. 54, 30 de agosto de 1794):444–47.

11. Since the statutes of most colleges did not include this statement or follow such a practice and since those of major universities such as Mexico and San Marcos barred only those vaguely referred to as having a "note of infamy," this cédula does not contradict itself with respect to education.

12. AGI, Caracas, 446. Real cédula, Madrid, 3 de junio de 1819.

13. Muñoz, *Recopilación,* passim.

14. *Nueva recopilación,* Lib. VIII, Tít. III, Ley 3.

15. Muñoz, *Recopilación,* Cap. VI, Sec. I, pp. 71–72.

16. Ibid., Cap. VI, Sec. II, p. 73. This supplementary provision is dated September 2, 1501, eight days before the order it was supposed to help carry out. The date is most likely a misreading for September 12, 1501.

17. AGI, Contratación, 5089. Real provisión, Burgos, 5 de octubre de 1511. This document is printed in several places, including Konetzke, *Colección,* I:30–31.

18. AHNM, Códices, 692 B; Códices, 684 al 725B, Cedulario Indico, Resoluciones y decretos reales durante los siglos XVI, XVII y XVIII, 42 tomos, IX, f. 72v. Real cédula al virrey de Nueva España, Madrid, 15 de octubre de 1535.

19. Muñoz, *Recopilación,* pp. 73–78. Auto del Real Protomedicato (Drs. Juan de Chavarri Azcona, Gaspar Bravo de Sobremonte, and Miguel de Alva), Madrid, 10 de noviembre de 1678.

20. Ibid., pp. 75–76. Papel del Consejo, Madrid, 26 de marzo de 1686.

21. Ibid., pp. 76–77. Informe del Protomedicato, Madrid, 5 de abril de 1686; Decreto del Consejo, Madrid, 29 de mayo de 1686.

22. Ibid., pp. 77–78. Real cédula al presidente y oidores de la audiencia y chancillería de la ciudad de Valladolid, Madrid, 25 de septiembre de 1691.

23. Ibid., pp. 80–81. Memorial del Protomedicato.

24. Ibid., pp. 81–85. Reales decretos, 23 de marzo y de 14 de mayo de 1726.

25. Ibid., p. 79.

26. Ibid., p. 91.

27. *Tractatus bipartitus de puritate, et nobilitate probanda, secundum statuta S. officii inquisitionis, regii ordinum senatus, sanctae Ecclesiae Toletanae, collegiorum, aliarumque communitatum Hispaniae* . . . (Lyons, 1637), to which the author appended an "Instrucción breve y sumaria para los comisarios y notarios de las informaciones de limpieza."

28. In the 1602 edition: Tít. XI, Const. 238, f. 41, p. 2; in the 1735 edition, Tít. XI, Const. 58, f. 69, p. 2.

29. *Constituciones de la Universidad de México,* Tít. XVII, Const. 236, p. 132. These stipulations go back to the seventeenth-century statutes and constitutions of the University of Mexico, for they were literally copied by Francisco Sarassa y Arce when he drew up his *Constituciones de la Real Universidad de San Carlos, aprobadas por la Magestad del Señor Rey Don Carlos II* (Guatemala, 1686 and 1783), Tít. XVI, Const. 196, f. 31, p. 1.

30. AGI, Indiferente General, 520, Lib. 10, f. 342. Konetzke, *Colección,* I:80–81.

31. Konetzke, *Colección,* I:391–92. Ordenanzas para el Gremio de Sombreros. Approved by the cabildo of Mexico, May 5, 1561.

32. Ibid., I:488. Ordenanzas de guanteros y agujeteros, México, 29 de abril de 1575. Approved by the viceroy, January 28, 1576.

33. Ibid., II, 1:108–109. Ordenanzas de los pasamaneros y orilleros, Cabildo, Lima, 19 de marzo de 1604.

34. Ibid., II, 1:280. Real cédula al presidente y oidores de la Real Audiencia de Panamá, San Lorenzo, 15 de octubre de 1623.

35. Ibid., III, 1:24. Real cédula que no se dan títulos de escribanos a mestizos y mulatos, Buen Retiro, 31 de agosto de 1750.

36. Ibid., III, 1:137–38. Real cédula al arzobispo de Lima, Madrid, 14 de febrero de 1717.

37. Ibid., II, 1:197, No. 132. Real cédula al virrey del Perú, San Lorenzo, 24 de abril de 1618.

38. AGI, México, 1070, Lib. 22, f. 49v in Konetzke, *Colección,* II, 2:542, No. 371. Real cédula al virrey de la Nueva España, Madrid, 6 de mayo de 1668.

39. *Memorias de los virreyes que han gobernado el Perú, durante el tiempo del coloniaje español,* 6 vols. (Lima, 1859), III:127. Virrey don José Armendáris, Marqués de Castel-Fuerte. (Hereinafter *Memorias de los virreyes.*)

40. José Pastor Larrinaga, *Apología de los cirujanos del Perú* (Granada, 1791).

41. *Recopilación de Indias,* Lib. I, Tít. XXII, Ley 57.

42. This interpretation is based upon the internal evidence of a royal cédula addressed to the viceroy and audiencia, university, and protomedicato, Buen Retiro, 27 de septiembre de 1752. *Memorias de los virreyes* (Virrey don Manuel Amat y Junient), IV:479.

43. Ibid., IV:480–81. Real cédula, Buen Retiro, 27 de septiembre de 1752.

44. AGI, Lima, 854. Expediente sobre legitimidad y limpieza de sangre de los estudiantes para ingresar en las universidades, colegios, y audiencias. Años 1767–70.

45. Ibid., 854. AHNM, Cedulario Indico, 32:117, f. 144. Real despacho, Madrid, 14 de julio de 1768.

46. See C. E. Paz-Soldán, *José Manuel Valdés, 1767–1843* (Lima, 1942), xxviii–xxxii.

47. Though most Peruvian medical historians such as Dr. Hermilio Valdés and Juan B. Lastres touch upon most Peruvian medical personalities, three authorities, though they sometimes contradict each other on small points, give a more complete impression of José Manuel Valdés: C. E. Paz-Soldán (see n. 46 above), José Antonio Lavalle, "El Doctor Don José Manuel Valdés, Apuntes sobre su vida y sus obras," *Gaceta médica de Lima,* 47–52 (August–November, 1858) and Manuel de Mendiburu, *Diccionario histórico-biográfico del Perú,* 2nd ed., 11 vols. (Lima, 1931–35), XI:162–65. (Hereinafter Mendiburu, *Diccionario histórico-biográfico.*)

48. See, for example, AGNM, Universidad, Grados de Licenciados y Maestros en Artes, 1753–84. Testimonio de las informaciones de limpieza de sangre de los padres, abuelos, y bisabuelos de don Antonio Méndez Prieto, vezinos de esta Ciudad de México, según, y en la forma que dentro se contiene.

49. AGI, Santo Domingo, 1607. Real cédula a Juan Fernández Valiente, Buen Retiro, 26 de julio de 1755.

50. Ibid., 1607. El Rey a los Protomédicos de la Habana, Aranjuez, 21 de mayo de 1757.

51. Ibid., 1455, Consejo No. 10. Expediente de José Francisco Báez y Llerena, profesor de cirugía en la Habana, sobre aversele prohivido la continuación en el uso de este Arte, a pretexto de no ser hombre blanco declaradamente, y solicitud de que se mandase al Prothomedicato de Aquella Ciudad, le dejase seguir en su facultad, y dispensas al mismo tiempo el punto de limpieza que se notaba a sus padres.

52. Ibid., 1607. Real cédula para que José Francisco Báez Llerena, vecino de la Habana pueda usar y ejercer libremente su facultad de Cirujía en la forma que se expresa, Aranjuez, 1 de junio de 1760.

53. Ibid., 1463. Año 1772, Cámara, Núm. 8.

54. Ibid., 1463. Dictamen del fiscal, Madrid, 21 de febrero de 1773.

55. Ibid., 1463. Dictamen del fiscal, Madrid, 26 de abril de 1773.

56. One of the most famous cases was that involving the sons of the "Licenciado" D Manuel María de Arellano y Cervallo, 1762, in AGNM, Universidad, Informaciones de Limpieza de Sangre.

57. AGI, Santo Domingo, 1357. Expediente núm. 16 tocante a la instancia que por medio del gobernador de Cuba introdujó Juan de la Cruz y Mena, profesor de medicina y cirugía en la Villa del Bayamo, sobre que se habilitase a sus hijos para ser admitidos en Universidades a cursar Ciencias sin embargo de su humilde calidad.

58. Ibid., 1357. El gobernador de Cuba, D. Lorenzo de Madariaga a S.M.,

Bayamo, 16 de junio de 1761, con un testimonio y representación de Juan de la Cruz y Mena.

59. Ibid., 1357. Dictamen del fiscal, Madrid, 15 de junio de 1762.

60. Ibid., 1347. Real cédula a la Universidad de la Habana, Buen Retiro, 10 de julio de 1764. Also in AGI, Santo Domingo, 889.

61. Ibid., 1457. Año de 763, Consejo, No. 7, Instancia de Miguel José de Avilés, s.l., s.f. 1763.

62 Ibid., 1457. Informe del fiscal, Madrid, 22 de junio de 1763.

63. Ibid., 911. Real cédula al Protomedicato de la Ciudad de San Cristóbal de la Habana, San Ildefonso, 29 de julio de 1763.

64. Ibid., 911. Real cédula para que Miguel José de Avilés, pardo libre, pueda ejercer libremente su arte de cirugía, Madrid, 24 de diciembre de 1766. This expediente is also in AGI, Santo Domingo, 1458. Año 1766, Consejo, No. 15.

65. Muñoz, *Recopilación,* pp. 151–52.

66. The petitioner received this news officially June 28, 1788. This expediente is to be found in AGNM, Hospitales, 144 (Archivo de Hacienda), and is printed in Velasco Ceballos, *La cirugía,* pp. 451–62.

67. ACB, Médicos y Abogados, 6, f. 526f–26v. Cartagena, 9 de junio de 1806.

68. Ibid., 6, f. 496. Cartagena, 29 de agosto de 1806.

69. All these testimonials are dated Cartagena, August 29, 1806, except that of Irogoyen, which is dated August 25. Ibid., 6, fs. 493–517f.

70. Ibid., 6, f. 510. Testimonio de Joaquín Francisco Fidalgo, Cartagena, 30 de agosto de 1806.

71. Ibid., 6, f. 510. Testimonio de Colonel Blas de Soria, Cartagena, 20 de agosto de 1806.

72. Ibid., 6, fs. 526v–28v. Informe del protomédico Licenciado Juan de Arias, Cartagena, 5 de agosto de 1806.

73. Ibid., 6, fs. 517f–20f. Santiago Padilla al virrey, Cartagena, 30 de agosto de 1806.

74. *Nueva Recopilación,* Lib. III, Tít. XVI, Ley 1, parra. 9; Ley 7, parra. 29.

75. ACB, Médicos y Abogados, 6, f. 537f.

76. Ibid., 6, fs. 537f–58f.

77. Ibid., 6, f. 560v.

78. Archivo General de la Nación, Caracas (hereinafter AGNC), Títulos de médicos, Tomo Unico. Real cédula que los pardos que ejerzan la medicina con Real aprobación, puedan concurrir a la enseñanza de anatomía, Aranjuez, 21 de junio de 1793.

79. Ibid. Francisco Colina solicitando se la admita a examen para el ejercicio de médico. Año de 1798.

80. Ibid. Dictamen del fiscal, D. Quintana, Caracas, 2 de marzo de 1798.

81. Ibid. Expediente No. 6, fs. 69–126. The names and highest academic titles of these physicians and surgeons are given here.

82. The list includes cédulas of February 10, 1795, July 12, 1796, September 22, 1797, October 24, 1801, and April 7, 1805. The cédula of 1805 is printed in Konetzke, *Colección,* II, 3:814–16.

83. AGI, Caracas, 446. No. 44. Año de 1806. La Universidad de Caracas, Rdo.

Obispo, y otros sobre oposición a admitir en sus aulas a los Pardos dispensados de estas calidades, y pretensiones en solicitud de estas y otros puntos acerca de honrar hasta cierto grado a los mulatos y zambos.

84. AGI, Guatemala, 421. Real cédula para que Mariano Fernández pueda abrir botica pública en la antigua Guatemala dispensandole al efecto la calidad de pardo, Isla de León, 7 de febrero de 1811. (Minuta.)

85. Ibid., 421. Real cédula para que Francisco Fernández pueda ejercer la facultad de Farmacia dispensandole al efecto la calidad de pardo, Isla de León, 7 de febrero de 1811.

86. AGI, Indiferente General, 1551, f. 29v. Al secretario de Guerra y Justicia: Pidiendole la Real Cédula de gracias al sacar del extinguido Consejo de Yndias, sobre dispensa de la calidad de Pardo en la Antigua Guatemala a Mariano Fernández, Boticario de la misma, Cádiz, 11 de marzo de 1813.

87. To document this new liberalization, see various documents in AGI, Indiferente General, 550.

8. The Handling of Charity

1. Muñoz, *Recopilación,* Cap. XIII, Art. I, p. 158.

2. *Nueva recopilación,* Lib. III, Tít. XVI, Ley 3, p. 301.

3. On August 5, 1644, for example, a clerk in a Spanish hospital made this typical entry: "Ciruelas p. almorzar los pobres doce libras a seis mrs." (Plums to feed the poor, twelve pounds at six maravedís.) Archivo del Hospital de San Bernabé y San Antolín, Palencia. Limros de gastos de 1644.

4. Muñoz, *Recopilación,* Cap. XIII, Art. IX, pp. 167–68.

5. Ibid., Cap. XIII, Sec. IX, p. 167.

6. AHFM, Protomedicato, 12:16, fs. 1–12. Año de 1818.

7. Carreño, *Efemérides,* II:796. Claustro de 6 de febrero de 1800.

8. AGNC, Títulos de médicos, Tomo Unico. Testimonios de los aranceles de médicos, cirujanos, y boticarios. Año de 1800.

9. Muñoz, *Recopilación,* Cap. XIII, Art. IX, p. 168.

10. AEAM, Médicos y boticas, 1, fs. 1–7. Cabildos de 4 de julio, 20 y 26 de septiembre, 8 de octubre de 1776; Informe del Real Protomedicato, México, 14 de octubre de 1776.

11. *Gazeta de México,* VI (No. 28, 28 de abril de 1794): 224–26, Bando de 14 de mayo de 1777, and AGNM, Bandos, 10, published in Velasco Ceballos, *La cirugía,* pp. 431–32.

12. *Reglamento formado de orden del Exmo. Señor Virrey Conde de Revilla Gigedo para el gobierno que ha de observarse en el alumbrado de las calles de México* (México, 1790). Approved by the viceroy on April 7.

13. Published in Velasco Ceballos, *La cirugía,* pp. 463–68.

14. Ibid., pp. 464–67.

15. Ibid., pp. 467–69. Dictamen del fiscal, México, 18 de noviembre de 1790; Decreto del virrey, México, 19 de noviembre de 1790. The case had begun on September 2, 1790.

16. AGNM, Hospitales, 144, printed in ibid., pp. 471–80. On April 23, 1794,

Revilla Gigedo renewed Bucareli's ban of May 14, 1777, and the penalties established on May 26, 1793.

17. Medina Collection, National Library, Santiago de Chile. *Orden superior de Don Félix María Calleja del Rey. Dado en el Real Palacio de México a 4 de Abril de 1815.*

18. AHNM, Inquisición, México, 1732. Tercera pieza.

19. The documentation in this case is found in AGNM, Protomedicato, 3:4. Expediente instruido en averiguación del motivo porque tres médicos no salieron a auxiliar a una enferma a las 12 de la noche. Años 1795–96.

20. AGI, México, 1313A. Informe de los doctores García Jove, Rada, Eguía y Muro, y el bachiller Cuevas, México, 11 de enero de 1796.

21. AHIAH, Hospital de Naturales, 84:10, fs. 143–56r. Acuerdos del Virrey Branciforte, 1794–96. Año de 1796.

22. AGNM, Matrimonios, 7:107. Informe certificación Dictamen del doctor Máximo Afán de Rivera, 15 de febrero de 1762.

23. Ibid., 12:4. Informe del Br. Mariano García, México, 8 de marzo de 1755.

24. Muñoz, *Recopilación,* Cap. XIII, Art. IX, p. 168.

25. AGI, Indiferente General, 676. *Despacho del Ministerio de lo Interior al Presidente de la Junta Superior Gubernativa de Medicina y Cirugía,* Madrid, 4 de julio de 1834. Reales cédulas, decretos y circulares, 1834–51.

26. AGI, México, 1299. Decreto del virrey, México, 30 de abril de 1760.

27. AHIAH, Hospital de Naturales, 105:19, fs. 210–28.

28. AGI, México, 400. Real cédula al Virrey de la Nueva España previniéndole lo que ha de ejecutar para que el cirujano del Hospital Real de S. Juan de Montesclaros de la Veracruz asista con puntualidad a la curación de sus enfermos, Madrid, 20 de septiembre de 1704.

29. AGG, A1. 4, 16436, 2265. El artículo movido por el Sr. Síndico de esta Ciudad, para que examinen los cirujanos. Año de 1762.

30. AGG, A1. 25, 1702. Cirujanos y curanderos, autos acordados, Guatemala, 9 de enero de 1799 y 23 de febrero de 1801.

31. AHIAH, Hospital de Naturales, 77:7. Antonio de Arroyo al virrey, México, 16 de mayo de 1763; Dictamen del asesor, México, 25 de mayo de 1763.

32. Ibid., 104:36, fs. 205r–7v. Reglas que se deban observar en el Hospital de la entrada de algún herido. Año de 1815.

33. *Letters from Spain,* 2nd ed. (London, 1825), p. 257. (Hereinafter White, *Letters from Spain.*)

34. Muñoz, *Recopilación,* Cap. 1, pp. 21, 25–26. When discussing this subject in the first chapter of his *Recopilación,* Muñoz acknowledges his indebtedness to a work of Andrés Tiraquelo.

35. The phrase was "siendo esto tan vulgar. . . ." *Aprobación* of Dr. Francisco Pascual y Miralles, in Muñoz, *Recopilación,* s.f.

36. White, *Letters from Spain,* p. 257.

37. Leonardo Gutiérrez-Colomer, "Médicos y farmacéuticos con Hernán Cortés," *Revista de Indias* 8 (January–June 1948):337.

38. More than a century and a half later, interestingly, as an assertion of the royal patronage, the viceroy followed a royal decree to have the arms of "the

archepiscopal mitre" chiseled from the facade of the building and the royal arms substituted. AGNM, Reales cédulas (Dup.), 44, 603: fs. 536–38. Real orden al obispo, México, 17 de mayo de 1701.

39. Mendiburu, *Diccionario histórico-biográfico*, IX:327; Eguiguren, *Catálogo histórico*, p. 53.

40. Eguiguren, *Catálogo histórico*, pp. 57–60; AGI, Lima, 543. *Constituciones*, Tít. VI, Const. 102.

41. AGI, Lima, 543. *Constituciones*, Tít. VI, Const. 102; Eguiguren, *Catálogo histórico*, p. 53.

42. AGI, México, 780. El P. Fray Juan Antonio de Avila a S.M., s.l., s.f.

43. Ibid., 780. Informe del Fiscal, Madrid, 26 de septiembre de 1753.

44. Ibid., 780. Confirmación del título . . . , San Lorenzo, 3 de noviembre de 1753.

45. AHFM, Protomedicato, 4:4, fs. 1–12. Oficio primero del justicia mayor, Pedro de Herrera Leyva, Aguascalientes, 9 de noviembre de 1791: Fr. Pedro de Cardozo al subdelegado y intendente Pedro de Herrera, Aguascalientes, 10 de noviembre de 1791; Segundo oficio de Pedro de Herrera Leyva al Fr. Pedro de Cardozo, Aguascalientes, 17 de diciembre de 1791.

46. AGNM, Reales cédulas (Dup.), 106:253, fs. 469–70. Real cédula al virrey de la Nueva España, San Lorenzo, 20 de octubre de 1775.

47. AGI, México, 660. Consejo No. 5; AGNM, Reales cédulas (Dup.), 136, fs. 253–54. Real cédula al virrey Antonio María Bucareli, Aranjuez, 18 de junio de 1775.

9. Pride and Preferment

1. Muñoz, *Recopilación*, p. 27.

2. Ibid., pp. 27–32.

3. Flores, *La historia de la medicina en México*, II:122.

4. Muñoz, *Recopilación*, pp. 63, 67–69. The decree was dated January 9, 1749.

5. AHNM, Consejos, 6839, No. 35. El Consejo con motivo de unas letras de inhibición expedidas por el auditor de guerra de Barcelona . . . sobre el conocimiento de una causa contra el Dr. Thomás Claraso, dice a V. M. su parecer, Madrid, 20 de enero de 1748.

6. AGI, Indiferente General, 551. Dn. Josef Espaillat professor de la medicina en la Universidad de Salamanca: sre. q. se le confiera la plaza de Médico en el Hospital Militar de Pto. Rico, 10 de octubre de 1812.

7. Ibid., 463. Real cédula a los oficiales de Real Hacienda de Nueva España, Madrid, 15 de junio de 1685.

8. AGI, Santo Domingo, 987. Real cédula al gobernador de Caracas, Aranjuez, 23 de abril de 1786.

9. AGI, Lima, 798. José Pastor Larrinaga a V.A., Lima, 5 de octubre de 1811.

10. *Diario de Lima de Juan Antonio Suardo (1629–1639)*, Publicado con introducción y notas por Rubén Vargas Ugarte, S.J., 2 vols. (Lima 1936), II:76–77, 100. (Hereinafter, Suardo, *Diario de Lima*).

11. Lanning, *Reales cédulas,* No. 177, bis, pp. 141–42.

12. Flores, *La historia de la medicina en México,* II:184.

13. AGG, Libro de Claustros, 1790–1808, fs. 44v–45. Claustro pleno de 13 de septiembre de 1794.

14. AGG, A1.3–18, 13121, 1953. Acerca de otorgar el tratamiento que corresponde al Dr. José Felipe Flores. Año de 1795. See Lanning, *The Eighteenth-Century Enlightenment,* pp. 273–74.

15. *Memoria sobre una invención fácil y sencilla para extraer las criaturas clavadas en el paso sin riesgo de su vida, ni ofensa de la madre, y para extraer la cabeza que ha quedado en el útero separada del cuerpo* (Guatemala, 1798).

16. AGG, A1.3–1, 12234, 1882, fs. 140–41, 146–47. Real cédula a la universidad de San Carlos, Aranjuez, 24 de junio de 1803; Libro de Claustros, 1790–1808. Claustros de 4 de junio de 1803 y 5 de diciembre de 1803.

17. AGG, A1.3, 4414, 49. Consulta del Escribano de Cámara acerca del tratamiento que debe darse al Dr. Narciso Esparragoza, Cirujano Honorario de Su Majestad.

18. AGI, Lima, 543. *Constituciones,* Tít. IV, Const. 3.

19. AGNM, Universidad, Libro de Claustros, 1801–17. Claustro pleno, 13 de febrero de 1805.

20. AGI, Indiferente General, 551. Los doctores en Medicina del gremio y claustro de la Universidad de Caracas, Caracas (26 de abril de 1820), solicitan que V.M. les declare opción al rectorado de la misma Universidad y que en los actos públicos tengan su lugar entre los Doctores en otras facultades segun la antigüedad de sus grados.

21. AGNM, Claustros, 1788–1801. Claustro mayor, 4 de abril de 1791.

22. Ibid. Real cédula al rector y junta de la Real y Pontificia Universidad de México, San Lorenzo, 18 de noviembre de 1790, in Lanning, *Reales cédulas,* No. XXVI, pp. 325–26.

23. *Recopilación de Indias,* Lib. VII, Tít. VI, Ley 15 and royal cédulas dated 1741, 1746, and 1748.

24. Ibid., Lib. VI, Tít. VI, Ley 15.

25. AGI, Santo Domingo, 521. El rector y claustro de la Universidad de la Habana, s.f., s.l. (Se vió en el Consejo, 12 de julio de 1754); Testimonio de autos del rector de la Universidad de la Habana, La Habana, 26 de marzo de 1754.

26. Ibid., 910. Real cédula al obispo de Cuba, Buen Retiro, 5 de septiembre de 1754; Real cédula al obispo auxiliar de Cuba, Buen Retiro, 5 de septiembre de 1754.

27. AGI, México, 1086. Real cédula a la audiencia de México, Buen Retiro, 3 de agosto de 1754.

28. AGNM, Claustros, 1771–79. Claustro pleno de 10 de septiembre de 1771.

29. Flores, *La historia de la medicina en México,* II:447.

30. Juan del Valle y Caviedes, *Obras de Don Juan del Valle y Caviedes: Introducción y notas de Rubén Vargas Ugarte, S.J.* (Lima, 1947). (Hereinafter Valle y Caviedes, *Obras.*) This work is permeated with caustic attacks on medical practitioners, called "idiotic doctors *(médicos idiotas)*" at one juncture, p. 140.

31. Ibid., p. 213. Professor John Fein of Duke University graciously assisted me with the translation (ed.).
32. Ibid., passim.
33. Ricardo Palma, *Tradiciones peruanas,* 6 vols. (Madrid, n.d.), I:170, writing of the fourth decade of the seventeenth century, described the physician of Lima thus: "He wore black woolen knee breeches, velveteen shoes with stone buckles, velvet coat and waistcoat and, hanging in the latter, a huge silver chain with most beautiful seals. If we add that he wore chamois gloves, the reader will recognize the perfect type of Aesculapius of that epoch."
34. Informe inédito del doctor don Francisco Javier Errazuriz al cabildo de Santiago sobre los aranceles por que debian cobrar los médicos sus servicios, Santiago, 27 de noviembre de 1781. Transcribed completely in Alejandro Fuenzalida Grandón, *Historia del desarollo intelectual en Chile (1541–1810)* (Santiago, 1903), pp. 472–78.
35. A similar list in the Sala de Manuscritos, Biblioteca Nacional, Lima, Perú, was prepared by the leading professor of medicine at the University of San Marcos de Lima and the medical examiner of the viceroyalty, Juan José de Castillo, and others. Tarifa y puntual aprecia que para el seguro expendio de los medicamentos Galénicos y Chymicos mas usuales en las Oficinas Pharmacéuticas de esta Reino, Lima, 1756.

10. *Government and the Apothecary*

1. *Nueva recopilación,* Lib. I, Tít. VII, Ley 13; Muñoz, *Recopilación,* Cap. II, Art. I y II; Cap. XIV, Art. IX.
2. See, for example, AGI, México, 1103. Real cédula a D. Antonio Fernández Méndez, Madrid, 1 de septiembre de 1704.
3. *Nueva recopilación,* Lib. III, Tít. XVI, Ley 9; Pragmática de Felipe II, San Lorenzo, 2 de agosto de 1593; Muñoz, *Recopilación,* Cap. XIV, Art. III; Cap. XV, Art. VIII.
4. Muñoz, *Recopilación,* Cap. I, p. 26, n. 79.
5. Ruiz Moreno, *La medicina,* p. 43.
6. The crown found it necessary to recognize that if there were two physicians or two druggists in a town, and the fathers and sons did not have to deal with each other, they might both practice. If the fathers and sons were in different towns, the law likewise did not affect them. Muñoz, *Recopilación,* Cap. XIV, Art. II, p. 170; Cap. XV, Art. VIII, p. 198. Real provisión, Aranjuez, 23 de junio de 1743.
7. *Nueva recopilación,* Lib. III, Tít. XVI, Ley 5; Muñoz, *Recopilación,* Cap. XIII, Art. III, p. 160; Cap. XV, Art. VIII, p. 198.
8. Muñoz, *Recopilación,* Cap. XIII, Art. II, p. 159.
9. Ibid., Cap. XV, Art. VIII, p. 196. Instrucción de los visitadores y Real Provisión, Aranjuez, 23 de junio de 1743.
10. Ibid., Cap. XIV, Art. XIII, p. 180.
11. Ibid., Cap. XV, Art. VIII, p. 196. Instrucción de los visitadores y Real Provisión, Aranjuez, 23 de junio de 1743.

12. Ibid., Cap. XIV, Art. XIV, p. 181; Cap. XV, Art. VIII, p. 196.

13. Ibid., Cap. XIV, Art. LI, p. 171.

14. *Nueva recopilación,* Lib. III, Tít. XVI, Ley 9.

15. The Castilian mark of one-half pound had eight ounces, each ounce eight drams, each dram three scruples, and each scruple twenty-four grains. Since the ounce in this mark had thirty-six grains more than in the Salerno mark, "which had been in use up until now," all "weight measures" in pharmacies had to be adjusted to the Castilian mark. In regular measures *(mensurales),* the pound had ten ounces of oil, weighed by the ounces of the Castilian mark, and the liquid ounce *(onca de caber)* six drams and two scruples of the same mark.

16. *Nueva recopilación,* Lib. III, Tít. XVII, Ley 10; Muñoz, *Recopilación,* Cap. XIV, Art. VI, pp. 163–77.

17. *Nueva recopilación,* Lib. III, Tít. VIII, Ley 11.

18. Muñoz, *Recopilación,* Cap. XXI, Art. I, p. 359.

19. *Pharmacopoeia Matritensis Regii, ac supremi Hispaniarum Protomedicatus auctoritate, jussu atque auspiciis elaboarata* (Madrid, 1739, 1762). I have used the 1762 edition.

20. Muñoz, *Recopilación,* Cap. XIV, Art. IV, pp. 173–75. Decreto del Tribunal del Real Protomedicato, El Pardo, 28 de enero de 1739.

21. Ibid., pp. 171–76. Carta auxiliatoria del Consejo de Castilla, Madrid, 6 de febrero de 1739.

22. Félix Palacios, *Palestra farmacéutica, chimico-galénica* . . . (Madrid, 1706, 1723, 1730, 1737, 1753, 1763, 1778, 1792, and 1797). Hereinafter Palacios, *Palestra.)* The 1763 edition appears to be essentially the same as that of 1723, the edition that responded to criticisms of that first published in 1706.

23. Ibid., p. 4.

24. Ibid., pp. 45, 659.

25. Ibid., p. 125.

26. Ibid., p. 659.

27. Ibid., passim.

28. Félix Palacios, *La Pharmacopea triunfante de las calumnias y imposturas que en "Hipócrates defendido" ha publicado D. Miguel Boix* (Madrid, 1713).

29. Jorge Basilio Flores, *Mesue defendido contra D. Félix Palacios; muy útil para todos los profesores de la medicina* (Murcia, 1721).

30. Palacios, *Palestra,* pp. 41, 59.

31. Ibid., front matter, no pagination.

32. The *Pharmacopoeia Matritensis* appeared first in 1739. Another edition appeared in 1762, followed by the *Pharmacopoeia Hispana* (Madrid, 1784, 1794, 1797, 1803, and 1817), which returned to the title *Pharmacopoeia Matritensis* in 1823. The Spanish pharmacopoeia thereafter appeared under other titles in 1865, 1884, 1905, 1915, 1926, and 1930.

33. A good example is the *Farmacopea Bateana* . . . (Pamplona, 1763).

34. Hospital del Pozo Santo, Sevilla, Legajo 459. Libros de recibo y gasto del Hospital de la Sangre, 10 a 17 de julio de 1605.

35. AHNM, Universidades, 135. Alcalá de Henares, enero de 1571 a marzo de 1572.
36. Hospital de Tavera, Toledo. Despensa, 18 de mayo de 1561.
37. Ibid. Despensa, 25 de abril de 1568; Despensa, 7 de abril de 1592.
38. AHNM, Universidades, 1025f. Colegio de San Lucás y San Nicolás de la Universidad de Alcalá, 17 de abril de 1591.
39. Hospital de Tavera, Toledo. Despensa, 12 de noviembre de 1576.
40. Hospital del Pozo Santo, Sevilla, Legajo 461. Libros de recibo y gasto del Hospital de la Sangre, 4 de octubre de 1626.
41. Ibid., Legajos 454 y 455. Libros de recibo y gasto del Hospital de la Sangre, Año de 1564; 26 de enero de 1573.
42. *"Uña de la gran bestia"* was the Spanish term.
43. The *nigrum graecum,* based on the excrement of the rat, was processed in the same way.
44. Palacios, *Palestra,* pp. 132, 644, 646, 656, 657, 698–704.
45. Hospital de Tavera, Toledo. Despensa, 20 de junio de 1588.
46. *Siete partidas,* Partida 8, Tít. 9, Ley 7; Muñoz, *Recopilación,* Cap. XIV, Art. XVIII, p. 185.
47. Hospital de Tavera, Toledo. Despensa, 20 de junio de 1588.
48. *Siete partidas,* Partida 5, Tít. 5, Ley 17.
49. Muñoz, *Recopilación,* Cap. XIV, Art. XIX, p. 186.
50. Ibid., Cap. XIII, Art. III, p. 160.
51. Suardo, *Diario de Lima,* I:149.
52. AGI, México, 1299. Certificación de José María Leal, México, 30 de julio de 1791.
53. AHFM, Protomedicato, 4:13. Dr. Pedro de Carbajal al Tribunal del Protomedicato, Guanajuato, 1 de junio de 1795.
54. Beltrán, *Protomedicato de Buenos Aires,* pp. 232–33, 244.
55. AGNM, Historia, 461, f. 15. Real Protomedicato al virrey, México, 31 de agosto de 1788.
56. These were Mexico City 34, Guadalupe 1, Puebla 11, Atlixco 1, Chalco 2, Tezcoco 2, Toluca 3, Córdoba 1; Guanajuato 4, Querétaro 5, San Miguel el Grande 3, San Luis Potosí 2, Zacatecas 3, Zelaya 1, Yrapuato 1; Xalapa 2, Perote 1, Orizaba 2, Veracruz 5, Oaxaca 5, Guadalajara 4, Pátzcuaro 1; Pachuca 1, Real del Monte 1, Tulanzingo 2, Durango 1, Valladolid 4, Guautitlán 1, Zimapán 1; total 105.
57. *Nueva recopilación,* Lib. III, Tít. XVI, Leyes 7 y 9.
58. The Pragmatic of 1588 assigned these outside duties to the senior examiner. Muñoz, *Recopilación,* Cap. XV, Art. II, p. 188.
59. *Nueva recopilación,* Lib. III, Tít. XVI, Leyes 2 y 3.
60. Muñoz, *Recopilación,* Cap. XV, Arts. II–VI, pp. 188–91.
61. Ibid., Cap. XV, Art. XI, pp. 200–204. Decreto de la cámara, Madrid, 5 de noviembre de 1742.
62. Ibid., Cap. XV, Art. VII, pp. 204–7. Real cédula al Real Protomedicato, Aranjuez, 14 de mayo de 1750.
63. The laws of the Indies, falling back upon a decree of Charles V dated in

1538, required viceroys, presidents, and governors to have the drugstores of their districts inspected whenever they thought necessary, and if the inspector found bad medicines, he had not only to pour them out but also to eliminate them in such a way that they could not be used again. *Recopilación de Indias,* Lib. V, Tít. VI, Ley 7. This law, though, was hardly operative in 1540.

64. AEAM. Actas del cabildo, 5 de octubre de 1540.

65. Ibid., 23 de enero de 1570.

66. AGI, México, 387. Real cédula al virrey de Nueva España, Madrid, 27 de noviembre de 1624.

67. Ibid., 387. Real cédula al virrey de Nueva España, Madrid, 12 de julio de 1628.

68. Ibid., 1100. Real cédula a la audiencia de México, Madrid, 22 de mayo de 1680.

69. AGI, Indiferente General, 1551. Real cédula para que los Prothomédicos del Prothomedicato de la Ciudad de México hagan las visitas de las Medicinas, y Boticas con limitación y en la forma, que arriva se expresa, Madrid, 26 de agosto de 1694.

70. Muñoz, *Recopilación,* n.p., in prefatory matter. Aprobación hecha de comisión del Real y Supremo Consejo de Castilla, Madrid, 15 de mayo de 1750; Certificación del Secretario de Cámara del Rey, Madrid, 10 de julio de 1750.

71. Ibid., pp. 192–99.

72. AHFM, Protomedicato, 2:11. Título e instrucción de los visitadores nombrados por este Real Protomedicato. . . . Año de 1790.

73. See Muñoz, *Recopilación,* Cap. XV, Parra. IX, p. 200.

74. This formula for inspection is based upon the "Instrucción de los visitadores" contained and endorsed in the *Real cédula circular,* Aranjuez, 23 de agosto de 1743. Muñoz, *Recopilación,* Cap. XV, Art. VIII, pp. 192–99. The Mexican protomedicato, though it began to insist upon this version toward the end of the eighteenth century because it gave the tribunal the exclusive jurisdiction it so ardently sought, most of the time issued its own instructions to the individual inspector in order to cope with special conditions.

75. *Nueva recopilación,* Lib. VIII, Tít. III, Leyes 3 y 4.

76. Muñoz, *Recopilación,* Cap. XV, Art. VIII, p. 195. Real cédula circular, Aranjuez, 23 de junio de 1743. P. D. Rodríguez Rivero, *Historia médica de Venezuela hasta 1900* (Caracas, 1931), p. 133.

77. AGNM, Universidad, 52, fs. 172–73. Auto de 21 de enero de 1693. I am indebted to Dr. Francisco Fernández del Castillo for the discovery of the documents relating to this case in the archives of the University of Mexico and for publishing them in his *La Facultad de Medicina,* pp. 191–201.

78. *Nueva recopilación,* Lib. III, Tít. XVI, Leyes 2 y 4.

79. Muñoz, *Recopilación,* Cap. XVII, Art. VII, pp. 336–42.

80. AHFM, Protomedicato, 1:5, fs. 1–18. Expediente sobre el nombramiento e instrucción como visitador de Puebla y sus alrededores, a favor del Dr. Bruno Francisco Sánchez, por jubilación del bachiller Tomás Bernardo de Otáñez. Año de 1775.

81. Ibid., 2:4. Expediente formado a instancia del Dr. Dn. Joseph Torres Médico en la Ciudad de Puebla sobre que se la continue en el empleo de visitador.
82. Ibid., 2:3. Dictamen del fiscal, México, 7 de junio de 1782.
83. Ibid., 4:9. Expediente de don Rafael Ceballos, arrendatario de la botica del Hospital Real. Año de 1815.
84. Ibid., 3:2. Joseph Mariano Pino al virrey, México, 18 de junio de 1794.
85. Ibid. Pedro Valenzuela al virrey, México, 3 de julio de 1794.
86. Ibid. Protomedicato al Virrey Revilla Gigedo, México, 3 de julio de 1794.
87. Ibid. Virrey Branciforte al Real Protomedicato, México, 1 de septiembre de 1796.
88. AHFM, Protomedicato, 10:9. Vicente Cervantes, Sebastián Morón, y Ignacio de León al virrey, México, 23 de febrero de 1809.
89. AGI, Indiferente General, 1349. Silvestre Collar a José Antonio Caballero, Madrid, 11 de noviembre de 1802.
90. Ibid., 1349. Expediente de la Junta Superior de Farmacia en que solicita se la autorice para que por medio de sus comisionados haga las visitas de las boticas de Indias de dos en dos años. Años 1801–6.
91. AGI, Lima, 798. Petición de Dn. Antonio Ximénez Salinas, Cádiz, 12 de marzo de 1813.

11. *Government and Surgery*

1. García Icazbalceta, *Obras,* I:76.
2. *Actas de cabildo de México,* XVI, 436; XVII, 453.
3. AGNM, Reales cédulas (Dup.), 2:73, f. 110. Real orden, México, 8 de agosto de 1634.
4. Ibid., 16:312, fs. 155v–56. Real orden, México, 19 de julio de 1620.
5. J. M. Reyes, "Historia de la medicina . . . ," *Gaceta médica de México,* I:256.
6. Hospital de Nuestra Señora Santa María de Esgueva, Valladolid. Libros de Despensa, 35, f. 58.
7. Muñoz, *Recopilación,* Cap. XIII, parra. V, p. 163. By the end of the seventeenth century, Latin physicians trained in medicine and in accredited universities enjoyed the right to prescribe.
8. AGI, México, 1094. Real cédula al virrey y audiencia de Mexico, Madrid, 10 de julio de 1621.
9. Orden del Dr. Juan de Salcedo, 29 de noviembre de 1795 en Fernández del Castillo, *La Facultad de Medicina,* pp. 136–37.
10. AGNM, Reales cédulas (Dup.), 22:125, f. 175. Real orden, México, 19 de julio de 1662 (Dup.), 24:42, fs. 55–56v. Real orden del Marqués de Mancera, México, 7 de julio de 1665. In 1775 the professor of prima of medicine drew an annual salary of 500 pesos and the professor of surgery and medicine 400. *Constituciones de la Universidad de México,* Tít. X, Const. 111 y 113, pp. 56, 57.
11. Lanning, *Academic Culture,* p. 57.

12. AGI, Indiferente General, 1551. Informe de la Contaduría General, Madrid, 16 de octubre de 1793.

13. AGG, A1. 4–1766. –18.013.–2379. Instancia del síndico del ayuntamiento . . . , Guatemala, 9 de julio de 1766.

14. See *Causa médico criminal que en este Real Protomedicato del Perú han seguido los profesores de la facultad de medicina contra los cirujanos, pharmacéuticos, phlebotómicos, etc., sobre contenerlos en los términos de sus respectivas profesiones* (Lima, 1764). (Hereinafter *Causa médico criminal.*)

15. AGNM, Reales cédulas (Dup.), 24:42, fs. 55–56v. Real orden, México, 7 de julio de 1665.

16. The application of Spanish law to American medical problems was possible, and in certain crises, actually done. A lengthy pragmatic of Philip II issued in 1593, however, was serious enough to attract attention even in America. For one thing, it actually provided that the examiners of the royal protomedicato not proceed to examine a candidate in surgery without having present a surgeon of outstanding repute "in this court." And, apparently to avoid connivance, the same one might not be called in every time. *Nueva recopilación,* Lib. III, Tít. XVI, Ley 9, parra. 8. This potential pragmatic also set up the requirements for examination of a "Latin surgeon." Henceforth, candidates to practice surgery had to complete three courses in medicine, after getting the degree of bachelor of arts, which presumed sufficiency in Latin, and after they had had two years of internship in surgery. For four years, and four years only, the protomédicos might license surgeons without these qualifications provided they came from places having no surgeons at all. *Nueva recopilación,* Lib. III, Tít. XVI, Ley 9, parra. 9.

17. Ibid., Lib. III, Tít. XVI, Ley 9, parra. 10.

18. The change to five years that was authorized in Spain in 1603 was apparently not known in Havana when this petition came under consideration.

19. AGI, Santo Domingo, 1123. Real cédula al gobernador de la isla de Cuba, Cuenca, 28 de febrero de 1604.

20. AGI, Buenos Aires, 229. Expediente de Auxiliatoria para ser examinado de cirujano, Madrid, 10 de marzo de 1779. D. Antonio Ventura de Taranco a D. Miguel de San Martín Cueto, Madrid, 17 de mayo de 1779.

21. *Nueva recopilación,* Lib. I, Tít. VII, Ley 13.

22. See the numerous applications and files in AHIAH, Protomedicato, T-4, 12.

23. AGNM, Indice de Bandos, Hospital de Naturales. Bando del virrey Marqués de Croix, México, 10 de abril de 1770.

24. AGNM, Bandos, 7. Bando del virrey Marqués de Croix, México, 10 de abril de 1770.

25. *Nueva recopilación,* Lib. III, Tít. XVI, Ley 10; *Recopilación de Indias,* Lib. V, Tít. VI, Ley 2. The latter commands the enforcement of the former.

26. AGI, Indiferente General, 11. Consulta del Consejo de Indias, Madrid, 3 de marzo de 1784. The protomedicato had simply proposed that internships be allowed outside the Royal Indian Hospital.

27. AGNM, Reales cédulas (Dup.), 127:167, fs. 320–22. Real cédula al virrey de la Nueva España, Madrid, 10 de abril de 1784.

28. AHIAH, Hospital de Naturales, 103:47, f. 177; *Gazeta de México,* XIV (No. 93, 7 de noviembre de 1807):736–37.

29. AGI, México, 412. El Consejo de Indias pasa a las reales manos de S.M. una carta de los oficiales reales de México, Madrid, s.f., 1719.

30. AGNM, Reales cédulas (Dup.), 138:165, f. 262–62v y 142:75, fs. 96–97. Real orden al virrey de Nueva España, San Lorenzo, 14 de noviembre de 1787. Real orden al virrey de Nueva España, Madrid, 20 de febrero de 1789.

31. Ibid., 145:44, f. 56–56v. Real orden al virrey de Nueva España, Madrid, 20 de enero de 1790.

32. Ibid., 164:83, f. 101–1v. Real orden al virrey de Nueva España, Aranjuez, 27 de mayo de 1796.

33. Ibid., 171:186, f. 234–34v.

34. Ibid., 207, fs. 326–27. Real orden al Secretario de Estado y del Despacho de la Gobernación, Cádiz, 20 de noviembre de 1812.

35. Ibid., 212:164, f. 214–14v y 215:204, fs. 247–48. Real orden circular, Madrid, 22 de mayo de 1815. Decreto del virrey, México, 22 de marzo de 1816. Real orden al virrey de la Nueva España, Madrid, 17 de mayo de 1816.

36. AGNM, Estado, 224. Expediente relativo a la supresión de los empleos de protomédico y cirujano mayor de los ejércitos.

37. AGI, Indiferente General, 62. Pretensiones de D. Domingo Rusi, México, 15 de abril de 1761 y 6 de noviembre de 1765.

38. Ibid., 62. D. Domingo Rusi a D. Julián de Arriaga, México, 15 de abril de 1763.

39. Ibid. Informe de don Diego Porcel, Madrid, 15 de septiembre de 1763.

40. Ibid. El Comandante General D. Juan de Villalba al rey, México, 2 de mayo de 1765.

41. Ibid. Real orden a D. Juan de Villalba y Angulo, San Ildefonso, 1 de octubre de 1765.

42. Ibid., 1310. Petición de don Juan Borrell, Madrid, 29 de julio de 1766.

43. AGI, Guatemala, 439. Título a D. Francisco Sánchez Martín en que S. M. le nombra cirujano del puerto de Omoa . . . , El Pardo, 18 de enero de 1778.

44. AGI, México, 2660. *Real orden de establecimiento de Seminario o Colegio de Practicantes de Cirugía a los oficios principales de Marina,* San Lorenzo el Real, 18 de noviembre de 1748. Sent to the president of the Casa de Contratación and the Intendente General of the Navy, Cádiz, 29 de noviembre de 1748.

45. AHNM, Consejos, 2081A. Autos hechos en el Consejo con motivo del exceso cometido por Eugenio Lázaro. . . . Informe del fiscal, Madrid, 19 de octubre de 1771.

46. Ibid., 2081A. Licenciado Félix Iñíguez a D. Pedro Virgili, San Ildefonso, 14 de enero de 1766, and enclosure.

47. Michael E. Burke, *The Royal College of San Carlos: Surgery and Spanish Medical Reform in the Late Eighteenth Century* (Durham, N.C., 1978), p. 149; Hernández Morejón, *Historia bibliográfica,* VI:241–45; Marcelino Menéndez y Pelayo, *La ciencia española (polémicas, proyectos, y bibliografía),* 3 vols. (Madrid, 1887–88), III:439.

48. AGI, Guatemala, 554. Juan González Bustillo al Bailio Frey D. Julián de Arriaga, Guatemala, 30 de julio de 1771. In the same legajo, see the detailed commentary on the lack of surgeons in Guatemala City. Expediente del Presidente interino de Guatemala sobre la falta de cirujanos que experimenta la ciudad. Año de 1772.

49. Ibid., 554. Expediente sobre los medios propuestos por el Ayuntamiento de la ciudad de Guatemala para pagar los sueldos consignados a los dos cirujanos que de orden de S.M. se remitieron a la misma ciudad. Años 1772 a 1774. The internal evidence of this expediente only shows that the king named D. Domingo Villaverde, "who will sail from Cádiz," at 1,200 pesos a year, and that the second, at 800 pesos a year, "would follow." There is no proof that they sailed.

50. Flores, *La historia de medicina en México,* II:335.

51. David A. Howard, *The Royal Indian Hospital of Mexico City,* Special Studies No. 20, Center for Latin American Studies, Arizona State University (Tempe, 1980), p. 46.

52. AGI, Indiferente General, 62. Consulta del Consejo de Indias, Madrid, 3 de noviembre de 1767.

53. AGNM, Reales cédulas (Dup.), 92:169, fs. 296–97. Real cédula al virrey de Nueva España, Aranjuez, 20 de mayo de 1768.

54. AGI, Indiferente General, 62. Consulta del Consejo de Indias y consulta de la Cámara, Madrid, 1 de octubre de 1770.

55. Ibid., 62. "Despachense los correspondientes títulos, que se han echado de menos en México . . . ," 24 de diciembre de 1770.

56. AHIAH, Hospital de Naturales, 103:41. A printed *Aviso al público* announced that Andrés Montañer y Virgili would begin daily demonstrations in anatomy on February 3 and that José Vicente Maldonado would explain physiology.

57. Flores, *La historia de medicina en México,* II:160.

58. See graph on graduates in Lanning, *The University in the Kingdom of Guatemala,* p. 201.

59. AGNM, Reales cédulas (Dup.), 192:15, fs. 33–34v; AGNM, Protomedicato, 3:16. Real cédula circular sobre el arreglo de la cirugía y farmacia en los dominios de América, Aranjuez, 2 de marzo de 1804.

60. AGNM, Protomedicato, 3:16. Informe del Doctor Antonio Serrano, México, 21 de septiembre de 1804.

12. *Government and Phlebotomy*

1. Feijóo, *Teatro crítico,* I:107. Discurso V, Sec. VI.

2. When he proceeded on his favorite theory that any medical practice that did not work should be abandoned, as he did when he opposed excessive bloodletting, Feijóo was at his best. But when there was no such principle to guide him, as in evaluating the circulation and transfusion of the blood, he dealt with the subject whimsically, scorning the experiments of Richard Lower at

Oxford (1665). Benito Jerónimo Feijóo y Montenegro, *Cartas eruditas, y curiosas, en que por la mayor parte se continua el designio del teatro crítico universal* . . . , 5 vols. (Madrid, 1759–76):I, Carta XV.

3. I am indebted to Earl J. Hamilton for use of his personal notes on bloodletting in the archives of Spanish hospitals.

4. Hospital del Pozo Santo, Sevilla, Legajo 456. Libro de Recibo y Gasto del Hospital de la Sangre, gastos extraordinarios de la semana de 4 de julio de 1587.

5. Hospital de Tavera, Toledo. Despensa, miercoles, 30 de agosto de 1589.

6. Hospital del Pozo Santo, Sevilla, Legajo 459. Libros de Recibo y Gasto del Hospital de la Sangre, gastos extraordinarios de la semana de 27 de septiembre de 1609.

7. Two "barber-surgeons" in Valencia were under contract to come to the Hospital Inocens, Valencia, Rebudes y Dates de 1523–24. (No foliation.)

8. García Icazbalceta, *Obras*, I:72.

9. *Actas de cabildo de México*, I:119. Cabildo de 1 de febrero de 1527.

10. It named Juan Rodríguez de Mesa on January 4, 1591, January 4, 1593, and January 10, 1594. Ibid., X:47, 133; XI:58; XII:7.

11. The viceroy, the Duke of Albuquerque (1650–60) first appointed Sebastián de Anjeris, and the Marqués de Laguna continued him as "surgeon and barber" of "the jail of Mexico." AGNM, Reales cédulas (Dup.), 28:471, f. 374. Real orden, México, 22 de mayo de 1681.

12. Diego López de Salazar, January 8, 1610, January 8, January 10, 1613, January 4, 1616, January 2, 1617; Simón García, January 2, 1623, January 29, 1624; Domingo de Cabildo, January 10, 1625. *Actas de cabildo de México*, XVII:453; XVIII:37; XIX:9; XX:251; XXI:150; XXIV:364; XV:86, 220; XXVI:84.

13. *Libros de cabildos de Lima*, IX:73–74. Cabildo de 3 de agosto de 1579.

14. Ibid. Alvaro de Torres received a similar appointment three years later; IX:408, Cabildo de 14 de julio de 1581.

15. Ibid., IX:397. Cabildo de 9 de junio de 1581; see also IX:365; X:146, 389. That Pérez might also trim the viceroy's beard made him no less a bloodletter.

16. Suardo, *Diario de Lima*, I:85. 5 de julio de 1630.

17. Ibid., I:158. 29 de abril de 1631.

18. Ibid., I:162; I:263; y II:103. 25 de mayo de 1631, 18 de mayo de 1633, and 25 de octubre de 1635.

19. ACB, Médicos y Abogados, 3, fs. 576v–78v. Miguel de Isla al virrey, Bogotá, 1 de mayo de 1805.

20. AGI, Indiferente General, 473. Real cédula al gobernador de la isla de Cuba, Valladolid, 19 de junio de 1615.

21. AGNM, Universidad, 286. Grados de doctores y licenciados en medicina, III. Thesis of José Gracida y Bernal, 9 de agosto de 1784: Plethorae ad vasa curationem in sanguinis cita missione consistere, pro viribus defensare conabor.

22. AHIAH, Protomedicato, T-4, 12, fs. 257–64v. Expediente promovido por

don Agustín Domingo del Castillo, pretendiendo ser examinado en el arte de Flebotomiano. Año de 1810.

23. Flores, *La historia de la medicina en México,* II:178–79. In 1759 the fee was fifty-five pesos and in 1813 seventy-five. However, when the viceregal government gave permission to examine bloodletters in the provinces, it added a charge of five pesos when the examination took place twenty to forty leagues from Mexico City, seven pesos and four reales in places forty to sixty leagues distant, and ten pesos for examinations conducted at a distance of more than one hundred leagues.

24. AGNM, Civil, 11:3, f. 51v. Testimonio del Br. Juan Bermúdez de Castro.

25. AGNM, Protomedicato 3:7, fs. 41–42v. Protomedicato al Virrey Iturrigaray, México, 10 de septiembre de 1803.

26. Ibid., fs. 60v–67v. Dictamen del fiscal de la Real Hacienda, México, 14 de octubre de 1804; fs. 44–45v, Real cédula al virrey de la Nueva España, Aranjuez, 9 de junio de 1796; *Recopilación de Indias,* Lib. V, Tít. VI, Ley 6.

27. AGI, Ultramar, 733, parra. 40. Real cédula circular, Madrid, 3 de agosto de 1801.

28. AHFM, Protomedicato 3:11, fs. 1–14 y 4:1, fs. 1–23. Criminal a queja de Manuel de San Ciprián, Maestro Bárbero, contra Dn. Josef Carabantes, Ministro executor del Real Tribunal del Protomedicato, y el hijo de este, por injurias; Expediente formado de oficio del Real Tribunal del Protomedicato contra el Mrs. Flebotomiano José [*sic*] San Ciprián por tener aviertas dos tiendas de barbería e haver echo resistencia al tiempo de su prisión pr. no querer respetar y obedecer los preceptos del Tribunal.

29. Ibid., f. 1. Decreto del Virrey Revilla Gigedo, 9 de mayo de 1791. The internal evidence of this file suggests that on the morning of May 10 the viceroy inadvertently used the date of the previous day, for many witnesses in the case made declarations "today about ten thirty in the morning." José Ignacio Jiménez, the bailiff of the judge, refers to "the happening of the tenth."

30. AHFM, Protomedicato 4:1, fs. 1–2. Declaración del Real Protomedicato, México, 10 de mayo de 1791.

31. For the declaration of the protomedicato witnessses, see ibid.

32. Ibid., fs. 12–13v. Informe del Real Protomedicato, México, 11 de junio de 1791.

33. Ibid., f. 14–14v. Parecer del fiscal Alva, México, 21 de junio de 1791; Decreto del virrey, 22 de junio de 1791.

34. Ibid., fs. 16–17v. Declaración preparatoria de Manuel de San Ciprián, 9 de agosto de 1791.

35. AGNM, Protomedicato 3:7, f. 1–1v. El Gobernador Yntendente de Puebla consulta sobre el mejor arreglo del oficio de bárberos Gobernador Manuel de Flor al Virrey Azanza, Puebla, 23 de septiembre de 1798.

36. Ibid., fs. 2–3v. Informe del Real Protomedicato, México, 25 de octubre de 1798.

37. *Nueva recopilación,* Lib. III, Tít. XVIII, Ley 1; *Recopilación de Indias,* Lib. V, Tít. VI, Ley 6.

38. AGNM, Protomedicato 3:7, fs. 4–6. Parecer del fiscal de lo civil (Borbón), México, 6 de noviembre de 1798.
39. Based on *Nueva recopilación,* Lib. III, Tít. XVIII, Ley 1 (*única*).
40. AGNM, Protomedicato 3:7, fs. 6v–8. Dictamen del asesor general, México, 9 de marzo de 1799; Bando del Virrey Azanza, México, 29 de marzo de 1799.
41. AGNM, Universidad, 52, fs. 142–44v. This appeal is published in Fernández del Castillo, *La Facultad de Medicina,* pp. 202–5.
42. That Spain was also suffering from the distances between the seat of the protomedicato and those who desired to practice phlebotomy can be seen at some length in AHNM, Consejos, 6837, Núm. 11. Año 1746.
43. AGNM, Protomedicato 3:7, f. 25–25v. Informe del Tribunal del Protomedicato, México, 20 de febrero de 1800.
44. Flores, *La historia de medicina en México,* II:178.
45. AGI, Ultramar, 727. Real cédula [circular] de gracias al sacar, Aranjuez, 10 de febrero de 1795. At this date the extra fee for examining medical candidates of all categories in their own districts (*partidos*) was left at the discretion of the examining protomedicato "taking into account the circumstances and distances" in each case.
46. AGNM, Protomedicato 3:7, fs. 27v–28v. Informe de la Real Hacienda, México, 28 de marzo de 1800.
47. Ibid., f. 40–40v. Bando de 26 de 1803.
48. Ibid., f. 39–39v. Bando del Virrey Iturrigaray, México, 29 de agosto de 1803.
49. Though a *chino* was a combination of Indian and *lobo,* a cross of Indian and Black, this term is no doubt intended to apply to mixed bloods in general.
50. AGNM, Reales cédulas (Dup.), 18:7, f. 40. If these barbers were the Mexican variety of chinos, they could not have established their blood purity.
51. AGNM, Civil, 11:3, f. 51v.
52. AHFM, Protomedicato, 7:1, fs. 1–22. Diligencias practicadas de pedimento de Juan de Cárdenas de Espinosa, vecino de Otumba sobre que se le admita a examen de flebotomía.
53. Ibid., fs. 15v–16. Testimonio de Visencio Antonio, Otumba, 3 de agosto de 1804.
54. Ibid., f. 7.
55. Ibid., fs. 21v–22.
56. AGI, Indiferente General, 1348. Consulta del Consejo de las Indias, Madrid, 27 de octubre de 1803.
57. Ibid., 473. Real cédula al gobernador de la isla de Cuba, Valladolid, 19 de junio de 1615.
58. Ibid., 1310. Petición de Juan Almeida, Madrid, 10 de diciembre de 1767.
59. AEAM, Médicos y Boticas, 1:1. Cabildo de 26 de septiembre de 1776. This distinction represents a change of signs.
60. ARAQ, Cuerpos Docentes. The deposition of Dr. Pedro Jiménez, Quito, October 1, 1813.
61. The ruling is dated November 18, 1813.
62. AHFM, Protomedicato, 9:1–5. Expediente formado contra el bárbero José María Orihuela, por ejercer oficio de flebotomiano (1818).

63. ANP, Protomedicato, Legajo Unico, Cuaderno 25. Año de 1818. Juan Zúñiga sobre que se le examine de flebotómico.
64. Lanning, *The Eighteenth-Century Enlightenment,* p. 78.
65. Feijóo, *Teatro crítico,* I:107–10. Discurso V, Sec. VI.
66. AHFM, Protomedicato, 7:16. Año de 1818. That there were only two physicians, as against ten surgeons and seven apothecaries who could qualify by the apprentice method, may be attributed to the ruin inflicted upon the university by the revolution then under way.

13. *Government and Obstetrics*

1. Hospital del Pozo Santo, Sevilla, Legajo 455. Libros de Recibo y Gasto del Hospital de la Sangre, 28 de abril de 1476. Hospital de Tavera, Toledo. Despensas, 5 de julio de 1588 y 10 de enero de 1596.
2. Hospital de San Bernabé y San Antolín, Palencia. Libros de gastos de 1581, 1627, y 1640.
3. *Nueva recopilación,* Lib. III, Tít. XVI, Ley 2.
4. Muñoz, *Recopilación,* Cap. XVI, Art. I, pp. 308–10.
5. Ibid., Cap. XVI, Art. II, pp. 309–13. Real cédula circular, Buen Retiro, 21 de julio de 1750.
6. Ibid., Cap. XVI, Art. III, p. 314.
7. *Cartilla nueva, útil y necesaria para instruirse las matronas que vulgarmente se llaman comadres, en el oficio de partear* (Madrid, 1759). (Hereinafter Medina, *Cartilla.*)
8. Ibid., Prólogo, Capítulo proemial.
9. Ibid., Capítulo proemial.
10. Ibid., Capítulo II.
11. Ibid., Capítulo III.
12. Ibid., Capítulo IV.
13. AGNM, Protomedicato 3:16. Informe al Virrey Iturrigaray, México, 21 de septiembre de 1804.
14. José Manuel Valdés, "Carta segunda de Erasistrato Suadel relativa a las precauciones que deben observarse en los partos en continuación de las publicadas en el Merc. Núm. 45," *Mercurio peruano* III (No. 102, 25 de diciembre de 1791):294.
15. José Manuel Valdés, "Disertación primera en la que se proponen las reglas que deven observar las mugeres en el tiempo de la prénez," *Mercurio peruano* II (No. 45, 5 de junio de 1791):88–95.
16. Joseph Erasistrato Suadel, "Disertación primera," *Mercurio peruano* II (No. 45, 5 de junio de 1791):89–95.
17. Joseph Erasistrato Suadel, "Carta segunda," *Mercurio peruano* III (No. 102, 25 de diciembre de 1791):296–97.
18. Flores, *La historia de medicina en México,* II:365.
19. Ibid., II:180.
20. Benavente Garcés, *El protomedicato en Chile,* pp. 78–80.
21. Ibid. Informe del Dr. José Antonio Ríos, Santiago, 8 de julio de 1790.

22. *Mercurio peruano,* III (No. 102, 25 de diciembre de 1791):295.

23. C. E. Paz-Soldán, "La obstetricía . . . ," *La reforma médica,* XXIX:658. Schools had been founded in Strasbourg (1737), Berlin (1751), Rome (1786), and Edinburgh (c. 1800).

24. José Ignacio Bartolache, *Mercurio volante con noticias importantes i curiosas sobre varios asuntos de Físico i Medicina* 5 (18 de noviembre de 1772):38. (Hereinafter Bartolache, *Mercurio volante.*)

25. Feijóo, *Teatro crítico,* I:68–73. Discurso V.

26. Bartolache, *Mercurio volante* 6 (25 de noviembre de 1772), quoted in Adrián Quirós Rodiles, "Breve historia de la obstetricia en Mexico," *Obstetricia y ginecología latino-americanas* III (1945):697–98. (Hereinafter Quirós Rodiles, "Breve historia.")

27. Quirós Rodiles, "Breve historia," pp. 693–94.

28. Described in ibid., p. 699.

29. Ibid., p. 698.

30. *Compendio de la medicina: o medicina práctica* (México, 1788), p. 157.

31. Quirós Rodiles, "Breve historia," p. 697.

32. José Manuel Rodríguez, *La caridad del sacerdote para con los niños encerrados en el vientre de sus madres difuntas y documentos de la utilidad y necesidad de su práctica* (México, 1772). (Hereinafter Rodríguez, *La caridad de sacerdote.*)

33. Francesco Emmanuele Cangiamila, *Embryologia sacra, sive de officio sacerdotum, medicorum et aliorum circa aeternam parvulorum in utero existentium salutem* (Palermo, 1758).

34. Flores, *La historia de medicina en México,* II:367–68. Bando de Virrey Antonio María de Bucareli, México, 21 de noviembre de 1772. Edicto del Arzobispo Alonso Núñez de Haro, México, 4 de diciembre de 1772.

35. Cangiamila insisted that the "irregularity" *in defectu lenitatis* was not valid except in incisions and mutilations of living bodies.

36. Rodríguez, *La caridad del sacerdote,* pp. 4–19.

37. Ibid., pp. 21–25.

38. Ibid., pp. 21–31.

39. Ibid., p. 33. This quibble is not unique; Feijóo concludes that "holding that there is no convincing reason why the male should be of the same species, as the species is determined by the mother," the cesarean should be performed and the fetus baptized absolutely. In support of his position, he cited the birth of Christ himself and, what was then new, that not only birds but mammals— "even man"—came from eggs. In case the mother was a beast and the father human, baptism should not be administered even under adverse conditions. *Teatro crítico,* VI:75–82. Discurso 1, Paradoxa xiv.

40. Rodríguez, *La caridad del sacerdote,* pp. 37–46. Corolarios I, II, y III.

41. Dr. D. Ignacio Segura, *Avisos saludables a las parteras para el cumplimiento de su obligación* (México, 1775).

42. *Gazeta de México,* II (No. 37, 19 de junio de 1787):374–75; X (No. 2, 11 de noviembre de 1799):10.

43. Quirós Rodiles, "Breve historia," p. 687.

44. *Gazeta de México,* VII (No. 35, 20 de junio de 1795):298.
45. Ibid., X (No. 2, 11 de noviembre de 1799):9–10.
46. Ibid., IX (No. 42, 29 de mayo de 1799):329–30.
47. Ibid., X (No. 27, 18 de noviembre de 1800):209.
48. Quirós Rodiles, "Breve historia," p. 687.
49. Don José Maximiliano Rosales de Velasco al virrey, México, 7 de julio de 1776. AGNM, Hospitales, 744, published in Velasco Ceballos, *La cirugía,* pp. 423–26.
50. Fray Pedro Mariano de Iturbide, *Compendio para que la operación cesárea se practique conforme a las obras del doctor Antonio Rodríguez y D. Francisco Cangiamila* (Guatemala, 1788). This item is entered in José Toribio Medina's *La imprenta en Guatemala (1660–1821)* (Guatemala, 2 vols. in 1, 1960), II: 1. no. 595, 210–11.
51. Medina, *Cartilla,* pp. 210–11. Breve y diminuto compendio de la obligación que hay de bautizar los fetos.
52. Arthur Robert Steele, *Flowers for the King* (Durham, N.C., 1964), pp. 139–40. (Hereinafter Steele, *Flowers for the King.*)
53. William Pratt Dale, "The Cultural Revolution in Peru, 1750–1820" (Ph.D. dissertation, Duke University, 1941), p. 95.
54. Francisco González Laguna, *El zelo sacerdotal para con los niños no nacidos* (Lima, 1781).
55. For a copy of this ban, see the original *El zelo sacerdotal* where it is undated, and Manuel Muñiz, "La medicina legal en el Perú (datos para su historia)" (Lima, 1886), pp. 256–57. (Hereinafter Muñiz, "La medicina legal.")
56. Muñiz, "La medicina legal," pp. 803–4.
57. Ibid., pp. 804–5.
58. The royal protomedicato had been divided into proto-medicato, proto-cirujanato, and proto-farmacéutico.
59. ARAQ, Cedulario, XV. Real cédula para que en los dominios e islas Filipinas se execute la operación cesárea, en la forma que previene la Instrucción que se acompaña, Madrid, 13 de abril de 1804. See also AGNM, Reales cédulas (Dup.), 192:35, fs. 108–9.
60. Modo de hacer la operación cesárea despues de muerta la madre. This document in ARAQ, Cedulario, XV, was signed by a commission of professors at the San Carlos College of Surgery in October, 1803.
61. A man of great personal curiosity and scientific bent, Esparragosa had trained first in Caracas and then fallen in with the first professor of medicine in the University of San Carlos de Guatemala, Dr. José Flores. This was the best thing that could have happened to him if he had looked over the whole empire, for Flores was a man with an experimental talent trying to forge ahead in anatomy, optics, electricity, and medicine.
62. Lanning, *The Eighteenth-Century Enlightenment,* p. 278.
63. *Gazeta de Guatemala,* II (16 de julio de 1798):284. Dr. Carlos Martínez Durán has published a facsimile of this illustration in his *Las ciencias médicas en Guatemala* (Guatemala, 1941), pp. 262–63, while a copy of Robert

Blake, a modern medical illustrator, is published by Lanning, *The Eighteenth-Century Enlightenment,* p. 279.

64. *Memoria sobre una invención fácil y sencilla para extraer las criaturas clavadas en el paso sin riesgo de su vida, ni ofensa de la madre, y para extraer la cabeza que ha quedado en el útero separada del cuerpo* (Guatemala, 1798).

65. AGG, A1. 3–1, 12236, 1882. Real cédula a la Universidad de Guatemala, Aranjuez, 24 de junio de 1803.

66. Archivo de la Facultad de Medicina de la Universidad de Madrid, Antiguo Colegio de San Carlos, Libro de Acuerdos (1787–1804), juntas of February 17, March 3, and March 17, 1803. I am indebted to Dr. Michael E. Burke for this reference.

67. Diego Carbonell, "Narciso Esparragosa y Gallardo sabio bueno y venezolano," *Gaceta médica de Caracas* XXVI (1929):286.

68. Quirós Rodiles, "Breve historia," pp. 681–82.

69. AGNM, Inquisición, 986:17, f. 193v. This document contains a denunciation of Juan Bautista Chirino by Dr. José Teodoro García de Arias, México, March 7, 1752.

70. A straightforward maternity house under the auspices of the Empress Carlotta was authorized only in 1865 by a decree promulgated in Puebla on June 7 of that year. Manuel S. Soriano, "Historia de la medicina en México: Origen de la Casa de Maternidad en México," *Boletín de ciencias médicas* IV (1913):100.

71. Quirós Rodiles, "Breve historia," pp. 692–93.

72. AEAM, Médicos y Boticas, 1:3. Informe del Real Protomedicato, México, 24 de mayo de 1793. (Signed by Dr. y Maestro José Giral and Dr. y Maestro José Ignacio García y Jove.)

73. Ibid., 1:3. Maestro Miguel Moreno y Peña al ilustre cabildo de México, s.f.

74. Ibid., 1:3. Decreto del Real Protomedicato, México, 9 de noviembre de 1793.

75. Ibid., 1:3. Informe del síndico del común, México, 25 de noviembre de 1794.

76. Ibid., 1:3. Parecer del procurador general, México, 20 de diciembre de 1794.

77. Ibid., 1:5 y 6.

78. Muñoz, *Recopilación,* Cap. XVI, parra. V, p. 316. Real orden al Tribunal del Protomedicato, Madrid, 6 de febrero de 1751.

79. AHFM, Protomedicato 10:12, fs. 1–2 (1816). The file is incomplete.

80. AHFM, Protomedicato 12:15, fs. 1–2 (1818). Expediente del examen (por comisión) como obstetriz, de María Francisca Ignacia Sánchez.

81. AHFM, Protomedicato 11:1 (1818). Nómina de médicos, farmacéuticos, cirujanos, flebotomianos y parteros examinados en 1818. The list included two physicians, nine surgeons, seven pharmacists, two phlebotomists, and two midwives.

82. In 1825, however, the professor of surgery and anatomy in Havana was actually staging examinations in obstetrics. See *Examenes públicos de obstetricia o arte de partear. . . .* (Havana, 1825).

83. "Lista de profesores de medicina, cirugía, farmacia, y flebotomía, residentes en el D. F., sacado del libro del Protomedicato (Año de 1830)," *Gaceta médica de México* XXXVI (1899):583.

14. *Medical Education, Learning, and Research*

1. See, for example, Lanning, *The University in the Kingdom of Guatemala*, pp. 211–13.
2. The discussion that follows on the establishment of chairs of medicine in the Royal and Pontifical University of Mexico is taken from the documents found in Fernández del Castillo, *La Facultad de Medicina*, pp. 86–138.
3. *Actas de cabildo de México*, VII:103, 468; VIII:20, 282, 327, 370, 379, 413, 473, 533; IX:242; X, 46.
4. The author of *La primera parte de los problemas, y secretos maravillosos de las Indias* (México, 1591).
5. For this story, see Lanning, *Academic Culture*, pp. 14–15, 20–21.
6. Eguiguren, *Catálogo histórico*, pp. 5, 23, 26, 29, 53, 57, 59.
7. Ibid., p. 59.
8. AGNC, Sec. 1, Indice de Gastos Públicos, 5:56. Plano que demuestra las cátedras que tiene en el día la Real y Pontificia Universidad de Caracas . . . , Caracas, 25 de noviembre de 1803. In 1795 President Pedro Carbonell had proposed adding the chair of vísperas of medicine and that of surgery and anatomy.
9. ACB, Médicos y Abogados, 6, fs. 832–34. Informe del Señor Rector don Fernando Caycedo y Flórez, excrito a solicitud del Virrey en que hace la historia de la cátedra de la Medicina del Colegio Mayor.
10. AGI, México, 390. Real cédula al virrey y audiencia de México, Madrid, 22 de noviembre de 1682; Real cédula a la audiencia de Manila, Madrid, 22 de noviembre de 1682.
11. See Leslie España Bauzón, *Deficit Government: Mexico and the Philippine Situado (1606–1804)* (Tokyo, 1981), pp. 50–76.
12. Convento Dominicano, Quito, Archivo, XXV. Informe de la Real Audiencia sobre la fundación de tres cátedras de jurisprudencia y una de medicina, Quito, 14 de diciembre de 1691.
13. AGI, Quito, 196. Constituciones del Real Colegio de San Fernando de la Ciudad de Quito . . . (1694), Título XII, Constitución y estatuto 29.
14. This mismanagement guaranteed that neither debts nor interest were collected. If the small endowment bequeathed to the University of San Carlos de Guatemala had yielded six per cent interest compounded annually, it would have amounted to the startling sum of 1,523,378 pesos when the university paid its first salary. Lanning, *The University in the Kingdom of Guatemala*, p. 66.
15. AGI, Guatemala, 674. Expediente sobre la creación de universidad en el Seminario Conciliar de la Ciudad de León de Nicaragua, 1812–20. Dictamen del fiscal, Cádiz, 12 de abril de 1812.
16. Ricardo Archila, *Historia de la medicina en Venezuela: época colonial* (Caracas 1961), p. 264.
17. AGI, Santo Domingo, 889. Real cédula a maestrescuela de la Universidad de Caracas, San Lorenzo, 21 de octubre de 1765.

18. Ibid., 490. Estatutos de la Universidad de San Gerónimo de la Habana (Año de 1733), Tít. IV, Art. 20.

19. Suardo, *Diario,* I:157.

20. See, for example, AGNM, Universidad, 26. Libro de claustros, desde 1779 hasta 1788, specifically, the claustro de conciliarios, 20 de octubre de 1785.

21. For the formalities involved in these substitutions, see Lanning, *The University in the Kingdom of Guatemala,* pp. 166–69.

22. Federico González Suárez, *Historia general de la República del Ecuador,* 7 vols. (Quito, 1903), VII:29.

23. See, for example, AGNM, Universidad, 287. Informaciones de práctica de medicina, 1800–1804, passim.

24. See AGI, Lima, 583. *Constituciones,* Tít. 25.

25. Repeated instances of this practice occurred in the University of San Carlos de Guatemala.

26. Flores, *La historia de medicina en México,* II:87.

27. AGNM, Universidad, 471–73. Libro de asignación de puntos en medicina. Aforísmos de Hipócrates, prognósticos, epidemias.

28. AGNC, Sec. 1, Gastos Públicos, 5, f. 512. Informe del Dr. Felipe Tamariz, Caracas, 28 de abril de 1803.

29. Archivo del Colegio de Rosario, Bogotá. Informe de Miguel de Isla, Bogotá, 12 de diciembre de 1803.

30. AGNC, Sec. 1, Gastos Públicos, 5, f. 512. Informe del Dr. Felipe Tamariz, Caracas, 28 de abril de 1803.

31. Flores, *La historia de medicina en México,* II:140.

32. AGNM, Universidad, 21, Gobierno, 1771–74. Positiones ex universa medicina theoretica . . . , thesis of José Paredo, die XX. Mensis Junii Ann. M. DCC. LXXI.

33. ACG, 246–48. Inventario de avaluos de bienes que quedaron por muerte del Doctor Manuel Trinidad de Avalos y Porras, protomédico de este reino. Año de 1776. (This item has been moved to the AGG.)

34. For details, see Lanning, *Academic Culture,* pp. 133–34, and *The Eighteenth-Century Enlightenment,* pp. 285–89.

35. Andrés Piquer, *Institutiones medicae ad usam scholae valentinae* (Madrid, 1762).

36. *Real provisión de S.M. y señores del consejo en la qual se da regla para preservar las regalias de la corona, y de la nación en las materias, y cuestiones que se defiendan y enseñan en las universidades de estos reynos; con la creación de censores regios en ellas, y demás que contiene,* Madrid, 6 de septiembre de 1770.

37. *Teatro crítico,* VIII, Discurso IV, pp. 42–43.

38. See, for example, George M. Addy, *The Enlightenment in the University of Salamanca* (Durham, N.C., 1966), p. 42, and Madariaga, *The Rise of the Spanish American Empire,* p. 37.

39. AGNM, Reales cédulas (Dup.), 195:165. Real cédula al virrey de la Nueva España, Aranjuez, 8 de junio de 1805.

40. AGNM, Universidad, 28, Libros de Claustros, 1808–17. Claustro mayor de 26 de agosto de 1806.

41. Lanning, *The Eighteenth-Century Enlightenment,* pp. 32, 35–43, 96, 102.

42. AGG, A1. 3–12, 12819, 1930. Printed theses of Luis Franco and Mariano Antonio de Larrave, March 28, 1798.

43. The wrangle does little credit either to the protomédico or to the curandero. When the suffering woman, in the throes of dangerous parturition, was found with a blood-soaked pigeon in her loins, Larrinaga saw his fame rise as the man responsible for revealing this singular discovery to the world. On the other hand, Unánue took the tack, natural enough in a man of science, that it was not possible for a woman to give birth to a pigeon.

44. The documentation presented by the young Spanish medical historian, José Aznar López, *El Doctor José de Flores: una vida al servicio de la ciencia* (Guatemala, 1960), pp. 49–56 (hereinafter Aznar López, *José de Flores*), supports the contention of Carlos Martínez Durán, *Las ciencias médicas en Guatemala,* 2nd ed. (Guatemala, 1945), pp. 289–90, that as Flores's figures could be taken apart and reassembled, they preceded those of the Abbé Fontana.

45. AGG, Libro de claustros, 1790–1808. Clautro pleno de 17 de septiembre de 1792, fs. 21–22.

46. *Específico nuevamente descubierto en el Reino de Guatemala por la curación del horrible mal de cancro* (Guatemala, 1781).

47. AEAM, Lagartijas, 1:1. Br. Juan Manuel de Venegas al virrey, México, 20 de junio de 1782.

48. AEAM, Lagartijas, 1:1. Dictamen del Licenciado don Manuel Antonio Moreno, México, 8 de septiembre de 1782.

49. AEAM, Lagartijas, 1:1. Parecer de don Andrés Montañer y Virgili, México, 11 de septiembre de 1782.

50. AEAM, Lagartijas, 1:1. Observaciones hechas por don Antonio Velázquez de León . . . por mandado del señor virrey, septiembre de 1782.

51. AEAM, Lagartijas, 1:1. Dictamen del Dr. Francisco Rada, México, 27 de septiembre de 1782.

52. AGI, Indiferente General, 1551. El Dr. dn. Josef Flores: Título de Primer Protomédico de la ciudad, y Reino de Guatemala. En 21 de junio de 1793.

53. Aznar López, *José de Flores,* p. 77.

54. The royal audiencia made a special point of conceding this treatment in 1805. See ibid., p. 68.

55. AGI, Indiferente General, 551, f. 26v. El Protomédico José Flores sobre la pensión que disfrutaba de dos mil pesos sobre el fondo de Comunidades de Yndios de aquel Reyno, 24 de abril de 1813.

56. Aznar López, *José de Flores,* p. 102.

57. Ibid., p. 105.

58. Ibid., pp. 115, 117–19.

59. Ibid., pp. 122–25. Here Aznar López publishes Flores's own instructions for shipping, apparently the scientist's only publication.

60. Ibid., pp. 131–39.

61. AGG, A1. 3–8, 12588, 1904. Ynforme [del Consulado] relativa a la erección de una escuela de matemáticas que por falta de fondos no se realizó, Guatemala, 28 de diciembre de 1804. Signed by Gregorio de Urruela, el Marqués de Ayzinena, and Lorenzo Moreno.

62. AGI, Indiferente General, 1558. Informe del Dr. José Flores, Madrid, 28 de febrero de 1803.

63. Ibid., 551, f. 27. José Limonta a los secretarios de las cortes, Cádiz, 24 de abril de 1813.

64. Ibid., 551, f. 18–18v. José de Limonta al Secretario Interino del Despacho de Hacienda, Cádiz, 9 de diciembre de 1812; José de Limonta a José de Flores, Cádiz, 17 de diciembre de 1812.

65. Ibid., 551, f. 36–36v. José de Limonta al Capitán General de Guatemala, Cádiz, 2 de julio de 1813. Aznar López, *José de Flores,* pp. 106, n. 30, 162. For Flores's elaborate but vehement exposition of his own case, dated July 15, 1813, see pp. 162–66.

66. Aznar López, *José de Flores,* pp. 163, 167, 169.

67. Eguiguren, *Catálogo histórico,* pp. 58, 60.

68. Manuel de Odriozola, *Documentos históricos del Perú en las épocas del coloniaje despues de la conquista y de la independencia hasta la presente. Colectados y arreglados por el Coronel de Caballería de Ejército, fundador de la independencia, Manuel de Odriozola. . . .* 10 vols. (Lima, 1863–77), VII:536. (Hereinafter Odriozola, *Documentos históricos del Perú.*)

69. *Observaciones sobre el clima de Lima* (Lima, 1806).

70. With the virtual disappearance of the archives of San Marcos, the data of Unánue's academic career are very thin. In an examination of anatomy, published in 1796 by the director of the Royal Amphitheater of Anatomy, Unánue, and the students, Pedro and Remigio Zarria, Manuel Seguién, José Pezet, Miguel Venegas, and Manuel Rioseco, his name appeared. Unánue was presiding when in 1798 Pezet presented his bachelor's thesis, and also in 1799 when Remigio Zarria brought forward his thesis for the licentiate. In 1800 he approved Dr. Villalobos's method for curing tabardillo and sanctioned in the following year José Manuel Valdés's study on uterine cancer. Between 1803 and 1807 he presided over the acts of the following medical theses: Félix Devoto (bachelor's), March 16, 1803; José Urreta (bachelor's), July 4, 1804; Pedro José Colmenares (bachelor's), June 1807; José Manuel Valdés (licentiate), June 1807. Valdizán, *La facultad de medicina de Lima,* II:13–14.

71. Ibid., II:14.

72. "Necrología del doctor don Miguel Tafur," *El genio de Rimac,* Lima, December 10, 1833.

73. *Mercurio peruano,* V (No. 180, 19 de julio de 1792), n. 161.

74. Odriozola, *Documentos históricos del Perú,* VI:538.

75. In addition, he used the services of José María Dávila, José Puente, José Manuel Valdés, Luis Bueno, José Vergara, and Baltazar Villalobos.

76. For example, see "Precauciones para conservar la salud en el presente otoño," *Mercurio peruano,* I (No. 275), n. 30.

77. This document is reproduced in toto in Valdizán, *La facultad de medicina de Lima,* III: 59–65.

78. Ibid., II: 24–26, n. 33.

79. Archivo del Colegio de Medicina y Cirugía de San Fernando, Lima. Libro de matrículas de 1808 hasta 1817.

80. AGI, México, 1028. Informe (de la Contaduría General) sobre establecimiento de un Nuevo Colegio de Medicina y Cirugía en Lima, con el título de San Fernando, Cádiz, 2 de marzo de 1812.

15. *The Government, Protomedicato, and Public Health*

1. Madariaga, *The Rise of the Spanish American Empire,* p. 191.

2. AGNM, Civil, 11:3, fs. 1–198. Testimonio de los informes de los proto-médicos de esta capital, y otros individuos de la misma facultad en la prueba dada por el Exmo. Sor Conde de Revilla Gigedo en su residencia pública. The names of these witnesses and the citations of their informes are Dr. y Mro. José Ignacio García Jove, 8 de agosto de 1796, fs. 1–3v; Dr. y Maestro José Francisco Rada, 12 de agosto de 1795, fs. 3v–13; Dr. Gabriel de Ocampo, 22 de julio de 1796, fs. 13–27; Br. Mariano Arnáez, 20 de junio de 1796, fs. 27–33v; Lic. Manuel Moreno, 19 de junio de 1796, fs. 33v–38v; Br. Juan Bermúdez de Castro, s.f., fs. 38v–69v; Br. Matías Antonio Flórez, 3 de junio de 1796, fs. 69v–82; Vicente Cervantes, 8 de julio de 1796, fs. 82–98.

3. James Manfredini, *The Political Role of the Count of Revillagigedo Viceroy of New Spain, 1789–1794* (New Brunswick, N.J., 1949), p. 3.

4. AHIAH, Hospital de Naturales, 84:9, fs. 112r–114v. Bando del Virrey Conde de Revilla Gigedo sobre la limpieza de la ciudad, México, 31 de agosto de 1790.

5. As an example of Revilla Gigedo's mastery of detail, he observed that the clock-time of this operation should vary one hour with the season of the year.

6. Ibid., 84:9, fs. 112r–114v. Bando del Virrey Conde de Revilla Gigedo sobre limpieza de la ciudad, México, 31 de agosto de 1790, Arts. 1–2.

7. AGNM, Civil, 11:3, fs. 8, 36. Informe del Dr. y Mro. José Francisco Rada; Informe del Lic. Manuel Moreno.

8. AGNM, Universidad, 66. Libro de Gobierno, desde 1800 hasta 1812; Pedro de Basave al Dr. José Vicente Sánchez, México, 15 de junio de 1796. Lanning, *Academic Culture,* p. 119.

9. *Gazeta de México* VIII (No. 1, 12 de enero de 1796): 2–6.

10. This incident is detailed in various documents in AGNM, Historia, 153:15, fs. 1–53. Comisión conferida al Sor. Oidor don Guillermo de Aguirre para averiguar el origen de la fetidez que se introdujó en México en la noche del día 23 y madrugada del 24 del corriente mes de marzo de 1810.

11. "Memoria de medicina doméstica, mandada publicar de orden de S.M.," *Gazeta de México* XII (No. 57, 20 de diciembre de 1805): 178.

12. AHNM, Consejos, 51690. Aranjuez, 25 de mayo de 1795, en "Decisiones reales que en materias de Indias se expedieron en el año de 1795," f. 27, no. 14.

13. *Concertatio medica de balsami copaibae in infantum convulsionibus praestantissimo uso, quam pro gradu bacclaureatus obtinendo. . . .* (Lima, 1807).

14. AGNM, Bandos, 19:15, f. 26. Bando del virrey el Marqués de Branciforte, Orizaba, 25 de marzo de 1797.

15. Lanning, *Academic Culture,* p. 125.

16. *Gazeta de México* I (No. 9, 5 de mayo de 1784):73–74.

17. Regimen curativo del sarampión formado de orden del Superior Gobierno por el Real Tribunal del Protomedicato para la gente del pueblo pobre, y sin proporciones de médico que les asista," ibid. XII (No. 7, 29 de febrero de 1804):54–56.

18. Ibid. II (No. 47, 18 de diciembre de 1787):466–67.

19. Ibid. VII (No. 56, 20 de octubre de 1795):482.

20. Ibid. II (No. 38, 10 de julio de 1787):384.

21. Ibid. II (No. 40, 21 de agosto de 1787):398.

22. There is other evidence that the Spaniards as well as literate Mexicans understood that, even by colonial standards, the early decay and loss of teeth were owing to a lack of hygiene as well as any "act of God." At approximately this same juncture, the government unhesitatingly approved the request of "José" Orsi, an Italian dentist from Verona, to remain in Mexico because his "services were useful." AHFM, Reales cédulas y ordenes, 174:173, f. 220–20v. Real orden al virrey de Nueva España, San Lorenzo, 25 de noviembre de 1799.

23. *Gazeta de México* II (No. 29, 27 de febrero de 1787):307.

24. Dr. Francisco Fernández del Castillo and Alicia Hernández de Torres give a summary of the expediente covering this case AHFM, Protomedicato, 1:17, fs. 1–16 in their *El Tribunal del Protomedicato en la Nueva España, según el Archivo Histórico de la Facultad de Medicina,* pp. 39–41. (Hereinafter Fernández del Castillo y Hernández Torres, *El Tribunal del Protomedicato.*)

25. AHFM, Protomedicato, 1:7. Testimonios de Francisco Xavier Angulo, México, 9 y 20 de marzo de 1787.

26. AHFM, Protomedicato, 1:7, Decreto del Protomedicato, México, 27 de julio de 1787 in Fernández del Castillo y Hernández Torres, *El Tribunal del Protomedicato,* p. 41.

27. AHFM, Protomedicato, 4:23, f. 11v. Virrey Branciforte al Real Protomedicato, México, 25 de diciembre de 1797.

28. Ibid., 4:23. Manuel del Castillo, delegado del virrey, al Real Protomedicato, México, 13 de noviembre de 1806.

29. Ibid., 4:23, f. 1–1v. Virrey Iturrigaray al Real Protomedicato, México, 5 de diciembre de 1807.

30. *Gazeta de México* VI (No. 2, 21 de enero de 1794):14; VI (No. 3, 10 de febrero de 1794):22–23.

31. *Consuelo de los navegantes en los estrechos conflictos de falta de ensaladas y otros víveres frescos en las largas navegaciones. . . .* (Madrid, s.f.).

32. *Consideraciones político-médicas sobre la salud de los navegantes* (Madrid, 1769).

33. AGI, Indiferente General, 1315. Informe del Tribunal del Protomedicato, Madrid, 14 de agosto de 1771.

34. Ibid. Los Directores de la Real Compañía Guipúzcoana de Caracas al Excmo. Sr. Bailio Fr. D. Julián de Arriaga, Madrid, 4 de septiembre de 1771.

35. Ibid. Madrid, 31 de octubre de 1791.

36. In 1768 Santiago de Cárdenas sought the support of the viceroy of Peru for his proposal "to fly messages to and from headquarters" when communications broke down during the attempt to "dislodge" the British from the Falkland Islands. Steele, *Flowers for the King,* pp. 67–68.

37. *Mercurio peruano* II (No. 50, 26 de junio de 1791):131–33.

38. AGNM, Protomedicato, 1:7. Decreto del virrey, México, 16 de marzo de 1816.

39. AGNM, Protomedicato, 1:7. Pedimento del fiscal, México, 19 de abril de 1816.

40. AGNM, Reales cédulas (Dup.), 83:24. Real cédula al virrey de la Nueva España, Buen Retiro, 13 de julio de 1763.

41. AGNM, Protomedicato, 1:7. Parecer del asesor general, México, 7 de mayo de 1816.

42. AGNM, Protomedicato, 1:7. Decreto del virrey, México, 7 de mayo de 1816.

43. AHNM, Consejos, 111934. D. Josef García de Burunda el Illmo. Sr. Conde de Campomanes, Decano Gobernador del Consejo, Madrid, 21 de septiembre de 1785.

44. AGI, Santo Domingo, 890. Real cédula a D. José Diguja, gobernador que fué de la provincia de Cumaná, Aranjuez, 22 de junio de 1766. Real cédula al obispo de Puerto Rico, Aranjuez, 22 de junio de 1766.

45. AHNM, Consejos, 51689. Real cédula al virrey de Nueva España, Madrid, 28 de diciembre de 1781.

46. AGNM, Epidemias, 1:1, f. 442–42v. Lista de los Socorros que han entrado en su Caja para Caridad de la presente epidemia de viruelas, México, 29 de noviembre de 1797.

47. AGNM, Epidemias, 6:7, f. 578. *Resumen general* . . .

48. AGNM, Epidemias, 1:1, f. 452. México, 11 de diciembre de 1797.

49. Lanning, *Academic Culture in the Spanish Colonies,* p. 120.

50. Lanning, *The Eighteenth-Century Enlightenment,* p. 251.

51. Cooper, *Epidemic Disease,* pp. 56–69. Cooper's excellent discussion provides many of the basic details concerning the course of various epidemics in Mexico City for the late eighteenth and early nineteenth centuries.

52. *Gazeta de México* I (No. 7, 24 de marzo de 1784):54–55.

53. *Instrucción que puede servir para que se cure a los enfermos de las viruelas epidémicas, que ahora se padecen en México* . . . (México, 1779) in AGNM, Bandos, 11:30, fs. 80–83v.

54. *Método curativo, que puede contribuir para precaver en mucha parte las desgracias que ocasiona la actual epidemia de viruelas a los pobres que las pa-*

decen en los pueblos y campos, y carecen de médicos que gobiernen prudentamente su curación . . . (Puebla, 1779).

55. AGI, Indiferente General, 1335. *Disertación físico-médica, en la cual se prescribe un método seguro para preservar a los pueblos de viruelas hasta lograr la completa extinción de ellas en todo el reino, su autor D. Francisco Gil, cirujano del Real Monasterio de S. Lorenzo y su sitio, e individuo de la Real Academia Médica de Madrid* (Madrid, 1784). (Hereinafter Gil, *Disertación físico-médica.*) Also in AGNM, Epidemias, 7.

56. AGI, Indiferente General, 1335. Orden General remitiendo impresos sobre el modo de preservar a los pueblos de viruelas, Aranjuez, 15 de abril de 1785.

57. Richard H. Shryock, *Medicine and Society in America: 1660–1860* (Ithaca, N.Y., 1962), pp. 83–84.

58. Gil, *Disertación físico-médica*, p. 30.

59. Ibid., pp. 43–44.

60. AGNM, Historia, 460. Real Protomedicato al Virrey Manuel Antonio Flórez, México, 14 de febrero de 1788.

61. *Gazeta de México* IV (No. 25, 11 de enero de 1791):243.

62. AGNM, Bandos, 19:12, fs. 19–21v. Circular reservada de 28 de febrero de 97, por el expresado Sr. Marqués, que para evitar la propagación de la peste, dicta providencias con que ha de cortarse la comunicación de los contagiados y han de usarse otros precauciones, México, 1797.

63. As the viceroy republished his *Disertación físico-médica* in 1797, this work may be said to have been the guide in the struggle against smallpox until the introduction of vaccine.

64. AGNM, Bandos, 19:83, fs. 127–46. *Instrucción para inocular las viruelas, y método de curarlas con facilidad, y acierto* (Puebla de los Angeles, 1797).

65. For a detailed discussion of the course of the epidemic, see Cooper, *Epidemic Disease*, pp. 86–156.

66. In addition to the archbishop, this "general" or "principal" junta had two members named by the dean and ecclesiastical cabildo, the superintendent don Cosme Mier, two regidores of the town council, one from the Tribunal del Consulado, and another from the Cuerpo de Minería. AGNM, Epidemias, 1:1, f. 498.

67. For the membership of this commission, see AHIAH, Hospital de Naturales, 84:15, f. 176v. The signatures were Alonso, Arzobispo de México, Juan Francisco de Campos, Antonio Rodríguez de Velasco, Cosme de Mier y Tres Palacios, Joseph Ruiz de Conejares, Felipe Teruel, Antonio de Basoco, Manuel García Zevallos, and Luis Gonzaga de Ibarra.

68. Cooper, *Epidemic Disease*, pp. 115–47. Actually, many of the steps taken by the Junta Principal had already been suggested or put into effect by Archbishop Alonso prior to the establishment of the Junta Principal in late October.

69. For examples of this practice, see the *Relación de méritos* . . . México, 1814, of Dr. Manuel José de Flores, who says that in the year 1798 the president of the protomedicato assigned him as physician to the second ward

(*cuartel*), "which he served to the satisfaction of the Real Junta de Caridad."
AGNM, Epidemias, 13:6, f. 125v.

70. AGNM, Epidemias, 6:7, f. 447. García Jove al Virrey Branciforte, México,
13 de noviembre de 1797.

71. AGNM, Epidemias, 6:7, f. 449. Resumen de las partes de 19 de noviembre
de 1797; García Jove al Virrey Branciforte, México, 20 de noviembre de
1797.

72. AGNM, Epidemias, 6:7, f. 511. Resumen de las partes de 4 de diciembre de
1797; García Jove al Virrey Branciforte, México, 4 de diciembre de 1797.

73. AGNM, Epidemias, 6:7, f. 569. Resumen de las partes del Dr. García Jove,
México, 11 de diciembre de 1797; García Jove al Virrey Branciforte, México,
11 de diciembre de 1797.

74. AGNM, Epidemias, 6:7, f. 586. *Resumen general de las sociedades de caridad, que para socorro de los contagiados de la epidemia del año de 1797 . . .
formado de los ocho Estados parciales . . .* , México, 17 de febrero de 1798.
(Hereinafter *Resumen general.*)

75. AGNM, Epidemias, 6:7, f. 586. The editor of the *Resumen general,* taking
his figures from the *Guía de forasteros,* explains that of the 12,221 deaths
in the city, 5,153 had died of other disease leaving 7,068 attributable to
smallpox. He explained the discrepancy between this figure and the 4,451
reported by the charitable societies, by pointing out that these societies did
not report those dying in hospitals, casas de comunidades, and private houses,
as well as those in outside towns in charge of city parishes. Only twenty-one
persons "among the many inoculated," were included in this mortality table.

76. AGNM, Epidemias, 6:7, f. 587. Estado general . . . , 2 de febrero de 1798.

77. Ibid., 6:7, f. 586. *Resumen general* . . . , Nota 2.

78. Ibid., 6:7, fs. 578–85. Estados de los cuarteles mayores, números 1–8.

79. Ibid., 1:1, fs. 484–502. Extracto certificado por el Notario y Escribano Real
Juan Vicente de Vega, de todo lo replacionado con las órdenes y medidas
que se observaron durante la Epidemia de Viruelas, México, 12 de febrero
de 1798.

80. Ibid., 16:8, f. 2, Art. 8. Circular de 28 de febrero de 1797 sobre providencias
para viruelas.

81. Ibid., 1:1, f. 501.

82. Alexander von Humboldt, *Political Essay on the Kingdom of New Spain,* ed.
by Mary Maples Dunn (New York, 1972), pp. 39–40.

83. AGNM, Epidemias, 1:1, f. 373. Estado que manifiesta los virolentos naturales los que de ellos han fallecidos, los inoculados, 10 de septiembre a 21
de octubre de 1797.

84. See Edward Jenner, *An Inquiry Into the Cause and Effects of the Variolae
Vaccinae* . . . (London, 1798); *Further Observations on the Variolae Vaccinae or Cow Pox* (London, 1799); and *A Continuation of Facts and Observations Relative to the Variolae Vaccinae or Cow Pox* (London, 1800).

85. Francisco Fernández del Castillo, *Los viajes de Don Francisco Xavier de
Balmis: Notas para la historia de la expedición de España a América y Fili-*

pinas (1803–1806) (México, 1960), p. 21. (Hereinafter Fernández del Castillo, *Los viajes de Don Francisco Xavier de Balmis*.)

86. Works more than adequate for establishing the story and gleaning the truth concerning this "around-the-world" expedition are the following: S. F. Cook, "Francisco Xavier Balmis and Introduction of Vaccination in America," *Bulletin of the Institute of the History of Medicine of Johns Hopkins University* XI (1942):543–60; XII (1942):70–101. Gonzalo Díaz de Yraola, *La vuelta al mundo de la expedición de la vacuna* (Sevilla, 1948). Fernández del Castillo, *Los viajes de Don Francisco Xavier de Balmis*. Aníbal Ruiz Moreno, *Introducción de la vacuna en América, expedición de Balmis* (Buenos Aires, 1947).

87. *Gazeta de México* XII (No. 12 [Suplemento]):93–96.

88. AGNM, Reales cédulas (Dup.), 197:168, fs. 250–53. Real orden al virrey de la Nueva España, San Lorenzo, 15 de octubre de 1806.

89. AGNM, Epidemias, 10:7, fs. 72–86v. Francisco Xavier de Balmis al Virrey Iturrigaray, México, 5 de septiembre de 1804.

90. AGI, Indiferente General, 1558. José Antonio Caballero al presidente de Guatemala, Aranjuez, 20 de mayo de 1804.

91. Ibid., 1558. *Reglamento para la propagación y estabilidad de la vacuna en el reyno de Guatemala. Dispuesto, de orden de S.M., por el Superior Gobierno del mismo reyno* (Nueva Guatemala, 1805).

92. Fernández del Castillo, *Los viajes de Don Francisco Xavier de Balmis*, p. 271.

93. J. L. Moreau de la Sarthe, *Traité historique et pratique de la vaccine* . . . (Paris, 1801), translated by Francisco Xavier de Balmis into Spanish as *Tratado histórico y práctico de la vacuna que contiene en compendio el origen y resultados de las observaciones y experimentos sobre la vacuna con un examen imparcial sobre sus ventajas y de las objecciones que se le han puesto por J. L. Moreau* . . . (Madrid, 1803).

94. AGI, Indiferente General, 1558. Copias de actas celebradas en la Junta Central de Vacuna de Caracas; Carta del Capitán General de Caracas, núm. 93, en que incluye el Reglamento de la Junta Central de Vacuna.

95. Informe del Dr. José Antonio Ríos y Dr. Fray Pedro Manuel Chaparro al capitán general de Chile, Santiago de Chile, 11 de abril de 1807 in Benavente Garcés, *El protomedicato en Chile,* pp. 82–84.

96. *Actuaciones literarias de la vacuna en la Real Universidad de San Marcos* (Lima, 1807), prólogo.

97. AGI, Indiferente General, 1558. Brevísimo resumen. . . .

98. AGNM, Reales cédulas (Dup.), 202:138, f. 241–41v. Real orden a la audiencia gobernadora de Nueva España, Real Isla de León, 20 de marzo de 1810; Superior orden del Virrey Venegas, México, 10 de diciembre de 1810.

ᓚ Bibliography of Works Cited

Archives and Manuscript Collections

CHILE
José Toribio Medina Collection, National Library, Santiago.

COLOMBIA
Archivo Colonial, Bogotá. Médicos y Abogados, 4–6; Reales Cédulas, 34.
Archivo del Colegio de Rosario, Bogotá.
Archivo Histórico Nacional, Bogotá. Cedulario de Ayala 48, 85; Colegios 1.
Biblioteca Nacional, Sala de Manuscritos, Bogotá. Manuscritos 169, 174, 202.

ECUADOR
Archivo de la Real Audiencia de Quito, Quito. Cuerpos Docentes; Cedulario XV.
Convento Dominicano, Quito. Archivo XXV.

GUATEMALA
Archivo Colonial de Guatemala, Guatemala City. Numbers 246–48. (Subsequently
    moved to the Archivo General de Gobierno.)
Archivo General de Gobierno, Guatemala City. A1.3, A1.3–1, A1.3–8, A1.3–12,
    A1.3–18, A1.4, A1.4–18, Libro de Claustros, 1790–1808.

MEXICO
Archivo del Ex-Ayuntamiento de México, Mexico City. Actas del Cabildo; Lagar-
    tijas, 1; Médicos y Boticas, 1.
Archivo General de la Nación Mexicana, Mexico City. Bandos 7, 10, 11, 19–20;
    Civil 11; Epidemias 1, 6, 10, 13, 16; Estado 224; Historia 153, 460–61;
    Hospitales 144; Indice de Bandos, Hospital de Naturales; Inquisición 986;
    Matrimonios 7, 12; Protomedicato 1–4; Reales Cédulas (Duplicados) 2, 14,
    16–18, 22, 24, 28–30, 33–34, 36, 40, 43–45, 47, 88, 92, 106, 127, 138, 145,
    151, 164, 170–71, 173, 192, 195, 197, 202, 207, 209, 212; Universidad 19,
    22, 25–26, 28, 52, 66, 71, 279–83, 286–87, 471–73; Grados de Bachilleres
    en Medicina; Grados de Licenciados y Maestros en Artes 1753–84; Informa-
    ciones de Limpieza de Sangre; Libros de Claustro 1771–79, 1779–88, 1788–
    1801, 1801–17.
Archivo Histórico de la Facultad de Medicina de la Universidad de México, Mexico
    City. Protomedicato 1–4, 6–7, 10–12; Reales Cédulas y Ordenes, 174.
Archivo Histórico del Instituto Nacional de Antropología e Historia, Mexico City.
    Protomedicato T-4, 12; Hospital de Naturales 77, 84, 103–5, 144.

PERU

Archivo del Colegio de Medicina y Cirugía de San Fernando, Lima. Libro de Matrículas de 1808 hasta 1817.

Archivo Nacional del Perú, Lima. Protomedicato, Legajo Unico.

Biblioteca Nacional, Sala de Manuscritos, Lima. Tarifa y puntual aprecia que para el seguro expendio de los medicamentos Galénicos y Chymicos más usuales en las Oficinas Pharmacéuticas de esta Reino, Lima, 1756.

SPAIN

Archivo de la Facultad de Medicina de la Universidad de Madrid, Madrid. Antiguo Colegio de San Carlos, Libro de Acuerdos (1787–1804).

Archivo Histórico Nacional, Madrid. Cedulario Indico 9, 33; Códices 684–725B, 692B; Consejos 1018, 6837, 6839, 51689–90, 111934; Inquisición, México, 1732; Ultramar 1610; Universidades 135, 1025f.

Archivo General de Indias, Sevilla. Contratación 5089; Gobierno: Buenos Aires 20, 229, 256, 273, 335; Caracas 241, 446; Chile 265; Lima 309, 337, 543, 583, 686, 798, 854, 914; México 16, 36, 325, 387, 389–91, 393–95, 397, 401, 403, 407, 412, 416–17, 419, 429, 432, 446, 471, 571, 660, 776, 780, 789, 1028, 1070, 1079, 1081, 1086, 1091, 1094, 1097, 1100–1103, 1108, 1111, 1115, 1138–39, 1299, 1313A, 1457, 1751, 1754, 1767, 1769, 1771, 1776, 2260, 2660; Quito 196, 356; Santo Domingo 426, 489–90, 495, 521, 874, 879, 881–83, 885, 887, 889–90, 893–94, 898, 905, 907–8, 910–11, 915–18, 1122–23, 1138, 1347, 1357, 1455, 1457–58, 1463, 1551; Indiferente General 3, 7, 11, 16, 18, 36, 62, 418–21, 463, 473, 478, 500, 550–51, 640, 668, 673, 734, 1291, 1310, 1315–16, 1330, 1335, 1339, 1344, 1348–49, 1551, 1558, 2660; Justicia 199; Ultramar 727, 733.

Hospital del Pozo Santo, Sevilla. Legajos 454–56, 459, 461.

Hospital de Nuestra Señora Santa María de Esgueva, Valladolid. Libros de Dispensas.

Hospital de San Barnabé y San Antolín, Palencia, Libros de Gastos.

Hospital de Tavera, Toledo. Libros de Dispensas.

Hospital Inoncens, Valencia. Rebudes y Dates de 1523–24.

VENEZUELA

Archivo General de la Nación, Caracas. Títulos de Médicos, Tomo Unico; Indice de Gastos Públicos; Gastos Públicos 5.

Publications

Actas de cabildo del ayuntamiento de México. 54 vols. México, 1889–1916.

Actas del cabildo de Caracas. 11 vols. Caracas, 1943–69.

Addy, George M. *The Enlightenment in the University of Salamanca.* Durham, N.C., 1966.

Aranzel de el Protomedicato. México, 1759.

Archila, Ricardo. *Historia de la medicina en Venezuela: época colonial.* Caracas, 1961.

Aznar López, José. *El Doctor José de Flores: una vida al servicio de la ciencia.* Guatemala City, 1960.

Bartolache, José Ignacio. *Mercurio volante con noticias importantes i curiosas sobre varios asuntos de Físico i Medicina.* México, 1772–73.

Bauzón, Leslie España. *Deficit Government: Mexico and the Philippine Situado (1606–1804).* Tokyo, 1981.

Beltrán, Juan Ramón. *Historia del Protomedicato de Buenos Aires.* Buenos Aires, 1937.

Benavente Garcés, Ricardo. *El protomedicato en Chile.* Santiago de Chile, 1929.

Bolton, Herbert E. *Coronado on the Turquoise Trail, Knight of Pueblo and Plains.* Albuquerque, N.M., 1949.

Burke, Michael E. *The Royal College of San Carlos: Surgery and Spanish Medical Reform in the Late Eighteenth Century.* Durham, N.C., 1978.

Cangiamila, Francisco Emmanuele. *Embryologia sacra, sive de officio sacerdotum, medicorum et aliorum circa aeternam parvulorum in utero existentium salutem.* Palermo, 1758.

Carbonell, Diego. "Narciso Esparragosa y Gallardo, sabio, bueno y venezolano." *Gaceta médica de Caracas* 26 (1929).

Cárdenas, Juan de. *La primera parte de los problemas y secretos maravillosos de las Indias.* México, 1591.

Carreño, Alberto María. *Efemérides de la Real y Pontificia Universidad de México.* 2 vols. México, 1963.

Causa médico criminal que en este Real Protomedicato del Perú han seguido los profesores de la facultad de medicina contra los cirujanos, pharmacéuticos, phlebotómicos, etc., sobre contenerlos en los términos de sus respectivas profesiones. Lima, 1764.

Caviedes, Juan del Valle y. *Obras de Don Juan del Valle y Caviedes: Introducción y notas de Rubén Vargas Ugarte, S. J.* Lima, 1947.

Compendio de la medicina: o medicina práctica. México, 1788.

Constituciones de la Real y Pontificia Universidad de México. México, 1775.

Cook, Sherburne F. "Francisco Xavier Balmis and Introduction of Vaccination in America." *Bulletin of the Institute of the History of Medicine of Johns Hopkins University* 11 (1942):543–60 and 12 (1942):70–101.

Cooper, Donald B. *Epidemic Disease in Mexico City, 1761–1813: An Administrative, Social, and Medical Study.* Austin, Tex., 1965.

Corbella, Antonio. *Disertación médico-churugica en la qual se trata. . . .* Madrid, 1794.

———. *Tratado de las enfermedades mas principales agudas y crónicas del pecho. . . .* Madrid, 1795.

Dale, William Pratt. "The Cultural Revolution in Peru, 1750–1820." Ph.D. Dissertation, Duke University, 1941.

Dávila, Fernando, et al. *Aranzeles de los tribunales, juzgados y oficinas de justicia, gobierno, y real hacienda, que comprehende la Ciudad de México, Capital de Nueva España.* México, 1759.

Díaz de Yraola, Gonzalo. *La vuelta al mundo de la expedición de la vacuna.* Sevilla, 1948.

Diccionario de la lengua castellana, compuesto por la Real Academia Española. Madrid, 1783.

Eguiguren, Luis Antonio. *Catálogo histórico del claustro de la Universidad de San Marcos, 1576–1800.* Lima, 1912.

——, ed. *Diccionario histórico cronológico de la Real y Pontificia Universidad de San Marcos y sus colegios.* 3 vols. Lima, 1940–51.

Escobar del Corro, Johannes. *Tractatus bipartitus de puritate, et nobilitate probanda, secundum statuta S. officii inquisitionis regii ordinum senatus, sanctae Ecclesiae Toletanae, collegiorum, aliarúmque communitatum Hispaniae. . . .* Lyons, 1637.

Esparragosa y Gallardo, Narciso. *Memoria sobre una invención fácil y sencilla para extraer las criaturas clavadas en el paso sin riesgo de su vida, ni ofensa de la madre, y para extraer la cabeza que ha quedado en el útero separada del cuerpo.* Guatemala, 1798.

Examenes públicos de obstetricía o arte de partear. Havana, 1825.

Feijóo y Montenegro, Benito Jerónimo. *Cartas eruditas, y curiosas, en que por la mayor parte se continua el designio del teatro crítico universal. . . .* 5 vols. Madrid, 1759–76.

——. *Teatro crítico.* 2nd edition, 8 vols. Madrid, 1773–81.

Fernández del Castillo, Francisco. *La Facultad de Medicina según el Archivo de la Real y Pontificia Universidad de México.* México, 1953.

——. *Los viajes de Don Francisco Xavier de Balmis: Notas para la historia de la expedición de España á América y Filipinas (1803–1806).* México, 1960.

——, y Hernández Torres, Alicia, eds. *El Tribunal del Protomedicato en la Nueva España según el Archivo Histórico de la Facultad de Medicina.* México, 1965.

Fernández de Recas, Guillermo S. *Medicina: Nómina de bachilleres, licenciados y doctores, 1607–1780 y guía de méritos y servicios, 1763–1820.* México, 1960.

Flores, Francisco A. *Historia de la medicina en México desde la época de los indios hasta la presente.* 3 vols. México, 1868–88.

Flores, Jorge Basilio. *Mesue defendido contra D. Félix Palacios: muy útil para todos los profesores de la medicina.* Murcia, 1721.

Flores, José de. *Específico nuevamente descubierto en el Reino de Guatemala por la curación del horrible mal de cancro.* Guatemala, 1781.

Fuenzalida Grandón, Alejandro. *Historia del desarollo intelectual en Chile (1541–1810).* Santiago de Chile, 1903.

García Icazbalceta, J. *Obras de D. J. García Icazbalceta.* 10 vols. México, 1896–99.

Gazeta de Guatemala. Vol. II.

Gazeta de México. Vols. I, II, IV, VI–X, XII.

González Laguna, Francisco. *El zelo sacerdotal para con los niños no nacidos.* Lima, 1781.

González Suárez, Federico. *Historia general de la República del Ecuador.* 7 vols. Quito, 1903.

Gutiérrez-Colomer, Leonardo. "Médicos y farmacéuticos con Hernán Cortés." *Revista de Indias* 8 (January–June 1948):331–37.

Hamilton, Earl J. "Wages and Subsistence of Spanish Treasure Ships, 1503–1660." *The Journal of Political Economy* 37 (August 1929): 430–45.

Hernández Morejón, Antonio. *Historia bibliográfica de la medicina española.* 7 vols. Madrid, 1842–52.

Howard, David A. *The Royal Indian Hospital of Mexico City.* Tempe, Ariz., 1980.

Humboldt, Alexander von. *Political Essay on the Kingdom of New Spain.* Ed. by Mary Maples Dunn. New York, 1972.

Iborra, Pascual. "Memoria sobre la institución del real protomedicato." *Anales de la Real Academia de Medicina* 6 (1885):183–592.

Iturbide, F. Pedro Mariano de. *Compendio para que la operación cesárea se practique conforme a las obras del doctor Antonio Rodríguez y D. Francisco Cangiamila.* Guatemala, 1788.

Jenner, Edward. *A Continuation of Facts and Observations Relative to the Variolae Vaccinae or Cow Pox.* London, 1800.

———. *An Inquiry Into the Cause and Effects of the Variolae Vaccinae. . . .* London, 1798.

———. *Further Observations on the Variolae Vaccinae or Cow Pox.* London, 1799.

Konetzke, Richard, ed. *Colección de documentos para la historia de la formación social de Hispanoamérica (1493–1810).* 3 vols. in 5. Madrid, 1953–62.

Lanning, John Tate. *Academic Culture in the Spanish Colonies.* New York, 1940.

———. *The Eighteenth-Century Enlightenment in the University of San Carlos de Guatemala.* Ithaca, N.Y., 1956.

———. "Legitimacy and *Limpieza de Sangre* in the Practice of Medicine in the Spanish Empire." *Jahrbuch für Geschichte von Staat, Wirtschaft und Gesellschaft Lateinamerikas* 4 (1967):46–52.

———. *Pedro de la Torre: Doctor to Conquerors.* Baton Rouge, La., 1974.

———, ed. *Reales cédulas de la Real y Pontificia Universidad de México de 1551 a 1816.* México, 1946.

———, ed. *Reales cédulas de la Real y Pontificia Universidad de San Carlos de Guatemala.* Guatemala, 1954.

———. *The University in the Kingdom of Guatemala.* Ithaca, N.Y., 1955.

Lardizabal, Vicente. *Consideraciones político-médicas sobre la salud de los navegantes.* Madrid, 1769.

———. *Consuelo de los navegantes en los estrechos conflictos de falta de ensaladas y otros viveres frescos en las largas navigaciones. . . .* Madrid, n.d.

Larrinaga, José Pastor. *Apología de los cirujanos del Perú.* Granada, 1791.

Las siete partidas del sabio rey, Don Alfonso el IX. . . . 4 vols. Barcelona, 1843–1844.

Lastres, Juan B. *Hipólito Unánue.* Lima, 1955.

———. *Historia de la medicina peruana.* 3 vols. Lima, 1951.

Lavalle, José Antonio. "El Doctor Don José Manuel Valdés, Apuntes sobre su vida y sus obras." *Gaceta médica de Lima* (August–November 1858):47–52.

Libros de cabildo de la ciudad de Quito. 26 vols. Quito, 1934–60.

Libros de cabildos de Lima. 20 vols. Lima, 1935–62.

"Lista de profesores de medicina, cirugía, farmacia, y flebotomía, residentes en el D. F., sacado del libro del Protomedicato (Año de 1830)." *Gaceta médica de México* 36 (1899).

Madariaga, Salvador de. *The Rise of the Spanish American Empire.* New York, 1947.

Manfredini, James. *The Political Role of the Count of Revillagigedo Viceroy of New Spain, 1789–1794.* New Brunswick, N.J., 1949.

Martínez Durán, Carlos. *Las ciencias médicas en Guatemala.* Guatemala, 1941.

Medina, Antonio. *Cartilla nueva, útil y necesaria para instruirse las matronas que vulgarmente se llaman comadres, en el oficio de partear.* Madrid, 1759.

Medina, José Toribio. *La imprenta en Guatemala (1660–1821).* 2 vols in 1. Guatemala, 1960.

Memorias de los virreyes que han gobernado el Perú, durante el tiempo del coloniaje español. 6 vols. Lima, 1859.

Menéndez y Pelayo, Marcelino. *La ciencia española (polémicas, proyectos, y bibliografía).* 3 vols. Madrid, 1887–88.

Mendiburu, Manuel de. *Diccionario histórico-biográfico del Perú.* 2nd ed. 11 vols. Lima, 1931–35.

Mercado, Luis. *Institutiones chirurgicae jussi regio factae. . . .* Madrid, 1594.

———. *Institutiones medicae. . . .* Madrid, 1594.

———. *Instituciones que Su Magistad mandó hazer al doctor Mercado. . . .* Madrid, 1599.

Mercurio peruano. Vols. I–III, V.

Método curativo que puede contribuir para precaver en mucha parta las desgracias que ocasiona la actual epidemia de viruelas a los pobres que las padecen en los pueblos y campos, y carecen de médicos que gobiernen prudentemente su curación. Puebla, 1779.

Moreau de la Sarthe, J. L. *Traité historique et pratique de la vaccine. . . .* Paris, 1801. Translated into Spanish by Francisco Xavier Balmis as *Tratado histórico y práctico de la vacuna que contiene en compendio el origen y resultados de las observaciones y experimentos sobre la vacuna con un examen imparcial sobre sus ventajas y de las objeciones que se le han suertas por J. L. Moreau.* Madrid, 1803.

Muñoz, Miguel Eugenio, ed. *Recopilación de las leyes, pragmáticas, reales decretos, y acuerdos del Real Proto-Medicato.* Valencia, 1751.

Navarrete, Martín Fernández de, ed. *Colección de los viages y descubrimientos que hicieron por mar los españoles desde fines del siglo XV. . . .* 5 vols. Madrid, 1825–37.

"Necrología del doctor don Miguel Tafur." *El genio de Rimac* (Lima, December 10, 1833).

Novísima recopilación de leyes de España. 6 vols. Madrid, 1805–7.

Nueva recopilación (Recopilación de las leyes destos reynos. . . .) 3 vols. Madrid, 1640.

Odriozola, Manuel de, ed. *Documentos históricos del Perú en las épocas del coloniaje después de la conquista y de la independencia hasta la presente. . . .* 10 vols. Lima, 1863–77.

Padden, Robert C. *The Hummingbird and the Hawk.* Columbus, O. 1967.

Palacios, Félix. *Palestra farmacéutica chimico-galénica.* . . . Madrid, 1706, 1723, 1730, 1737, 1753, 1763, 1778, 1792, 1797.

―――. *La Pharmacopea triunfante de las calumnias y imposturas que en "Hipócrates defendido" ha publicado D. Miguel Boix.* Madrid, 1713.

Palma, Ricardo. *Tradiciones peruanas.* 6 vols. Madrid, n.d.

Palmer, Thomas W., Jr. *Guide to the Law and Legal Literature of Spain.* Washington, D.C., 1913.

Paz-Soldán, Carlos Enrique. *José Manuel Valdés, 1767–1843.* Lima, 1942.

Pharmacopoeia Matritensis Regii, ac supremi Hispaniarum Protomedicatus auctoritate, jussu atque auspiciis elaboarata. Madrid, 1739, 1762.

Piquer, Andrés. *Institutiones medicae ad usem scholae valentinae.* Madrid, 1762.

Quirós Rodiles, Adrián. "Breve historia de la obstetricia en México." *Obstetricia y ginecología latino-americanas* 3 (1945).

Reales ordenanzas generales de los colegios y escuelas de cirugía. México, 1799.

Recopilación de leyes de los reynos de las Indias. . . . 3 vols. Madrid, 1681.

Reglamento formado de orden del Exmo. Señor Virrey Conde de Revilla Gigedeo para el gobierno que ha de observarse en el alumbrado de las calles de México. México, 1790.

Reyes, J. M. "Historia de la medicina. Estudios históricos sobre el ejercicio de la medicina." *Gaceta médica de México* 1 (1865).

Rodríguez, José Manuel. *La caridad del sacerdote para con los niños encerrados en el vientre de sus madres difuntas y documentos de la utilidad y necesidad de su práctica.* México, 1772.

Rodríguez Rivero, P. D. *Historia médica de Venezuela hasta 1900.* Caracas, 1931.

Ruiz Moreno, Aníbal. *Introducción de la vacuna en América, expedición de Balmis.* Buenos Aires, 1947.

―――. *La medicina en la legislación medioeval española.* Buenos Aires, 1946.

Schäfer, Ernst. "Los Protomedicatos en Indias." *Anuario de Estudios Americanos* 3 (1946): 1040–46.

Segura, Ignacio. *Avisos saludables a las parteras para el cumplimiento de su obligación.* México, 1775.

Shryock, Richard. *Medicine and Society in America: 1660–1860.* Ithaca, N.Y., 1962.

Soriano, Manuel S. "Historia de la medicina en México: Origen de la Casa de Maternidad en México." *Boletín de ciencias médicas* 4 (1913).

Steck, Francis Borgia, ed. and trans. *Motolinía's History of the Indians of New Spain.* Washington, D.C., 1951.

Steele, Arthur R. *Flowers for the King.* Durham, N.C. 1964.

Suardo, Juan Antonio. *Diario de Lima de Juan Antonio Suardo (1629–1639). Publicado con introducción y notas por Rubén Vargas Ugarte, S.J.* 2 vols. Lima, 1936.

Unánue, Hipólito. *Observaciones sobre el clima de Lima.* Lima, 1806.

Valdés, José Manuel. *Concertatio medica de balsami copaibae in infantum convulsionibus praestantissino uso, quam pro gradu baccalaureatus obtinendo.* . . . Lima, 1807.

Valdizán, H. *La facultad de medicina de Lima, 1811–1911.* Lima, n.d.

Velasco Ceballos, Rómulo, ed. *La historia de la cirugía mexicana en el siglo XVIII.* México, 1946.

White, Joseph Blanco. *Letters from Spain.* 2nd edition. London, 1825.

Woodham, John E. "Hipólito Unánue and the Enlightenment in Peru." Ph.D. Dissertation, Duke University, 1964.

Index